短期集中！オオサンショウウオ先生の

医療統計セミナー
論文読解レベルアップ30

京都大学 臨床統計学講座
田中司朗

滋賀医科大学 医療統計学部門
田中佐智子

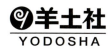

本書は小誌レジデントノート連載「論文を"正しく"よむ い・ろ・は～オオサンショウウオの統計集中講座」（2015年6月～11月，全6回）に加筆・修正を加え，単行本化したものです．

【注意事項】本書の情報について

　本書に記載されている内容は，発行時点における最新の情報に基づき，正確を期するよう，執筆者，監修・編者ならびに出版社はそれぞれ最善の努力を払っております．しかし科学・医学・医療の進歩により，定義や概念，技術の操作方法や診療の方針が変更となり，本書をご使用になる時点においては記載された内容が正確かつ完全ではなくなる場合がございます．また，本書に記載されている企業名や商品名，URL等の情報が予告なく変更される場合もございますのでご了承ください．

◆ 推薦のことば ◆

　このたび，私の尊敬する生物統計学者である，田中司朗先生，田中佐智子先生のご夫妻が臨床医向けに執筆した本著を推薦できることは，至上の喜びであります．田中先生ご夫妻は，東京大学の疫学・生物統計学教室（大橋靖雄名誉教授）のご出身で，その後，ご縁があって，お二人とも私の主宰する京都大学の薬剤疫学の教室にて，教員として研究指導や教育にご尽力をいただいていました．私自身は，臨床医の経験ののち，基礎医学研究，米国での行政官を経て，現在は社会医学の領域で，医療データベース研究とその基盤整備を行っております．

　昨今，診療報酬請求（レセプト）情報，病院のDPCデータ，電子カルテ由来の診療情報，疾患登録など，各種のデータベースが構築され，大規模医療データベースを用いた臨床疫学，薬剤疫学研究を実施することが世界的な潮流となっています．2014年にはレジデントノート誌にて，医療現場に立脚した臨床研究の実例についてのシリーズを監修させていただいたこともあり[※]，このようなデータベース研究の分野は国内でも大きな注目を集めるようになっています．

　私の教室には，全国から多くの若手医師が大学院に入学し，大規模データベースを用いた臨床研究の世界に足を踏み入れてこられています．大学での取り組みのみならず，田中先生ご夫妻のご助力をいただいて，これまでの数年間に，神戸では年に3回，さらには，札幌，東京，横浜，博多など各地で，若手医師や薬剤師向けに臨床研究の初学者のためのセミナーやワークショップを開かせていただきました．その際にも，医療統計学に関する質問や苦手意識の声はよく聞かれます．

　田中司朗先生，田中佐智子先生は，上述のようなさまざまな教育コンテンツの開発や指導のご経験を踏まえて，この「短期集中！オオサンショウウオ先生の医療統計セミナー」では忙しい臨床医などにも無理なく読んで学習いただけるような工夫を取り入れられています．私も，もっと若いうちにこの本に出会っていれば…と，いまこの本を手に取っている読者を羨ましく思うところです．繰り返しになりますが，今後，各種の大規模医療データベースや疾患登録情報を用いた臨床疫学研究は，医学研究の中心となっていくと思います．そのなかで，医療統計の考え方，読み取り方を学んでいくことで，皆さんの臨床研究力と発想力が広がっていくことを祈念しています．

※シリーズ「臨床の疑問を解決する手段　臨床研究をはじめよう！」全6回（レジデントノート2014年1月号〜2014年11月号，隔月で掲載）

2016年9月

京都大学大学院医学研究科薬剤疫学 教授
川上浩司

◆ はじめに ◆

　ふしぎだと思うこと　これが科学の芽です
　よく観察してたしかめ　そして考えること　これが科学の茎です
　そうして最後になぞがとける　これが科学の花です

朝永振一郎（ともながしんいちろう）（1974年）
（物理学者，1906～1979年）

　桜の季節になると，京都大学にはたくさんの新入生が入学してきます．私が担当している講義「臨床試験」は，医師になった後に京都大学School of Public Health (SPH) に入った大学院生向けのものです．学生の多くは数年の臨床経験を積んでいて，臨床で生じるさまざまな疑問を解決するためにやってきます．そのような「科学の芽」を「科学の花」にしたいと思うのは当然のことです．しかし，講義を通じて知ってほしいと思っているのは，「科学の茎」にこそ真に学ぶべき価値があるということです．

　本書は，これから臨床論文を読もうとするすべての医師に向けて，京都大学SPHで用いている講義ノートに基づいて書きました．短く30講に区切られた形式と，数式を排除しケーススタディから学ぶスタイルを採用したのは，臨床現場の多忙さを配慮してのことです（本来，統計学は腰を落ち着けて学ぶべきものなのですが！）．

　ケーススタディには，2005～2015年にLancetやBMJなどに掲載された教科書的な5論文を採用しました．疾患領域は，腎疾患（第1～11講），循環器疾患（第15～19講），精神疾患（第20～24講），がん（第25～28講），歯科疾患（第29・30講）です．

　しかし，研究者を悩ませた事例もないと議論が深まりません．そこで，生存曲線の解釈が難しかった研究（第4講），主たる解析の後に3通りの統計解析を行ってしまった研究（第8講），リスク・ベネフィット両方の評価を試みた非劣性試験（第12講），製薬企業によるデータ隠しを指摘した研究（第15講），チェルノブイリ原発事故後のスクリーニング効果が論議をよんだ研究（第25講）も紹介しました．

　本書を通じて生物統計学 (biostatistics) を学ぶことで，臨床試験・メタアナリシス・疫学研究の基礎になっている方法論とその原理を理解し，論文で示されている統計解析の結果を読み取ることができるようになるでしょう．

　執筆を助けていただいたすべての人に感謝します．草稿の段階で貴重なご意見をいただいた箕浦孝晃氏，今井匠氏，レジデントノート誌の連載時から丁寧な編集をしていただいた冨塚達也氏，中川由香氏には深くお礼を申し上げます．

2016年9月

田中司朗，田中佐智子

ガイダンス

- 本書は，講義30コマ，演習問題，課題論文5本（別冊に収載）により構成されています．課題論文に沿って解説していきますので，最初に論文の抄録を読んで全体を把握してください．論文の参照箇所は講義中で随時お示ししていますから，講義を中心に読み進め，必要に応じて論文に戻る形で結構です．

- 講義の冒頭で「本講のテーマ」を掲げた後に，それについての解説がなされ，最後に「本講のエッセンス」としてまとめを行っています．本書をひととおり終えた後には，課題論文の通読にトライしてみてください．

- 解説の途中で，生徒とオオサンショウウオ先生の質疑応答があります．講義の補足となっていますので，合わせて読むようにしてください．

- 可能なかぎり数式は用いていません．いくつか大切なトピック〔Kaplan-Meier（カプラン・マイヤー）法，Wald（ワルド）検定，サンプルサイズの公式，最小化法，ランダム化に基づく統計的推測，メタアナリシス，誤分類によるバイアス，交絡と層別解析〕については，講義の後に「理解を深めるための計算」を用意しています．お急ぎなら，こちらは飛ばして読んでいただいても構いません．

- 生物統計学は，統計学，臨床試験，メタアナリシス，疫学といった学問分野にまたがっているため，全体を俯瞰しづらい面があります．図1に，本書に登場するキーワードを整理しました．プロペンシティスコアやネットワークメタアナリシスなど流行の手法や，データの品質管理・保証など知っておくべき話題もカバーしています．疾患サーベイランス，予後因子研究，診断研究，医療経済評価の手法は扱っていません．

- 本書では英語論文を読む助けになるよう，キーワード初出には日本語と英語を併記しています．外国人名は英語表記としました．図1のVanderWeele（ヴァンダーウィル），Shpitser（シュピツァー），Poisson（ポアソン），Cox（コックス），Bayes（ベイズ）は著名な統計学者・数学者です．

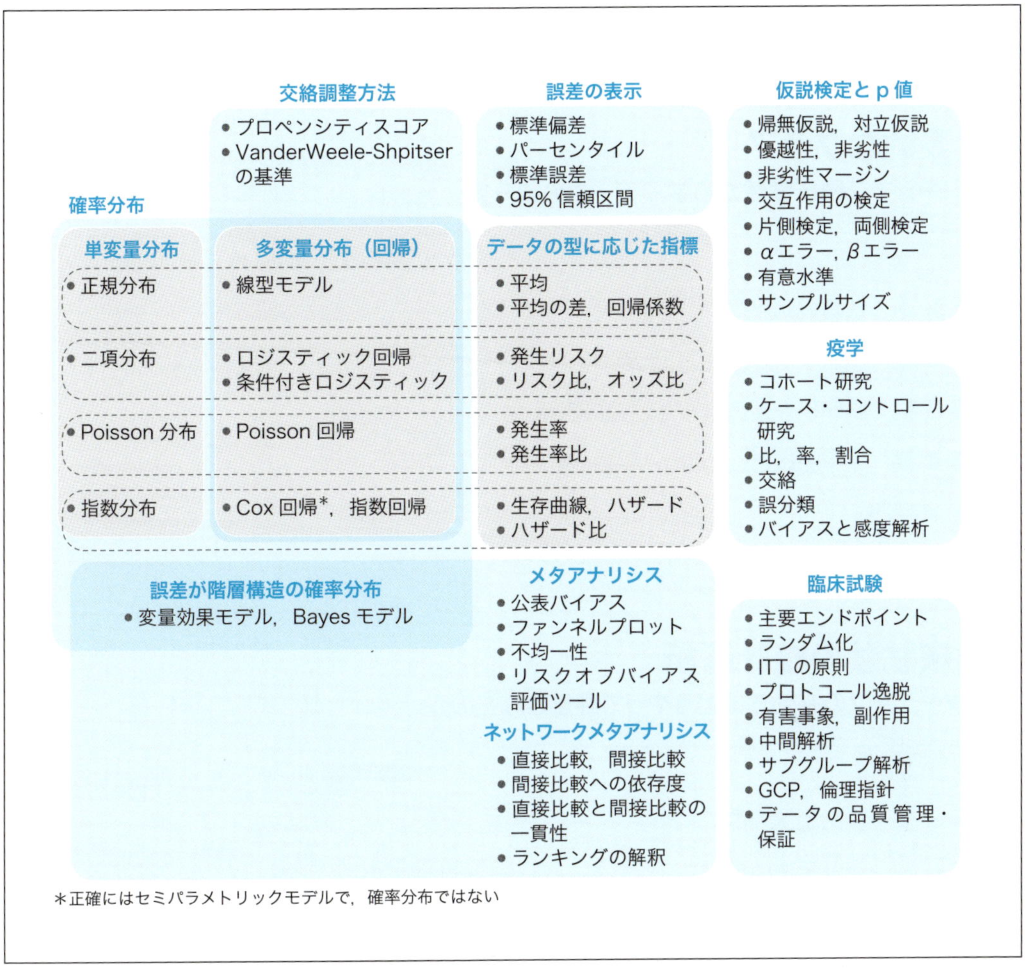

確率分布

単変量分布
- 正規分布
- 二項分布
- Poisson 分布
- 指数分布

多変量分布（回帰）
- 線型モデル
- ロジスティック回帰
- 条件付きロジスティック
- Poisson 回帰
- Cox 回帰*，指数回帰

誤差が階層構造の確率分布
- 変量効果モデル，Bayes モデル

交絡調整方法
- プロペンシティスコア
- VanderWeele-Shpitser の基準

誤差の表示
- 標準偏差
- パーセンタイル
- 標準誤差
- 95% 信頼区間

データの型に応じた指標
- 平均
- 平均の差，回帰係数
- 発生リスク
- リスク比，オッズ比
- 発生率
- 発生率比
- 生存曲線，ハザード
- ハザード比

メタアナリシス
- 公表バイアス
- ファンネルプロット
- 不均一性
- リスクオブバイアス評価ツール

ネットワークメタアナリシス
- 直接比較，間接比較
- 間接比較への依存度
- 直接比較と間接比較の一貫性
- ランキングの解釈

仮説検定と p 値
- 帰無仮説，対立仮説
- 優越性，非劣性
- 非劣性マージン
- 交互作用の検定
- 片側検定，両側検定
- α エラー，β エラー
- 有意水準
- サンプルサイズ

疫学
- コホート研究
- ケース・コントロール研究
- 比，率，割合
- 交絡
- 誤分類
- バイアスと感度解析

臨床試験
- 主要エンドポイント
- ランダム化
- ITT の原則
- プロトコール逸脱
- 有害事象，副作用
- 中間解析
- サブグループ解析
- GCP，倫理指針
- データの品質管理・保証

*正確にはセミパラメトリックモデルで，確率分布ではない

図1　本書で解説する生物統計キーワード
課題論文ごとのキーワードを，別冊に収録した各論文の冒頭ページに示しています．

目 次

- ◆ 推薦のことば　　　　　　　　　　　　　　　　　　　　　　川上浩司
- ◆ はじめに
- ◆ ガイダンス

I　代表的なグラフ
リツキシマブ臨床試験から学ぶデータの読み方

課題論文1　Iijima K, et al：Lancet, 2014［腎疾患］

- 第 1 講　抄録の読み方とPICO ……………………………………………… 14
- 第 2 講　患者取り扱いのフローチャート ………………………………… 19
- 第 3 講　臨床検査値の推移と誤差の表示 ………………………………… 25
- 第 4 講　生存曲線とKaplan-Meier法 ……………………………………… 31
- ◆ 演習問題 …………………………………………………………………… 39

II　臨床試験の統計解析
リツキシマブの有効性はどうやって評価されたのか

課題論文1　Iijima K, et al：Lancet, 2014［腎疾患］

- 第 5 講　論文読解のポイント ……………………………………………… 42
- 第 6 講　統計手法の選択 …………………………………………………… 45
- 第 7 講　生存時間解析 ……………………………………………………… 49
- 第 8 講　p値によるエラーの制御 ………………………………………… 53
- ◆ 演習問題 …………………………………………………………………… 63

III　臨床試験のデザイン
リツキシマブ臨床試験とダビガトラン非劣性試験を例に

課題論文1　Iijima K, et al：Lancet, 2014［腎疾患］

- 第 9 講　サンプルサイズの計算 …………………………………………… 66
- 第10講　中間解析 …………………………………………………………… 72

第11講	ランダム化	75
第12講	非劣性試験	81
◆ 演習問題		92

IV 臨床試験の基礎知識

| 第13講 | 臨床試験と規制 | 96 |
| 第14講 | データの流れと品質管理・品質保証 | 102 |

V メタアナリシス
抗凝固薬に関するエビデンスの統合

課題論文2　Ruff CT, et al：Lancet, 2014［循環器疾患］

第15講	メタアナリシスの大前提－偏りのない試験選択	108
第16講	メタアナリシスの本質は「平均値」	112
第17講	固定効果モデルと変量効果モデルの使い分け	115
第18講	サブグループ解析と交互作用の検定	119
第19講	試験ごとのバイアスの評価	124
◆ 演習問題		128

VI ネットワークメタアナリシス
17通りの双極性障害治療レジメンを比較するには

課題論文3　Miura T, et al：Lancet Psychiatry, 2014［精神疾患］

第20講	大流行のネットワークメタアナリシス	130
第21講	273通りのリスク比	133
第22講	間接比較への依存度	138
第23講	直接比較と間接比較の一貫性	141
第24講	ランキングの解釈	144
◆ 演習問題		146

VII コホート研究とケース・コントロール研究
放射線被曝問題でみる疫学研究の実際

課題論文4　Cardis E, et al：J Natl Cancer Inst, 2005 ［がん］

- 第25講　長年の議論に決着をつけたケース・コントロール研究 …………………………… 148
- 第26講　ケースとコントロールの選択と調査 …………………………………………………… 152
- 第27講　交絡とはリンゴとバナナを比較すること ……………………………………………… 159
- 第28講　回帰モデルを用いた交絡の調整 ………………………………………………………… 165
- ◆ 演習問題 …………………………………………………………………………………………… 171

VIII プロペンシティスコア
受動喫煙の影響を正しく推定するには

課題論文5　Tanaka S, et al：BMJ, 2015 ［歯科疾患］

- 第29講　プロペンシティスコアを用いた交絡の調整 …………………………………………… 174
- 第30講　バイアスと感度解析 ……………………………………………………………………… 182
- ◆ 演習問題 …………………………………………………………………………………………… 187

- ◆ オオサンショウウオ先生からのご挨拶 ………………………………………………………… 188
- ◆ 索 引 ……………………………………………………………………………………………… 190

contents

理解を深めるための計算

- 1. Kaplan-Meier 法 ……………………… 35
- 2. Wald 検定 ……………………………… 60
- 3. サンプルサイズの公式 ………………… 70
- 4. 最小化法 ………………………………… 77
- 5. ランダム化に基づく統計的推測 ……… 78
- 6. メタアナリシス ………………………… 113
- 7. 誤分類によるバイアス ………………… 157
- 8. 交絡と層別解析 ………………………… 163

知っとこ！（押さえておきたい用語の説明）

- ◆ PICO ……………………………………… 15
- ◆ 重篤な有害事象 ………………………… 15
- ◆ 有意差 …………………………………… 16
- ◆ p 値 ……………………………………… 16
- ◆ 指数分布と比例ハザード性 …………… 68
- ◆ ITT, FAS, PPS ………………………… 90

解説（理解が深まる知識の紹介）

- ◆ 3勝1敗のレトロゾール臨床試験 その1：
  治療のクロスオーバー ………………… 23
- ◆ 統計的推測 その1：仮想的反復 ……… 29
- ◆ 統計的推測 その2：
  中心極限定理と正規分布 ……………… 29
- ◆ 統計的推測 その3：ランダム誤差とバイアス … 34
- ◆ Kaplan-Meier 法の公式 ……………… 38
- ◆ データの型と確率分布 ………………… 47
- ◆ 3勝1敗のレトロゾール臨床試験 その2：
  4つのp値 ………………………………… 59
- ◆ 推定値が正規分布に従う ……………… 61
- ◆ ランダム化の実際 ……………………… 77
- ◆ ランダム化が許容されるとき ………… 77
- ◆ 統計的推測 その4：
  モデルベースとランダム化ベース …… 79
- ◆ 医薬品の臨床開発 ……………………… 98
- ◆ 倫理指針改訂のポイント ……………… 99
- ◆ 臨床統計家（生物統計家：biostatistician）とは … 100
- ◆ 公表バイアスを見つける手がかりは？ ……… 110
- ◆ メタアナリシスでも PICO は重要 …… 114
- ◆ 交互作用を検討するほかの状況 ……… 122
- ◆ ランダム誤差とバイアス ……………… 125
- ◆ 公表バイアスとネットワークメタアナリシス … 136
- ◆ 統計的推測 その5：
  Bayes 統計学と主観確率 ……………… 137
- ◆ 回帰モデルの誤特定 …………………… 156
- ◆ 測定の信頼性と妥当性 ………………… 156
- ◆ 95％信頼区間は必ず対称か？ ………… 169
- ◆ 回帰モデルでも95％信頼区間と
  p値を報告すべき ……………………… 169
- ◆ 交互作用は回帰モデルの用語 ………… 169
- ◆ 統計的推測 その6：
  モデルの誤特定と感度解析 …………… 169
- ◆ VanderWeele-Shpitser の基準と
  因果ダイアグラム ……………………… 180
- ◆ 回帰モデルの説明変数の選択 ………… 180

別冊　課題論文 & 演習問題の解答と解説

著者プロフィール

田中司朗　Shiro Tanaka

保健学博士，生物統計家．

東京大学疫学・生物統計学教室で学位取得後，京都大学探索医療センターにてメトレレプチン治験などの統計業務に従事．2012年より社会健康医学系専攻薬剤疫学分野，2017年より臨床統計学講座にて教育・研究を行う．主な担当科目は，臨床試験，臨床研究データ管理学，医学，医薬ビジネスや政策のための統計学．2014年度ベストティーチャー賞受賞．2016年にノースカロライナ大学チャペルヒル校に留学後，2017年より現職．

所属する多施設臨床試験グループは，JCCG（日本小児がん研究グループ；統計委員），JCOG（日本臨床腫瘍研究グループ；効果・安全性評価委員・プロトコール審査委員），A-TOP（骨粗鬆症至適療法研究会；実行委員）．主な学外活動は，日本薬剤疫学会評議員，日本骨粗鬆症学会評議員，日本学術振興会専門委員，PMDA（医薬品医療機器総合機構）専門委員，AMED（日本医療研究開発機構）課題評価委員，厚生労働省がん免疫療法ガイドライン作成のための検討委員．

田中佐智子　Sachiko Tanaka

保健学博士，生物統計家，薬剤師．

東京大学薬学部卒業後，東京大学大学院医学系研究科で学位を取得し，国立がん研究センターがん予防・検診研究センターにてがんの疫学研究の計画・統計解析に従事．東京理科大学工学部経営工学科を経て，京都大学医学研究科EBM研究センター，京都大学臨床研究総合センターにてアカデミア主導臨床試験に統計解析者として，研究計画，統計解析にかかわる．京都大学薬剤疫学分野を経て，2015年より滋賀医科大学医療統計学部門に在籍．また，2015年より，滋賀大学データサイエンス教育センターに，クロスアポイントメントとして在籍．

オオサンショウウオ先生プロフィール
臨床試験や疫学研究など，統計関連の業務や教育に従事しています．このような生物統計の専門家は，日本ではオオサンショウウオのような天然記念物と言われています．著者が属する京都大学や滋賀医科大学は，数少ない生物統計家の生息地です．

I

代表的なグラフ
リツキシマブ臨床試験から学ぶデータの読み方

課題論文1　Iijima K, et al：Lancet, 2014［腎疾患］
▶別冊　2〜11ページ

I 代表的なグラフ

課題論文1 Iijima K, et al：Lancet, 2014 ［腎疾患］

第1講 抄録の読み方とPICO

本講のテーマ

2～11ページ：
課題論文1

最初のケーススタディは，日本で行われた，難治性ネフローゼ症候群にリツキシマブが有効かどうかを調べた臨床試験です．まずはSummary（抄録）を読んでみましょう（図1）．

図1 リツキシマブ臨床試験のSummary（抄録）
（課題論文1より転載）

---

keyword

PICO，主要エンドポイント，p値

PICOを読み取ろう

臨床試験の概要は，
- Patients（患者）
- Intervention（介入）

- Comparison（比較対照）
- Outcomes（アウトカム，エンドポイント）

という4つの要素 **"PICO"** で整理できます．まずはこれらを読み取ることが大切です．

PICO

研究仮説をわかりやすく人に伝えるために，クリニカルクエスチョンとよばれる「問いかけ」の形がよく用いられます．臨床試験の場合，「どんな患者に（Patients），どんな介入を行うと（Intervention），何と比べて（Comparison），どうなるか（Outcomes）が知りたい」というのがクリニカルクエスチョンの基本形です．学会抄録など，手短に研究を説明したいときは，PICOを意識するとうまくいきます．

この試験では，Patientsは頻回再発型またはステロイド依存性ネフローゼ症候群患者48人，Interventionはリツキシマブ（375 mg/m²/週），Comparisonはプラセボ（偽薬）です．治療の結果であるOutcomesは無再発期間と有害事象の頻度・重篤度です．

重篤な有害事象

臨床試験では，**有害事象（adverse event）** と **副作用（side effectまたはadverse drug reaction）** を区別しています．有害事象は，医薬品が投与された患者に生じるあらゆる好ましくない医療上のできごとと定義されます．一方，副作用は，有害事象のうち医薬品と事象の発生との因果関係❶があるもののことです．ただし，因果関係をどこで線引きするかは難しい問題で，日本の規制当局は「因果関係を否定できないもの」を副作用として扱ってきましたが，欧米ではそれではノイズが多いということで「因果関係について合理的な可能性があるもの」としています．

さらに，**重症（severe）** と **重篤（serious）** も異なる意味をもちます．重症は，軽度（mild），中等度（moderate），高度（severe）のように，ある特定の疾患の進行度や症状の程度を表すために用いられます．一方，重篤な有害事象とは，
①死に至るもの
②生命を脅かすもの
③治療のための入院または入院期間の延長が必要であるもの
④永続的または顕著な障害・機能不全に陥るもの
⑤先天異常・先天性欠損をきたすもの
⑥その他の医学的に重要な状態
とされています．これは国際的に標準化された薬事行政上の基準で，例えば，有害事象の一部は国への報告義務がありますが，（重症度ではなく）重篤度と未知／既知の違いによって，報告ルールが異なります．

❶臨床医学における因果関係については第25講で解説します．

結果と結論は一対一

Summaryを読んでまず気がつくのは、**エンドポイント・解析結果・結論が一対一に対応する**ように論理構成されていることです。Findings（結果）には、エンドポイントと解析結果について

「リツキシマブ群の無再発期間中央値（267日）はプラセボ群（101日）に比べ有意に長かった（p＜0.0001）」

と書かれています。これがInterpretation（解釈）に書かれている"Rituximab is effective"という結論の根拠です。すなわち、**主要エンドポイント（primary endpoint）である無再発期間のp値により有効性を判定している**わけです。一方で安全性については、重篤な有害事象の発生割合に有意差はなく（p＝0.36）、それ以外の毒性も考慮したうえで"Rituximab is safe"と述べています。

 有意差

　学術論文で有意（significant）という場合には、ほとんどが「統計学的に有意」ということを意味します。無再発期間に差があったとしても、もしかしたらランダム誤差（系統的でないばらつき）のせいでたまたま差が生じたのかもしれない、と疑うのが、統計学的なものの見方です。統計学的有意差とは、ランダム誤差とはいえないほど大きな差のことで、これを判定するための道具がp値です。

p値

　この論文では、「リツキシマブはプラセボに比べ無再発期間を延長する効果がある」のか「効果がない」のか、**二者択一の判断をするため、仮説検定（hypothesis test）という統計手法を用いています**❷。p値は仮説検定において計算される指標です。多くの場合、p＜0.05であれば「統計学的に有意」とみなせます。ちなみに、p値を計算する仮説検定にはものすごくたくさんの種類があり、Fisher（フィッシャー）、Wilcoxon（ウィルコクソン）、McNemar（マクネマー）など、発明した統計学者の名前がついていることが多いです。

　この試験は48人とそれほど大規模ではありませんが、この結果、リツキシマブの適用拡大が認められ、患者に画期的新薬を届けられた、という意味で、「小粒でもピリリと辛い」試験といえます。

 ここまでで質問はありますか？

 主要エンドポイントって何ですか？

簡単にいうと，エンドポイント，アウトカムとは治療や介入の結果のことですが，大事なのは「主要」の2文字です．

エンドポイントが複数あると，「いいとこどり」ができてしまうのです．例えば，主要エンドポイントが1つ（生存期間）のときと，5つ（生存期間，QOL改善，無再発期間，有害事象の頻度，重篤度）のときを想像してみましょう．後者ではp値が5つ出てきて，それぞれp＜0.05で有意差があるかどうかを判定することにします．p値が1つだと，誤って有効と判定してしまう確率❸は5％ですが，5つあると「いいとこどり」によって，どこかの検定で有効と判断してしまう確率が5％から23％に増えてしまうことが知られています❹．

有効性を検証する臨床試験では，**最も関心のある結果を1つだけ設定して主要エンドポイントとよび，その結果から有効性を判定します**．それ以外は**副次エンドポイント（secondary endpoint）**とよばれます．

❸ αエラーといいます（第8講で解説）．
❹ $1 - 0.95^5 = 0.23$

例えば，有効性に関する主要エンドポイントと副次エンドポイントがあって，それぞれでp＝0.06とp＜0.05だったらどうなります？
副次エンドポイントのp値をもって薬は有効といえますか？

その場合，有効性を結論することはできません．これは，大学入試の合格基準を操作してはならないのと同じで，公平に判定するための一種のルールです．

じゃあ，その薬は効かないってことになるんですね

いえ，必ずしもそういうわけではありません．有意でなかった理由として，「薬に本当に効果がなかった」のか「別の理由で有意差が出なかった（データが少なかった，服薬遵守率が低かった，対象患者の選択がまずかった，など）」のか，いろいろなものが考えられます．

その場合，別の研究デザインで臨床試験が行われることもありますし，**メタアナリシス（meta-analysis）**❺という有力な手法もあります．メタアナリシスにより，ほかの臨床試験の結果と統合解析をすることで，より確実な結論が得られることがあります．

❺ 第15〜24講で解説します．

主要エンドポイントは1つだけ，というルールに例外はないんですか？

例外はあります．例えばアルツハイマー病治療薬の臨床試験では，認知機能と全般臨床症状を別々のスケールで測って，両方を主要エンドポイント（co-primary endpoints とよびます）にすることがふつうです．ただしその場合でも，「いいとこどり」を防ぐために専用の統計手法が必要になりますが，ここでは触れません．

もう1つ，複数のイベントを1つにまとめてしまう**複合エンドポイント（composite endpoint）**という考え方もあります．ダビガトラン臨床試験❻がその例で，脳卒中と全身塞栓症のいずれか先に起きたほうを，主要エンドポイントと設定しています．

❻第12講で解説します．

本講のエッセンス

- ☐ 抄録では，PICO（Patients, Intervention, Comparison, Outcomes）を読み取ることが重要です．
- ☐ 有効性を検証する臨床試験では，最も関心のある主要エンドポイントが1つだけ設定されます．
- ☐ 主要エンドポイントの解析結果と研究の結論は，一対一に対応します．

第2講 患者取り扱いのフローチャート

課題論文1 Iijima K, et al：Lancet, 2014［腎疾患］

p値にばかり目がいきがちですが，それ以前に確認しておくべきことがあります．解析対象となったのは何人でしょうか？

論文のResults（結果）を読むと，冒頭でFigure 2（図1）が示されています．「患者63人をスクリーニング」からスタートして，解析対象になったのは「リツキシマブ投与24人」と「プラセボ投与24人」の48人で，それ以前に15人が除外されたことがわかります．さらに，48人の解析対象集団のうち，リツキシマブ群で4人，プラセボ群で20人が治療を中止したことも示されています（明らかに偏りがあることに注意！）．

今回の解析対象集団は妥当なのでしょうか？例えば，治療中止の24人の患者

別冊 6ページ

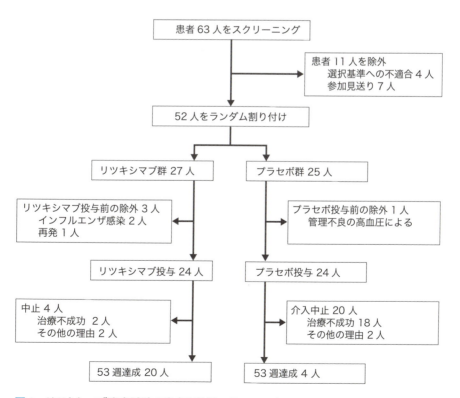

図1　リツキシマブ臨床試験の患者取り扱いのフローチャート
（課題論文1よりFigure 2を転載）

は，予定どおりの治療を受けていないのだから除外してはいけないのでしょうか？63人中15人が除外されていますが，どこからが除外すべきで，どこからが解析対象に含めるべきなのでしょうか？

> **keyword**
> ITTの原則，最大の解析対象集団，プロトコール遵守集団，プロトコール逸脱

患者取り扱いのルール

　臨床試験における患者の取り扱いは，国際的に合意されたルールがあって，**Intention-To-Treat（ITT）の原則**とよばれています．ITTの原則とは，一言でいうと「**ランダム化された全患者を，割り付けの結果どおりに解析すべき**」というものです．ランダム化の後に起こる計画からの逸脱（例えば治療中止）は，群間で偏っている可能性があります．それでも，せっかくランダムに治療を割り付けたのだから，両群で実験条件がそろうように扱う，というのがITTの原則です．

　ただし，「ランダム化された全患者」というのは厳しすぎる，という意見があり，現在最も一般的なルールは，「割り付けられた治療を一度も受けていない患者」と「データが全くない患者」だけは除外してよい，というものです（**図2**）．これらの患者のみを除外した集団を，**最大の解析対象集団（Full Analysis Set：FAS）**とよんでいます．これに加えて，プロトコール逸脱（protocol deviation）や試験治療不遵守の患者を除いた集団を**プロトコール遵守集団（Per-Protocol**

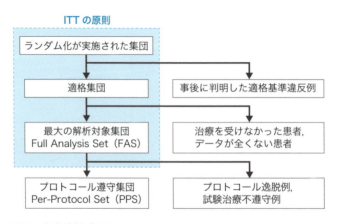

図2　解析対象集団の分類

Set：PPS）とよんでいます．

　プロトコール逸脱や試験治療不遵守によって，試験の結果がどのような影響を受けるかはよく問題になることですが，ITTの原則に従うFASが統計学的観点からは好まれます．FASに対して行う統計処理をITT解析，PPSに対して行う処理をPPS解析といいます．

FASかPPSか

　臨床試験の解析結果を読み取るときには，FASとPPSのどちらなのかを見落とさないようにしましょう．

　リツキシマブ臨床試験ではFASが採用されました．すなわち，治療をランダムに割り付けられた52人のうち，インフルエンザ感染，再発，高血圧のため治療を開始できなかった4人は除外され，治療を開始した48人すべてが統計解析に含められました．

6ページ，
Results第2段
落冒頭

 ここまでで質問はありますか？

 プロトコール逸脱って何ですか？

 具体的に，日本臨床腫瘍研究グループ（JCOG）が用いているプロトコール逸脱の分類を一例として紹介しましょう．このグループでは，
①プロトコール違反
②プロトコール逸脱
③許容範囲の逸脱
の3カテゴリーを用いています．

　①のプロトコール違反とは，試験実施計画書（プロトコール）に従って試験を実施しなかったケースのうち，臨床的に不適切で，逸脱の程度が大きいものです．プロトコール違反は，論文公表する際に原則として個々の違反の内容を記載することになっています．

　また，試験ごとに逸脱の許容範囲が設けられており，逸脱の程度が小さいもの（③に該当）についてはモニタリングレポートや論文などに示されません．

　②のプロトコール逸脱とは，プロトコール違反にも，許容範囲からの逸脱にも該当しないものです．

❶エンドポイントの評価へ影響するものや，系統的なものなど，複数の基準に該当するものをいいます．

 常にITTの原則に従うのが正しいんですね？

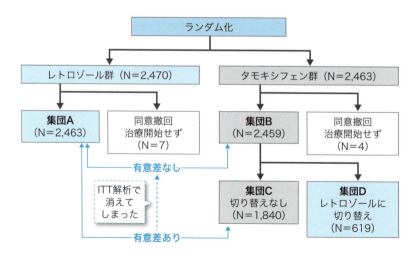

図3 レトロゾール臨床試験の5年追跡時点の解析における患者取り扱いのフローチャート
(文献3を参考に作成)

そういうわけでもありません．ITT解析は，両群に割り付けた治療以外の違いが，可能なかぎり生じないようにする保守的な方法なのです．

　ITT解析を行うと有意差が消えてしまった例として，レトロゾール臨床試験を紹介しましょう．詳細については後述の「解説」を読んでもらうとして，図3がレトロゾール臨床試験の患者取り扱いのフローチャートです．FASは，集団AとBですよね．ところが，この試験では，事情があってタモキシフェン群のうち619人が，タモキシフェンを投与開始した後にレトロゾールに切り替えてしまいました（集団D；クロスオーバー）．そうすると，タモキシフェン群の予後は，レトロゾール群に近づいてしまうと予想されますよね．この試験では，追跡5年時点で集団AとBの全生存期間が比べられたのですが，有意差はみられませんでした（p＜0.08）．

　一方で，集団Bのうち，集団Dをクロスオーバー時点で観察打ち切り[2]にする解析を行ったところ（一種のPPS解析です），こちらでは有意差があったのです．このように**ITT解析は，保守的で，群間差がつきにくい**といわれています．

[2] 第4講で解説します．

では，ITT解析とPPS解析の両方とも行えばいいんですね

それは一理あるのですが，いずれにしてもどちらが主たる解析なのかを事前に決めておく必要があります．これも「いいとこどり」を避けるための知恵です．

PPS解析のほうが好まれる状況もある，ということですか？

そのとおりです．そのような状況の1つは，通常とは逆に，差がないことを証明しようとする非劣性試験（non-inferiorty trial）❸です．非劣性試験では，ITT解析とPPS解析の両方を行うことが積極的に勧められています．もちろん主たる解析はどちらか一方なのですが．

❸第12講で解説します．

例えば，抗うつ薬の臨床試験だと，治療中止後は来院がなくて，うつ重症度の評価ができないこともあります．その場合，データがないから除外してもいいですか？

それはITTの原則に反します．判断材料の1つは，**その患者にエンドポイントに関係するデータが全くないかどうか**です．抗うつ薬臨床試験では，主要エンドポイント評価時点を8週目などと特定しますが，治療開始から8週の間にデータが1つでもあれば，8週目のデータが欠測だったとしても解析に含めます．

個人内で反復測定されているデータの解析では欠測の問題はつきもので，これを解決するため，**変量効果モデル（random-effects model）**とよばれる統計手法を用いることが一般的です❹．

❹第6講で解説します．

リツキシマブ臨床試験のように，再発などのイベントが起きるまでの期間（生存時間データ）がエンドポイントのときには，ITTの原則に従い，イベントが起きなかった患者も，「打ち切り（censoring）」として解析に含めなければいけません．

 3勝1敗のレトロゾール臨床試験 その1：治療のクロスオーバー

今回紹介したレトロゾール臨床試験の経緯を**表1**に示します．

BIG 1-98試験は，ホルモン感受性早期乳がん患者を対象に，レトロゾールとタモキシフェンを術後療法として比較したランダム化臨床試験です[1)～3)]．この試験は1998～2011年まで続いた長期試験で，追跡途中の主たる解析でレトロゾールの有効性が示されたため，タモキシフェン群のおよそ1/4の患者が，タモキシフェンからレトロゾールに切り替えました．このような治療のクロスオーバーは，明らかにランダム割り付けを崩すものですが，患者側の強い希望があればやむを得ません．

レトロゾール臨床試験では，有効性に関する結果が3つの論文で4回にわたり報告されています．この話の結末は，59ページの「解説」で．

表1 レトロゾール臨床試験の経緯

1998年3月	BIG 1-98試験の登録開始
2004年12月	2年追跡が完了し，主たる統計解析を実施 ・レトロゾール群の無病生存期間が有意に優る
2005年4月	プロトコール改訂 ・タモキシフェン群の患者へのレトロゾール提供を許容 ・その後，タモキシフェン → レトロゾールのクロスオーバーが頻発
2005年12月	第1報公表（NEJM論文），レトロゾール承認
2009年8月	第2報公表（5年追跡結果をまとめたNEJM論文） ・タモキシフェン単独投与群の1/4（619人）がクロスオーバー ・ITT解析の結果，全生存期間に有意差なし（p＝0.08）
2011年3月	第3報公表（JCO論文）

（文献1～3をもとに作成）

本講のエッセンス

☐ 解析対象集団がITTの原則に従っているかどうかを見過ごさないようにしましょう．

☐ 割り付けられた治療を一度も受けていない患者・データが全くない患者を除外した集団を，最大の解析対象集団（FAS）とよびます．これに加えて，プロトコール逸脱・試験治療不遵守を除いた集団を，プロトコール遵守集団（PPS）とよびます．

☐ プロトコール逸脱や試験治療不遵守によって，試験の結果がどのような影響を受けるかはよく問題になることですが，ITTの原則に従うFASが統計学的観点からは好まれます．

文献

1) BIG 1-98 Collaborative Group, et al：Letrozole therapy alone or in sequence with tamoxifen in women with breast cancer. N Engl J Med, 361：766-776, 2009

2) Breast International Group (BIG) 1-98 Collaborative Group, et al：A comparison of letrozole and tamoxifen in postmenopausal women with early breast cancer. N Engl J Med, 353：2747-2757, 2005

3) Colleoni M, et al：Analyses adjusting for selective crossover show improved overall survival with adjuvant letrozole compared with tamoxifen in the BIG 1-98 study. J Clin Oncol, 29：1117-1124, 2011

| I 代表的なグラフ | 課題論文1　Iijima K, et al：Lancet, 2014［腎疾患］|

第3講　臨床検査値の推移と誤差の表示

本講のテーマ

論文のFigure 4（図1）には，末梢B細胞数の平均の推移が時間軸に沿って示されています．リツキシマブ投与直後に末梢B細胞数が低下し，徐々にもとに戻ったことがわかります．ここで注目してほしいのは，平均の周りに示されているエラーバーです．これが誤差を表していることは想像に難くありませんが，その正確な意味は何でしょうか？

別冊 9ページ

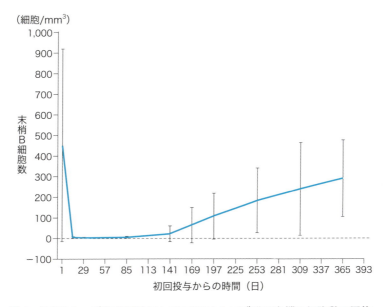

図1　リツキシマブ臨床試験におけるリツキシマブ群の末梢B細胞数の平均
（課題論文1よりFigure 4を転載）

keyword

エラーバー，標準偏差，パーセンタイル，標準誤差，95％信頼区間

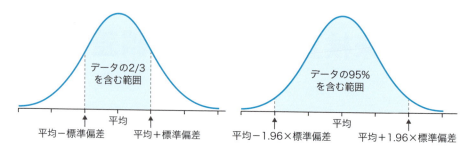

図2 正規分布と平均±標準偏差（左），平均±1.96×標準偏差（右）の関係

エラーバーの種類

　エラーバーはランダム誤差（系統的でないバラツキ）の程度を表すためのもので，以下の4つが使い分けられます．
- ±標準偏差（standard deviation：SD）
- パーセンタイル（percentile）
- ±標準誤差（standard error：SE）
- 95％信頼区間（confidence interval：CI）

エラーバーの関係性

これらには，標準偏差，95％信頼区間，標準誤差の順に狭くなるという性質があります．図の注釈を確認すると，エラーバーは標準偏差であることがわかります．

標準偏差

標準偏差はデータのバラツキを示す指標です．±標準偏差は，直感的にはおおよそ**データの2/3**が含まれる範囲と考えて間違いはありません．±1.96×標準偏差だと，おおよそ**データの95％**が含まれます❶．これらの目安は，データが正規分布に従うときにはかなり正確です（図2）．

❶臨床検査の正常範囲は，健常人の95％が含まれる区間ですよね．

パーセンタイル

　しかし，中性脂肪や尿アルブミンなどは，飛びぬけて高い値（外れ値）をとる患者がいますよね．外れ値があるデータは，正規分布の当てはまりが悪いので，平均±標準偏差ではなく，25％点から75％点までの範囲（四分位範囲）を示すことがあります．25％点や75％点は，パーセンタイルの一種です．x％点（xパーセンタイル）とは，データを小さい順に並べたとき，最小値から数えて全体のx％に位置する値のことです．例えば中央値は50％点のことで，データ全体の真ん中に位置する値です．25％点は小さいほうから数えて上位25％，75％点は上位75％に対応する値です．

図3 箱ひげ図の例
中央値と四分位範囲の代わりに平均±標準偏差を示すこともあります．

データのバラツキを表すために，最大値，75％点，中央値，25％点，最小値を「箱」と「ひげ」で表した，箱ひげ図もよく用いられます（図3）．

標準誤差

標準誤差は，平均などの推定値のバラツキを示す指標です．平均では「標準偏差/サンプルサイズ（症例数）の平方根」として計算され，サンプルサイズが大きくなるほど小さくなります．

95％信頼区間

95％信頼区間は「平均±1.96×標準誤差」として計算されます❷．

❷その意味は後述します．

 ここまでで質問はありますか？

 たくさん種類がありますが，よく使われるのはどれですか？

 そこがポイントですよね．この4つのうち，**臨床研究で最もよく用いられるのは95％信頼区間**です．統計学では，母集団のある値を推定するとき，95％以上の確率でその真の値を含む区間を推定する方法を，95％信頼区間と定義しています．

 すみません，95％信頼区間というのがよくわからないのですが…

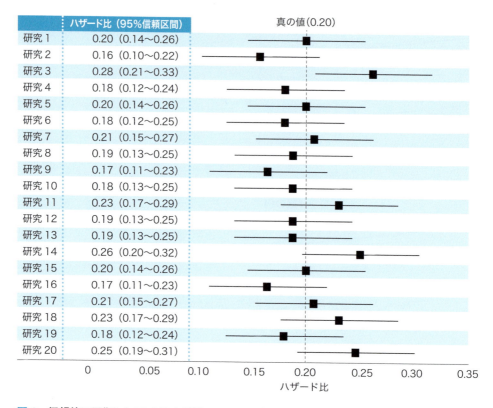

図4 仮想的に反復した20の臨床試験による95％信頼区間のシミュレーション

95％信頼区間などの統計用語は，数学的に定義されるものなのでわかりづらいのです．特に，95％信頼区間の意味についてはさまざまな哲学や学派があるのですが，ここでは直感的な説明をしましょう．

ハザード比の真の値が0.20である臨床試験があったとします（図4研究1）．それと同様の研究を，仮想的に20回繰り返した仮想的反復のシミュレーション結果が図4の研究2〜研究20です．研究ごとにリツキシマブ群とプラセボ群の無再発期間の差（ハザード比❸；■）とその95％信頼区間が計算されていて，その結果は95％信頼区間を意味するエラーバーで図示されています．個々のハザード比の値は，真の値である0.20（仮想的な設定値です）を中心にばらつきます．

一方で95％信頼区間は，多くは0.20を含んでいますが，0.20を含んでいないものが1つあります（研究3）．これは20回に19回（95％）は真の値を含むことを表しています．

実際には真の値はわからないし，研究は研究1の1回しか行われていませ

❸第7講で解説します．

ん．研究1からわかることは，ハザード比0.20（95％信頼区間は0.14〜0.26）という結果だけです．しかし，図4のように考えることで，同じ研究を繰り返したとき，どの程度ばらつくのかを想像することができます．

 では，なぜ図1では標準偏差を使っているんですか？

 おそらく，末梢B細胞数の分布の変動範囲を示したいという意図でしょうね．また，平均値は中央値よりも外れ値の影響を受けやすいので，末梢B細胞数では外れ値はそれほど影響しなかったのでしょう．外れ値が気になる場合には，中央値の上下に25％点から75％点までの範囲を示したはずです（図3のように）．

 それ以外に標準偏差を使うのは，どんなときですか？

 対象者がどのような特徴をもっていたのかを記述するときです．リツキシマブ臨床試験のTable 2でも，連続データのバラツキを表すために標準偏差を用いています．

別冊
7ページ

 解説 統計的推測 その1：仮想的反復

　図1と図4では，統計学的なものの見方が異なることに注意してください．図1は，24人から得られた末梢B細胞数の推移を表していて，反復の単位は「人」，確率変数は「末梢B細胞数」です．一方で図4は，反復の単位は「試験」，確率変数は「ハザード比」です．

　統計学が扱う「ランダム誤差」という言葉からイメージするのは，実際に測定された値1つ1つのバラツキかもしれません．しかし，統計学ではむしろ，実測値のバラツキではなくて，実測値から計算された推定値について，仮想的反復を行ったときの誤差分布を考えていることのほうが多いのです．標準偏差と標準誤差というよく似た用語は，もとの確率変数のバラツキと，推定値のランダム誤差を区別するためのものです．メタアナリシス❹は臨床試験のある種の反復ですから，仮想的反復をイメージする助けになるかもしれません．

❹第15〜24講で扱います．

 解説 統計的推測 その2：中心極限定理と正規分布

　統計学の研究テーマの1つは，仮想的反復を想定したときに平均などの推定値がどのような誤差分布に従うのか，ということです．一般に，誤差分布はサンプルサイズ（症例数）が小さいときと大きいときで分けて検討されます．なぜなら，サンプルサイズが大きいとき，かなり一般的な状況で，誤差分布は正規分布に収束するためです．

　よく知られている中心極限定理は，「独立同一な確率変数から平均を計算したと

き，サンプルサイズが大きいと，もとの確率変数がどんな確率分布であっても，その誤差は近似的に正規分布に従う」ということを示したものです．また，**回帰モデル[5]の回帰係数の推定値〔最尤推定（maximum likelihood estimation）といいます〕も，サンプルサイズが大きければ誤差は正規分布に従います．**

ここで注意してほしいのは，実際に測定された値1つ1つが正規分布に従うということは仮定されていないということです．例えば，Wald（ワルド）検定[6]は，測定値ではなくて，推定値が正規分布に従うことを前提にする手法です．これは，図1ではなくて図4のような仮想的反復における誤差分布のことをいっているのです．

[5] 第28講で解説します．

[6] 第8講で解説します．

本講のエッセンス

- □ エラーバーには±標準偏差，パーセンタイル，±標準誤差，95％信頼区間の4つが使い分けられます．
- □ 臨床研究で最もよく用いられるのは95％信頼区間です．
- □ 中央値，25％点，75％点などのパーセンタイルは，外れ値の影響を受けにくいという特徴があります．

I 代表的なグラフ

課題論文1　Iijima K, et al：Lancet, 2014［腎疾患］

第4講　生存曲線とKaplan-Meier法

本講のテーマ

　今回は，生存曲線を解釈できるようになるため，リツキシマブ臨床試験に加えて2つのケーススタディを取り上げます．図1A左と図1B左のグラフをご覧ください．この2つはいずれも，抗がん剤の臨床試験（ゲフィチニブ臨床試験[1]とシスプラチン臨床試験[2]）のもので，おのおののグラフには，異なる治療を受けた患者を追跡したとき生存していた割合を示す2本の生存曲線が描かれています．左上は，2本に差がありそうですがクロスしています．左下は，1本の曲線の生存確率だけが

A　ゲフィチニブ臨床試験の無増悪生存曲線

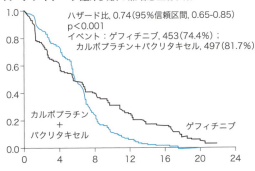
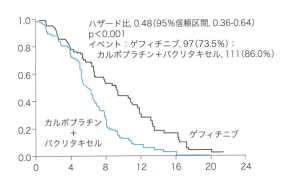

B　シスプラチン臨床試験の無病生存曲線

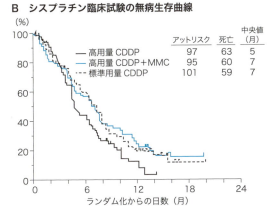
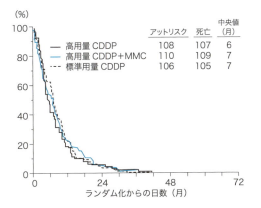

図1　差があるのかどうか判断が難しい生存曲線の例
Aはゲフィチニブ臨床試験（文献1より引用），Bはシスプラチン臨床試験（文献2より引用）．CDDP：シスプラチン，MMC：マイトマイシンC

低そうですが差は微妙です．はたしてどのような解釈が正しいのでしょうか？

> **keyword**
>
> Kaplan-Meier法，アットリスク数，打ち切り，脱落バイアス

生存曲線の読み取り方

8ページ

いよいよ，この試験の主たる解析結果であるFigure 3A（図2）です．このグラフは，**生存曲線またはKaplan-Meier（カプラン・マイヤー）曲線**とよばれており，各時点で再発せずに「生き残る」確率をプロットした，階段状のグラフです．

図から，リツキシマブ群の1年無再発確率と無再発期間中央値を読み取ってみましょう．**1年無再発確率は，横軸が365日のところ（図2↑）を読めばよいので，42％になります．無再発期間中央値は，50％の患者が生き残っている時点を読む**ことになります．つまり，縦軸が50％のところ（図2→）なので，267日です．

アットリスク数に注目

図2からリツキシマブ群のほうがプラセボ群よりも無再発確率が高いことがわかりますが，1年を越えたあたりで，リツキシマブ群で急激に再発が起きている（階段が下がっている）ことが気になりませんか？

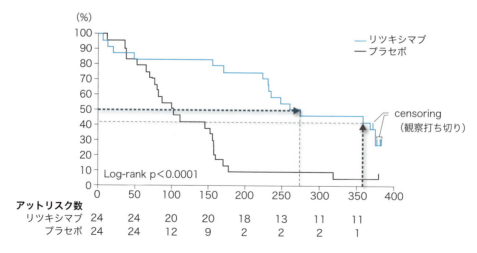

図2　リツキシマブ臨床試験におけるリツキシマブ群とプラセボ群の無再発曲線
（課題論文1よりFigure 3Aを転載．「censoring（観察打ち切り）」，引き出し線，矢印，破線は著者追記）

実は，これは重要ではありません．なぜなら，この試験は予定追跡期間が1年なので，その周辺では対象者の人数が少ないためです．このことを示しているのが，グラフの下にある**アットリスク数（number at risk）**です．アットリスク数は，各時点で，観察が継続している（再発も観察打ち切りも起きていない）人数のことで，24人からスタートして，350日時点では11人しかいません．そのため，**グラフの右端では誤差が大きいのです**．

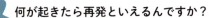

　ちなみに**観察打ち切り**は英語ではcensoringといい，図2では，打ち切りが発生した時点は曲線の上の「ひげ」で表されています．試験開始直後はひげがなく，終了したあたりにひげが集中していることにも注目してください．予定追跡期間の終了時期なので，打ち切りが起きているのです．

 ここまでで質問はありますか？

何が起きたら再発といえるんですか？

うっかりしていました．無再発期間のような生存時間データでは，**イベント時点と打ち切り時点の定義を確認することが重要**です．
　これは論文ではなくプロトコールにのみ書かれているのですが，この試験では，尿試験紙による早朝尿の尿タンパク2＋以上が連続3日続き，プレドニゾロン投与が必要になった時点を，再発時点としています．患者が来院しなかった等で再発がないことが確認できなかった最後の日が，打ち切り時点です．

試験開始直後にひげがあるとおかしいんですか？

ありえないことではないですが，あまり多いと不自然ですよね．Kaplan-Meier法は，打ち切りがランダムであることを前提にしています．増悪や副作用など，疾患の悪化に関係して打ち切りが生じた場合，Kaplan-Meier法を用いたとしても正しく生存曲線を推定することはできません．これは，**脱落バイアス（attrition bias）**の一種です．

❶第19講を参照ください．

図2では2本の生存曲線がありますが，この場合は1年目にどちらが高いかを比べればいいんですか？

別冊 3ページ,Summary のFindings 2〜4行目

いえ，必ずしもそうではありません．特定の時点（1年無再発確率など）を比較することもありますが，曲線全体を平均的に比較することのほうがむしろ一般的です．Summaryには，

「リツキシマブ群の無再発期間中央値（267日）はプラセボ群（101日）に比べ有意に長かった（p＜0.0001）」

と書かれていましたが，このp値はログランク検定（log-rank test）という手法によるもので，曲線全体を比較したものです．1年目などの特定の時点を比べているわけではありません．

❷第3講で扱いましたね．

❸第19講，第30講で取り上げます．

解説 ▶ 統計的推測 その3：ランダム誤差とバイアス

ランダム誤差❷は，基本的にはゼロを中心としたバラツキを想定しています．一方で，得られた推定値が真の値から系統的にずれていることを，バイアス❸といいます．別の言い方をすると，生存曲線などの推定値に過大評価や過小評価が生じること，と理解してもらっても構いません．臨床研究における統計学の目標は，ランダム誤差を制御し，バイアスを可能なかぎりゼロに近づけることです．

差の判断が難しいケース

さて，冒頭の図1に戻りましょう．これらは図2と違って，差があるのかどうか判断が難しいケースです．

治療反応性の高いサブグループが隠れている場合

冒頭の図1A左は，未治療でステージⅢB〜Ⅳの肺がん患者1,217人を対象に，ゲフィチニブとカルボプラチン＋パクリタキセル併用療法を比較したランダム化臨床試験の結果です[1]．主要エンドポイントは，腫瘍増悪または死亡までの期間（無増悪生存期間）です．図1A左では，**無増悪生存曲線がクロス**していて，6カ月まではゲフィチニブ群で無増悪生存確率が低く，それ以降は高くなっています．

なぜこのような現象が起きたのでしょうか？ それは，ゲフィチニブはEpidermal Growth Factor Receptor（EGFR）遺伝子突然変異が陽性の患者に，特に有効だからだと考察されました．図1A右は，EGFR陽性の261人における無増悪生存曲線を描いたものです．このサブグループでは，ゲフィチニブの無増悪生存曲線が全期間を通じて上回っていることがわかります．EGFR陰性の集団では，逆にゲフィチニブのほうが下回っていました．つまり，図1A左の解釈は，**6カ月あたりからEGFR陽性患者が増悪しないまま生き残っていることが，曲線に表れてきた**，ということになります．

ちなみにこの試験の結論は，ゲフィチニブはカルボプラチン＋パクリタキセル併用療法に比べ，有効であるというものでした．

中間解析の場合

図1B左は，別の臨床試験の**中間解析（interim analysis）**のものです[2]．この試験では，非小細胞肺がんを対象に，標準用量シスプラチンをコントロール群として，高用量シスプラチンと高用量シスプラチン＋マイトマイシンC併用療法という2つの試験治療が比べられました（三群比較試験）．主要エンドポイントは，無病生存期間です．中間解析は，期待イベント数の1/3，2/3が観察された時点に行うと予定されていました．

図1B左は第1回中間解析の結果ですが，期待に反して，試験治療の1つである高用量シスプラチン群の無病生存曲線が，一番下にあるのがわかります．これを検定してみると，「高用量シスプラチン群は標準用量シスプラチン群に勝てない」ということが，統計学的な有意差をもって示されました．つまり，高用量シスプラチンが逆転して有意に勝つ可能性はきわめて低いということです．

この中間解析結果に基づき，データモニタリング委員会は，**無益性（futility）**による登録中止を勧告しました．皆さんだったら，この試験を早期中止しますか？

図1B左は中間解析のものでしたが，図1B右は登録中止後にさらに患者を追跡したときの無病生存曲線です．この2つを比較すると，追跡後は中間解析時点のものと違い，差がほとんどないことがわかります．追跡調査を行うと，追加でイベント発生の情報が得られることになりますから，**生存期間は短くなり，生存曲線は左にシフト**します．つまり中間解析の結果は，不確実性が伴うものなのです．

そんな…中間解析の結果なんか信じられません！

そう思います．特に，あまり早い時期に有効性の中間解析を行うと，データが少なすぎて判断を誤りがちです．一方で，登録を開始したばかりの時期に安全性を確かめておくことは必要なのですが，そのような「安全性モニタリング」は中間解析と区別するのがふつうです．

一般に中間解析とは，試験途中で，ランダム化したグループ間を統計学的に比較することを意味します．

理解を深めるための計算1

Kaplan-Meier法

Kaplan-Meier法のポイントは以下の4つです．
- 時点ごとに順番に計算する
- イベント時点では生存確率が下がる

表1 リツキシマブ臨床試験におけるリツキシマブ群の無再発曲線の描き方

再発/打ち切り	××	××	××	××	××	××	××	××	××	××	××
時点	6	13	20	49	155	170	224	231	232	236	249
d	1	1	1	1	1	1	1	1	1	1	1
n	24	23	22	21	20	19	18	17	16	15	14
生存確率	1−1/24＝0.96	1−2/24＝0.92	0.88	0.83	0.79	0.75	0.71	0.67	0.63	0.58	0.54

再発/打ち切り	××	××	××	××	○○	××	××	○○	○○	○○	○○	○○	○○
時点	260	275	358	366	370	375	375	376	381	382	382	382	382
d	1	1	1	1	0	2		0	0	0	0	0	0
n	13	12	11	10	9	8		6	5	4	3	2	1
生存確率	0.5	0.46	0.42	0.38	0.38	0.38×(1−2/8)＝0.29		375日以降イベントが起きていないため0.29					

d＝その時点で再発した人数,n＝その時点で観察されている患者数.1つ1つの列は,リツキシマブ群24人の再発または打ち切りまでの期間を表す.××は再発した17人に,○○は打ち切りの7人に対応.

- 打ち切り時点では生存確率は下がらない
- 打ち切りの患者を分母(アットリスク数)から除く

● 実際の計算─リツキシマブ臨床試験を例に

表1にリツキシマブ群の24人の患者のデータを示します.これは,リツキシマブ群の患者24人を,再発または打ち切りまでの期間が短い順に並べたものです.

最初の患者は6日時点で再発しており,6日から375日にかけて全17人の患者で再発が観察され,それ以外の7人の患者は,370日,376日,381日,382日で観察が打ち切られていました.計算にはこのデータを使います.

＊　　＊　　＊

再発しか生じない366日までは簡単です.まず,6日時点では24人中に1人再発したので,1から再発確率を引いて,

6日生存確率＝1−1/24
　　　　　＝0.96

という計算になります.この,「1−イベント数/アットリスク数」という計算が基本です.次の13日時点では24人中に2人再発したので,

13日生存確率＝1−2/24
　　　　　　＝0.92

です.つまり,打ち切りが発生するまでは,単純な割合を計算すればよいのです.

図2のリツキシマブ群の250日を見てください.再発確率は,0.5(50％)より少し上ですよね.表1によると,249日までに11人が再発していることから,

249日生存確率＝1－11/24
　　　　　　＝0.54

で，計算が合うことがわかります．図2と表1で，その後0.54→0.46→0.42→0.38と推移していることを確認してみてください．初めて打ち切り患者が登場するのは370日時点ですが，この時点では「打ち切り時点では生存確率は下がらない」ので，370日生存確率は366日生存確率と同じ1－15/24＝0.38です．

　　　　　　＊　　　＊　　　＊

　問題は375日時点です．「打ち切りの患者を分母から除く」という考え方によると，375日時点で存在している患者は370日時点で打ち切りの患者を除いた8人ですから，8人中2人で再発したことになります．つまり，75％が生き残ったわけです．**したがって，370日時点の生存確率0.38と比べると，次の時点には75％だけ確率が下がるはずです**．これを計算してみると，

375日生存確率＝0.38×(1－2/8)
　　　　　　＝0.38×0.75
　　　　　　＝0.29

となります．したがって，0.38の次は0.29まで階段が下るグラフを描けばよいのです．打ち切りが何度出てきても，同じように分母から除く操作をして，時点ごとに順番に，その時点で生き残る確率を掛けていけばよいのです．

ここまでで質問はありますか？

イベントが定期的な検査のタイミングで起きる状況では，階段は等間隔になりますね？

そのとおりです．図1Aがガタガタ下がっていくのは，腫瘍増悪の画像判定のタイミングで曲線が下がるためです．イベントが死亡だとこうはなりません．

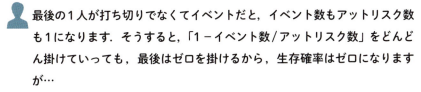
最後の1人が打ち切りでなくてイベントだと，イベント数もアットリスク数も1になります．そうすると，「1－イベント数／アットリスク数」をどんどん掛けていっても，最後はゼロを掛けるから，生存確率はゼロになりますが…

それも本当です．追跡期間が最も長い対象者がイベントを起こしたとき，生存曲線はゼロまで下がります．

解説 ▶ Kaplan-Meier法の公式

より一般的に，Kaplan-Meier法を数式で表してみましょう．i番目の時点のイベント数をd_i，アットリスク数をn_iで表します．x年生存確率は，「$1-d_i/n_i$」をx年に達するまで掛けた

$$x年生存確率 = \left(1 - \frac{d_1}{n_1}\right) \times \left(1 - \frac{d_2}{n_2}\right) \times \cdots$$

で計算されます．

本講のエッセンス

- ☐ 生存曲線（Kaplan-Meier曲線）をみる前に，イベント・打ち切り時点の定義と予定追跡期間・実際の追跡期間を確認しましょう．
- ☐ 何人がイベントで何人が打ち切りだったか，アットリスク数，打ち切りのタイミング（ひげ）を読み取ることも重要です．
- ☐ グラフの右端でアットリスク数が小さい部分では，誤差が大きくなります．
- ☐ 試験開始直後に打ち切りがあまり多いと，打ち切りがランダムではなくバイアスが生じているかもしれません．

文献

1) Mok TS, et al：Gefitinib or carboplatin-paclitaxel in pulmonary adenocarcinoma. N Engl J Med, 361：947-957, 2009
2) Gandara DR, et al：Evaluation of cisplatin intensity in metastatic non-small-cell lung cancer: a phase III study of the Southwest Oncology Group. J Clin Oncol, 11：873-878, 1993

次は演習問題です

I 代表的なグラフ

演習問題

問題1 課題論文4（Cardis E, et al：J Natl Cancer Inst, 2005）を読んで，以下の問いに答えなさい．

別冊
32〜41ページ

1 コホート研究やケース・コントロール研究では，PICOではなくPECO（Population, Exposure, Comparison, Outcomes）を用います．PECOはそれぞれ論文のどこに書いてあるか読み取りなさい．

2 Figure 2のエラーバーは，平均±標準偏差，平均±標準誤差，95％信頼区間のうちどれでしょうか？

3 平均±標準偏差，平均±標準誤差，95％信頼区間のうち，エラーバーの長さについて正しいのは，次のうちどれでしょうか？

ⓐ 95％信頼区間＞平均±標準偏差＞平均±標準誤差
ⓑ 95％信頼区間＞平均±標準誤差＞平均±標準偏差
ⓒ 平均±標準偏差＞平均±標準誤差＞95％信頼区間
ⓓ ⓐ, ⓑ, ⓒすべて誤り

問題2 試験治療群とコントロール群の脳卒中発生率を，Kaplan-Meier法を用いて比較する臨床試験を想定して，以下の問いに答えなさい．

1 脳卒中が発生したかどうかについて，どのようなタイミングで評価を行うべきでしょうか？

ⓐ 6カ月間隔で定期的に
ⓑ 可能なかぎり頻回に
ⓒ 予定された検査時点で
ⓓ 患者の希望に合わせて

2 Kaplan-Meier法を用いるべきなのは，どのような場合でしょうか？

　　ⓐ 追跡期間が正規分布するとき
　　ⓑ 脱落する対象者が多いとき
　　ⓒ 追跡期間が長いとき
　　ⓓ 対象者間で追跡期間が異なるとき

3 Kaplan-Meier法が妥当なのは，どのようなときでしょうか？

　　ⓐ 追跡期間が正規分布するとき
　　ⓑ 追跡不能の理由が疾患の悪化によらないとき
　　ⓒ 追跡期間が長いとき
　　ⓓ 試験治療群とコントロール群の間で比例ハザード性が成り立つとき

4 生存期間中央値を報告してよいのは，どのような場合でしょうか？

　　ⓐ 半数以上の対象者がイベントを起こしたとき
　　ⓑ 目安としてサンプルサイズが100人以上のとき
　　ⓒ すべての対象者が予定された追跡期間を完了したとき
　　ⓓ ⓐ, ⓑ, ⓒすべて誤りである

II 臨床試験の統計解析
リツキシマブの有効性はどうやって評価されたのか

課題論文1　Iijima K, et al：Lancet, 2014 ［腎疾患］
▶別冊　2〜11ページ

II 臨床試験の統計解析

課題論文1　Iijima K, et al：Lancet, 2014［腎疾患］

第5講　論文読解のポイント

本講のテーマ

別冊
5〜6ページ

今回は，読み飛ばされがちなMethods（方法）のStatistical analysis（統計解析）にチャレンジしてみましょう．図1は，その最初の2段落です．

Statistical analysis
On the basis of previous reports,[12,13,18] we assumed that 40% of the patients in the rituximab group and 10% of the patients in the placebo group would maintain remission 6 months after registration. 30 patients in each group would be needed to establish the superiority of the test treatment for the primary endpoint with 90% power at a 2·5% one-sided significance level under the assumption of exponential distribution of relapse-free survival time and proportionality of hazards.
　We used the log-rank test to analyse the primary endpoint and other time-to-event endpoints. We did an interim analysis (appendix) after 30 patients had relapsed, with a significance level set at 0·25% (one-sided). We summarised time-to-event data with the Kaplan-Meier method and estimated therapeutic effect hazard ratios (HRs) and their 95% CIs with Cox regression.

図1　リツキシマブ臨床試験のStatistical analysis（統計解析）の記述
（課題論文1より転載，ハイライトは著者追記）

●keyword

検出力，有意水準，サンプルサイズ，ログランク検定，Kaplan-Meier法，ハザード比，95％信頼区間，Cox回帰，中間解析

統計用語の整理と内容の確認

　一目見ただけでも，なじみのない統計用語のオンパレードですよね．最初に用語の整理をしながら，内容の確認をしたいと思います．図1でハイライトした用語を順にみていきましょう．

＊　　　＊　　　＊

まず，**検出力（power）**と**片側有意水準（one-sided significance level）**は仮説検定の用語です．最初の段落を訳すと，

> 「先行研究に基づいて，リツキシマブ群の患者の40％と，プラセボ群の患者の10％が，登録後6カ月時点で寛解を維持していると仮定した．無再発期間について指数分布と比例ハザード性を仮定したとき，試験治療の有効性を検出力90％，片側有意水準2.5％で示すために，1群30人の患者が必要であった」

となり，どのようにサンプルサイズ（症例数）を計算したのかが記述されています❶．

＊　　＊　　＊

第2段落目には，主要エンドポイントとその解析方法について書かれています．ここで**ログランク検定（log-rank test）**とは，第4講 図2のような2本以上の生存曲線を比較する手法で，Summary（抄録）のp＜0.0001もログランク検定のものです．この試験では，30人が再発した時点で**中間解析（interim analysis）**が行われていたようです❷．**Kaplan-Meier法（Kaplan-Meier method）**は，生存曲線を描くための手法でしたね❸．

また，リツキシマブの効果を定量的に評価するためには，生存曲線だけではなく，再発のリスクが何倍になったのかが知りたいですよね．それを表す指標が**ハザード比（hazard ratios）**です．また，推定されたハザード比のバラツキを表すのが**信頼区間〔95％CI（confidence interval）〕**です．このハザード比を計算する手法が**Cox（コックス）回帰（Cox regression）**です❹．リツキシマブ臨床試験の生存曲線からは，ハザード比は0.27（95％信頼区間0.14〜0.53）と計算されました．つまり，再発が1/3以下になった，ということです．

統計解析を読むポイント

Statistical analysis（統計解析）を読むときのポイントとして，独断と偏見で優先順位をつけると，以下のような順番になります．
①主要エンドポイントとその統計手法
②サンプルサイズの計算
③中間解析の有無とその統計手法

知らない統計手法があるとどうしてもそちらに目が行きがちですが，枝葉末節よりポイントを押さえておくべきです．

①が大切なのは，主たる結論と主要エンドポイントは対応関係にあるためです❺．また，主要エンドポイントの統計解析がどのような手法で行われたかも重要です❻．

②で注目すべきなのは，計算された症例数自体ではありません．実は，ここには**研究者が研究実施前にどのような研究結果を予想していたか**が書かれています．

> 「リツキシマブ群の患者の40％と，プラセボ群の患者の10％が，登録後6カ月

❶サンプルサイズの計算については第9講で解説します．

8ページ，Figure 3A

❷中間解析については第10講で解説します．

❸第4講をみなおしてください．

❹第7講で詳しく解説します．

❺第1講で述べましたね．

❻リツキシマブ試験に用いられた解析方法（生存時間解析）については，次回（第6講）に詳しく取り上げます．

時点で寛解を維持していると仮定した」
という部分ですね．リツキシマブは予想どおりの効果を示したわけですが，予想よりも効果が小さいことも大きいこともあるわけです．

③の中間解析では，**きちんと試験を完遂したのか，試験途中に何か計画の変更が行われたのか**を読み取らなければなりません．もしかしたら，この論文は中間解析の結果を報告したものかもしれないのですから．

本講のエッセンス

- 臨床試験論文のMethods（方法）を読むときには，まずは主要エンドポイントとその統計手法，サンプルサイズの計算，中間解析の有無とその統計手法を押さえましょう．
- また，統計解析では，統計手法の名前だけではなく，検出力や有意水準の数字も重要です．

第6講 統計手法の選択

課題論文1 Iijima K, et al：Lancet, 2014［腎疾患］

本講のテーマ

リツキシマブ臨床試験のSummary（抄録）に戻ってみましょう．そこには2つのp値が登場します．これらは別の種類の統計手法によるもので，無再発期間のp値（p＜0.0001）はログランク検定（log-rank test），重篤な有害事象のp値（p＝0.36）はFisherの正確検定（Fisher exact test）です．これらの統計手法は，どのように使い分けられているのでしょうか？

別冊 3ページ

keyword

連続データ，2値データ，計数データ，生存時間データ，反復測定，交絡の調整

統計手法の使い分け

統計手法の使い分けのポイントは，データの型，反復測定の有無，交絡調整の有無の3つです．表1に沿って解説していきましょう．

データの型

アウトカムはデータの型によって4種類に分類されます．すなわち，
- **連続データ**（例：血圧）
- **2値データ**（例：有害事象の有無）
- **計数データ**（例：骨折発生率）
- **生存時間データ**（例：再発までの期間）

です．データの型によって，正規分布や二項分布など確率分布が異なるので，それぞれ別の記述統計（グラフなどを作成してデータの傾向をつかむ手法）や仮説検定が用いられます．

連続データの場合，その分布が正規分布に従うときは対応のないt検定を，正規分布に従わないときはWilcoxon順位和検定（Wilcoxon rank-sum test）が用いられることが多いです．

表1　統計手法の選択

データの型	反復測定	交絡調整	適切な統計手法	備考
連続データ	なし	なし	対応のないt検定, Wilcoxon順位和検定	平均の比較
	個人内で2回測定	なし	対応のあるt検定, Wilcoxon符号付順位検定	対応のある2つの連続データの比較
	なし	あり	線型モデル	回帰モデルの一種
	2回以上	あり	変量効果モデル	回帰モデルの一種
2値データ	なし	なし	χ^2検定, Fisherの正確検定	割合の比較
	個人内で2回測定		McNemar検定	対応のある2つの2値データの比較
	なし	あり	ロジスティック回帰	回帰モデルの一種
	あり	あり	変量効果モデル	回帰モデルの一種
計数データ	2回以上	なし	χ^2検定	発生率の比較
	なし	あり	Poisson（ポアソン）回帰	回帰モデルの一種
	2回以上	あり	変量効果モデル	回帰モデルの一種
生存時間データ	なし	なし	ログランク検定	生存曲線の比較
	なし	あり	Cox回帰	回帰モデルの一種

個人内で反復測定があるか

　同じ患者に別の日に臨床検査を行うと，似たような検査結果になりますよね．これを反復測定といいます．例えば，第3講 図1の末梢B細胞数の推移は，1人の患者に複数回の測定値がある反復測定データです．反復測定データでは，**個人内の測定値は独立ではありません**．したがって，独立性を仮定している対応のないt検定やχ^2検定などは不適切です．

　2回以上の反復測定データの解析では，**変量効果モデル（random-effects model）**とよばれるやや高度な手法が用いられます．これらの方法は，データが独立ではないこと（データの相関）を考慮するものです．

　変量効果モデルは，個々の測定値のランダム誤差に加え，**もう1つのランダム誤差項（変量効果）をもつモデルのこと**です．変量効果モデルはメタアナリシスでも用いられます[1]．反復測定データでは，変量効果は「1人1人の患者の効果」を表しますが，複数の試験を統合解析するメタアナリシスでは，変量効果は「1つ1つの試験の効果」のことです．

[1] 第17講を参照ください．

交絡の調整が必要かどうか

　交絡因子（confounding factor）とは，治療とアウトカムとの関係をゆがめる第3の因子のことです[2]．仮に，アウトカムが2値データで，性・年齢（交絡因

[2] 第27講を参照ください．

子）が結果をゆがめているとしましょう．そのような場合，性・年齢の影響を調整した検定を行うために，ロジスティック回帰が用いられます❸．

❸第28講で解説します．

ランダム化臨床試験では，**比較する群間で実験条件がそろっているため，交絡の調整は不要**です．一方，**コホート研究やケース・コントロール研究では交絡の調整は必須**です．

リツキシマブ臨床試験の例

では，リツキシマブ臨床試験ではどうだったか確認してみましょう．

無再発期間は，データの型は生存時間データで，反復測定はなく，ランダム化臨床試験なので交絡調整は必要ありません．有害事象は，2値データで，反復測定はなく，交絡調整はありません．したがって，前者にはログランク検定が，後者にはFisherの正確検定が用いられています．

それでは，この論文ではなぜ χ^2 検定ではなくてFisherの正確検定なのですか？

χ^2 検定では，中心極限定理❹を利用して p 値を計算するのですが，サンプルサイズ（症例数）が小さいときには，計算された p 値があまり正確でないのです．一方，Fisherの正確検定は，第11講で解説する並び替え検定の一種で，起こりうるすべてのパターンを数え上げるため，サンプルサイズが小さくても p 値の計算が正確です．

❹第3講"「解説」統計的推測 その2"を参照ください．

目安として，1群あたりの有害事象発生数が5より小さいときには，Fisherの正確検定を用いるべきです．

そういえば，誰かが t 検定にするかWilcoxon順位和検定にするか，悩んでました

実は，データが正規分布に従っていたとしても，Wilcoxon順位和検定を用いても間違いではないのです．正しく差を検出する確率（検出力）が少し落ちるだけなので，**迷うようであればWilcoxon順位和検定などのノンパラメトリック法（確率分布を仮定しない統計手法）を使ってしまってもよい**です．

解説 データの型と確率分布

データの型によって想定される確率分布はさまざまです．代表的なものは，

- 正規分布（normal distribution，連続データの分布）
- 二項分布（binomial distribution，2値データの分布）
- Poisson分布（計数データの分布）

- 指数分布（exponential distribution，生存時間データの分布）

の4つです．

　データの分布になんらかの確率分布を仮定し，それに基づいて構成される統計手法をパラメトリックな手法とよびます．一方，確率分布を仮定しない統計手法はノンパラメトリックな手法といいます．

本講のエッセンス

- ☐ 統計手法は主に，データの型，反復測定の有無，交絡調整の有無によって使い分けられます．
- ☐ ランダム化臨床試験では，比較する群間で実験条件がそろっているため，交絡の調整は不要です．
- ☐ 一方，コホート研究やケース・コントロール研究では，交絡の調整は必須なので，統計解析には回帰モデルがよく用いられます．

| II 臨床試験の統計解析 | 課題論文1　Iijima K, et al：Lancet, 2014 ［腎疾患］

第7講　生存時間解析

本講のテーマ

Statistical analysis（統計解析）から，リツキシマブ臨床試験の主要エンドポイント（無再発期間）の解析には，Kaplan-Meier法，ログランク検定，Cox回帰が用いられていることがわかりました．この3つの統計手法は「生存時間解析三種の神器」とよばれています．これらを詳しくみていきましょう．

別冊
5ページ

keyword

生存時間データ，打ち切り，Kaplan-Meier法，ログランク検定，Cox回帰

生存時間解析三種の神器

Kaplan-Meier法❶は，生存曲線を描くための道具でした．残りのログランク検定は生存曲線に違いがあるかどうか二者択一の判断を行うための道具，Cox回帰は生存曲線の違いを**ハザード比（hazard ratio）**で定量化する道具です．この3つは，がんや循環器疾患など生存時間データを扱う論文で必ず出てきますから，セットで覚えておいてください．

❶第4講で出てきましたね．

なぜこれらが必要なのか

なぜ，生存時間データではこれらの方法が必要になるのでしょうか？
それは，**打ち切り（censoring）**があると単純な方法で解析できないからです．仮に打ち切りがなければ，再発までの期間はただの連続データですから平均を比べるだけで十分なのですが，打ち切りがあると平均が計算できません．追跡不能の患者では，再発までの正確な期間がわかりませんよね．また，再発の有無（2値データ）として解析すると，短い期間で再発が起こったかどうかという情報が反映されません．
そこで導入されたのが，**生存確率（survival probability）**と**ハザード（hazard）**という数学的概念です．

生存確率とハザード

割合，率，比の違い

生存確率とハザードの説明に入る前に，割合（proportion），率（rate），比（ratio）の3つの違いについて確認しておきましょう．

● 比

比とは，**ある量を別の量で割ったもの**のことです．例えば，BMIは体重を身長で割ったものですから，比の一種で，単位はkg/m^2です．

● 割合

割合は，**一部の数を全体の数で割ったもの**（言い換えると，分母が分子を含んでいるもの）ですから，比の一種です．しかし，割合は，①100％を超えない，②人数を人数で割っているためキャンセルして単位がない（無単位），という特徴があります．例えば，100人中5人が再発すると，再発割合は0.05ですよね．再発割合は，再発確率や再発リスクとよばれたりもします．

● 率

割合と区別してほしいのが率です．率は，ある現象が生じるスピードを示すものです．再発発生率は，**一定時間に再発が発生するスピード**のことで，人年法（イベントの発生した人数/観察人年[2]）で計算されます．人数を人数×年で割っているため，単位は1/年（より一般には1/時間）です．

「発生率」を時間の関数として扱ったものがハザード

生存曲線は横軸に時間をとったグラフでした[3]．つまり，生存曲線では，**「生存割合（生存確率）」を時間の関数**とみなし，いつの時点でどのくらい生存しているかをみていることになります．

これとは対照的に，ハザードは，**「発生率」を時間の関数**として扱ったもので，いつの時点でどのくらいのスピードで発生するのかをみています．発生率を調べた研究の多くで，イベントが発生するスピードは時間によらず一定と仮定しています．1年あたりの交通事故発生率などではこの考え方は正しいのですが，リツキシマブ投与後の再発は，時間によらず一定とは考えられません．したがって，この場合は時間の関数と考えるほうが適切です．

*　　　*　　　*

ハザード比は，まさに2群間のハザードの比ですが，必ずしもすべての状況で比例関係が成立するわけではありません．第4講 図1A左のように生存曲線がクロスしている場合は，時点によってハザード比が1より大きくなったり1より小さくなったりしています．

比例関係にあることを比例ハザード性とよんでいますが，**比例ハザード性が満**

---

[2] 観察された追跡期間の合計のこと．「人数×年」で計算します．

[3] 第4講でみましたね．

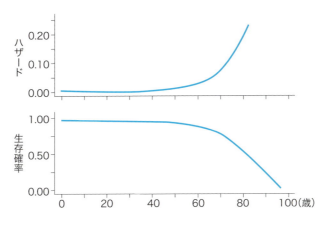

図1　日本人のハザードと生存確率

たされない場合，ハザード比により2本の生存曲線に差があったとしても，それを1つの数字で要約することはできません．また，比例ハザード性を満たす確率分布を，Cox回帰モデルまたは比例ハザードモデルとよんでいます[4]．

[4] 回帰モデルについては第28講で解説します．

ランダムな打ち切りが前提

第4講で述べたことの繰り返しになりますが，最後に大事な注意があります．
　生存時間解析はすべて，**打ち切りがランダムであること**を前提にしています．増悪や副作用など，疾患の悪化に関係して打ち切りが生じた場合，**脱落バイアス（attrition bias）**が生じます[5]．

[5] バイアスについては第19講，第25講で述べます．

　スウガクテキガイネンと聞いて，急に眠くなってきてしまいました…

具体例がないと興味が湧かないですよね．
　図1は，人口動態統計から推定した，日本人の年齢ごとの生存確率とそれに対応するハザードです．出生後数年で死亡するハザードは，10歳代に比べるとほんのわずかに高く，その後最低になり，60歳以降に急速に上昇します．同時に生存確率は低下し，100歳まで存命する人は数％です．

　図1は，年齢ごとに生き残っている割合から，ハザードを計算したってことですか？

そうです．このように，生存確率とハザードは数学的には一対一に対応し

ます❻.

❻単純な場合の関係式は第9講で出てきます.

本講のエッセンス

☐ 打ち切りに対処するための統計手法として,「生存時間解析三種の神器」といわれるKaplan-Meier法,ログランク検定,Cox回帰が用いられます.

☐ これらはすべて,打ち切りがランダムであること(脱落バイアスがないこと)を前提にしています.

☐ Cox回帰では,これに加え比例ハザード性が成り立っている必要があります.

第8講 p値によるエラーの制御

II 臨床試験の統計解析　　課題論文1　Iijima K, et al：Lancet, 2014［腎疾患］

本講のテーマ

Summary（抄録）に出てくるp値ですが，いったい何を表しているのでしょうか．統計学の教科書を紐解くと，図1のような正規分布が登場して，「p値は右すその青い面積である」と説明されることがあります．もちろんこれは正しいのですが，抽象的でわかりづらいという方のために，ここではもう少し具体的な話から始めます．

3ページ

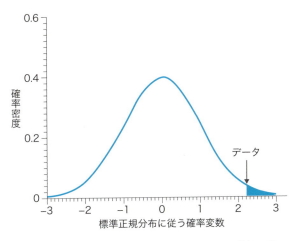

図1　標準正規分布に従う指標を用いたときの片側p値

keyword

p値, 仮説検定, 帰無仮説, 片側検定, 両側検定, 有意水準, αエラー, βエラー, 検出力, サンプルサイズ

p値の考え方──イカサマコインを例に

p値と仮説検定（hypothesis test）は，**研究仮説が正しいかどうかについて，二者択一の判断をするための統計手法**です．

なんだか難しそうなので，たとえ話で説明しましょう．コイン投げをして，6回連続で表が出たとします．このコインは，イカサマコイン（表が出る確率が1/2でない）でしょうか？

p値では次のように考えます．「表が出る確率は1/2」（このコインはイカサマコインではない）という仮説の下で，6回連続で表の確率は $(1/2)^6$ で0.0156（1,000回投げて15.6回）ですよね．6回連続で裏の確率は同じく0.0156です．すなわち，このようなデータが得られる確率は，足してp＝0.0312ときわめて低いことがわかります．

このような極端なデータが得られるのはおかしくはありませんか？「したがって，このコインにはイカサマがある」というのが，p値を用いて仮説（表が出る確率は1/2）を否定するときのロジックです．

仮説検定のステップ

リツキシマブ臨床試験に戻りましょう．仮説検定では3段階の手続きを行います．

ステップ1：仮説の設定

まず，仮説を設定します．

リツキシマブ臨床試験では，真実は「リツキシマブはプラセボに比べ無再発期間を延長する効果がある」と「効果がない」の2通りがありえます．仮説検定では，「効果がない」という仮説に注目して，**帰無仮説（null hypothesis）** とよびます（こちらが，「表が出る確率は1/2」に対応します）．

ステップ2：確率分布の導入

次に，帰無仮説の下でデータがどのように分布するかを調べます．

仮に，同じ対象者48人の試験を1,000回繰り返したと想像してみてください（図2）．無再発期間に差がなかったとしても，ランダム誤差のため，リツキシマブ群のほうがよい場合もあれば，プラセボ群のほうがよい場合もあるでしょうが，1,000回繰り返した結果は，差がないという結果を中心に分布するはずです．

ステップ3：p値の計算

そこで，この分布と実際に得られたデータとを比べ，p値を計算します．p値とは，**帰無仮説が正しい，つまり「生存曲線に差がない」という仮定の下で**，得られたデータよりも極端な差が観察される確率のことです．

1つ1つの生存曲線を実際の生存曲線と比べると，一番右のものと同じくらい差が開いています．したがって，この例では1,000回の繰り返しの中で4回だけ，データより極端な差が観察されたことになります．つまり，図から計算されるp値は，4/1,000＝0.004ということになります．

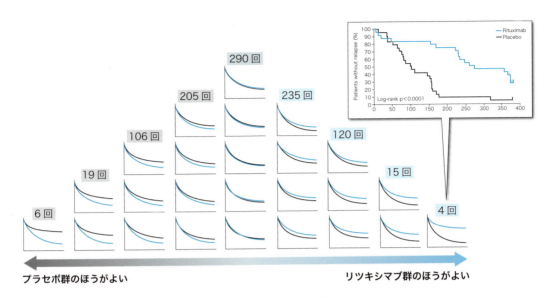

図2 仮想的に反復した1,000の臨床試験によるp値のイメージ

p値が大きいということは，当たり前のことが起きたという意味です．逆にp値が小さいと，極端なことが起きた，という意味です．そうすると，こんな極端なことはありそうもないから，生存曲線に差がないという仮定は間違いだ，という判断になるわけです．

p値を用いた判断は正しいか

さて，先ほどはp値の意味について説明しました．しかし本質的に重要なのは，p値を用いた判断に，どのような合理性があるのか，ということです．

判断を誤ってしまうケース：αエラーとβエラー

真実は「リツキシマブはプラセボに比べ無再発期間を延長する効果がある」と「効果がない」の2通りがあるといいました．一方で，試験の結果も$p<0.05$と$p\geq0.05$の2通りです．これらの組み合わせには2×2の4通りがあります（表1）．

このうち，臨床試験の結果から判断を誤ってしまうケースは2つです．つまり，効果があるのに$p\geq0.05$になってしまうケースと，効果がないのに（帰無仮説が正しいのに）$p<0.05$になってしまうケースです．仮説検定では，前者を**βエラー**（beta error），後者を**αエラー**（alpha error）とよんでいます．また，βエラーを1から引いたものを**検出力**（power）とよんでいます[1]．

αエラーとβエラーが生じる確率

αエラーとβエラーが生じる確率を考えてみましょう．理論的に考えると，サ

[1] つまり，βエラーは1から検出力を引いたものともいえます．

表1　仮説検定における2種類の判断の誤り（αエラーとβエラー）

試験の結果	真実	
	効果あり	効果なし
p≧0.05（有意差なし）	βエラー（1−検出力） （生産者リスク）	正しく判断できた
p＜0.05（有意差あり）	正しく判断できた	αエラー （消費者リスク）

ンプルサイズが大きくなるほど，ランダム誤差は小さくなります．αエラーとβエラーも同じで，サンプルサイズが大きいほど小さくなる（判断を誤りにくくなる）性質があります．

しかし，2つのエラーはトレードオフの関係にあります．サンプルサイズが一定だと，両方同時に小さくすることはできません．そこで通常は，**αエラーを優先して**，事前に決めた水準よりも小さく保たれるような**判定方式を用います**．これが仮説検定であり，この水準のことを有意水準とよびます．

p値と有意水準

実は，p＜0.05で判定することと有意水準を5％と設定することは，同じ意味です❷．p＜0.025だと，2.5％有意水準に対応します．

リツキシマブ試験でいうと，無再発期間のp値を0.025と比べる判定方式は，リツキシマブに効果がなくても，100回に2〜3回は**リツキシマブが**有効と判定します（つまりαエラーは2.5％）．

重篤な有害事象のp値を0.05と比べる判定方式はどうでしょう？こちらは両側検定なので，リツキシマブとプラセボに差がなくても，100回に5回は**リツキシマブとプラセボのどちらかが**有害事象が多いと判定します（αエラーは5％）．

❷証明は統計学の教科書に与えられています．

ここまでで質問はありますか？

別冊
5ページ

いつもp値を0.05と比べてますが，第5講でやったStatistical analysis（統計解析）には2.5％片側有意水準（one-sided significance level）と書かれています．この数値や「片側」ってなんですか？

スルドイつっこみです．**仮説検定には，片側（one-sided）検定と両側（two-sided）検定の2種類があります**．リツキシマブ臨床試験でいうと，片側検定では，リツキシマブ群のほうが無再発期間が長かったときのみ，有意と判定

します．一方で両側検定では，リツキシマブ群のほうが長かったときとプラセボ群のほうが長かったときのいずれの結果でも有意と判定します．

　Statistical analysis（統計解析）をよく読むと，主要エンドポイント（無再発期間）では片側有意水準2.5％を，副次エンドポイント（重篤な有害事象）では両側有意水準5％を採用した，と書かれています．つまり，**無再発期間のp＜0.0001は2.5％と比べるのが，重篤な有害事象のp＝0.36は5％と比べるのが，正しいのです．**

　また，**片側2.5％＋片側2.5％＝両側5％**です．したがって，片側有意水準2.5％と両側有意水準5％は，実質，同じ基準で判定していることになります（なんてヤヤコシイ！）．もし論文に特に断りが書かれていなければ，両側検定と5％有意水準を用いたと読むのが一般的です．というわけで，今回の解説では両側検定のときの数字で説明させてもらいました．

　では片側検定は忘れていいんですか？

　いえ，ほとんどの場合は両側検定なのですが，非劣性試験（non-inferiority trial）は例外的に片側検定を用います❸．

❸第12講で解説します．

　うーん，やっぱり両側片側のイメージが湧きません

　それでは，図2に戻って，確認してみましょう．
　以前解説したときは，右すそだけを考えていましたが，あのp値（4/1,000＝0.004）は片側検定のものです．**両側検定の場合，左すそと右すその両方を数えます．**図2によると，1,000回の繰り返しのなかで，6＋4＝10，つまり10回，データより極端な差が開いています．したがって，両側検定でのp値は10/1,000＝0.01になります．

　両側片側はわかってきましたが，いきなりαとかβとか確率とかが出てきて，さっぱり意味がわかりません

　たくさんの統計用語が登場しましたからね．まずは1つ1つの言葉をきちんと理解しましょう．p値，αエラー，有意水準は，すべて0.05という値と関連して用いられるので混乱しやすいのですが，これらの区別は概念を明確に整理するために不可欠です．

　その0.05の意味がわからなくなってしまったのですが，なぜ0.05なので

しょうか？

0.05は，もともとαエラーの確率を5％よりも小さく保つ，ということからきています．つまり，
① αエラーの確率を5％より小さくすることを，
② 有意水準5％とよんでおり，
③ それはp値が0.05よりも小さいときに有意と判断する
ことで達成されているのです．

そうですよね…．もう少しイメージが湧く説明をしていただけるとありがたいです

❹ 第4講を参照ください．

αエラーの具体例として，シスプラチン臨床試験❹があげられるかもしれません．
　この試験の第1回中間解析では，期待に反して「高用量シスプラチン群の無病生存確率は低いので，標準用量シスプラチン群に勝てない」ということが，有意に示されました（第4講 図1B左）．しかし，登録中止後にさらに患者を追跡したときの無病生存曲線では，差がほとんどなくなっていたのでしたね（第4講 図1B右）．この中間解析では，本当は差がないのに差があると判断してしまったわけです．もちろん，追跡期間が十分でなかったなど，ランダム誤差以外の要因もあるのですが．

ですが，結果的には高用量シスプラチンは効かなかったんですよね

まあそうです．しかし，2つのエラーは意思決定にかかわるので，その結果，何が起きるかを想像することは意味があることです．
　リツキシマブ臨床試験のような有効性を検証する試験では，αエラーは無効な薬が市販されてしまうことにつながります．いわば，「αエラー＝消費者リスク」といえます．一方で，βエラーは有効な薬なのに開発中止してしまうことを意味するため，「βエラー＝生産者リスク」といわれています．医療の立場から気になるのは，やっぱりαエラーのほうですよね．
　安全性の臨床試験や，リツキシマブ臨床試験では重篤な有害事象の検定の結果も報告されていますが，こちらでは逆で，「βエラー＝副作用を見過ごす消費者リスク」になります．

有意差がつかなかったらどうなりますか？例えば実薬AとBを比較する臨床

試験だったとして，AとBの効果は同等と結論に書かれることはあるんですか

それはルール違反で，「有意差がないこと」と「同等」は厳密に区別されています．「同等」や「劣らない」という結論を出すには，同等性（equivalence）試験や非劣性（non-inferiority）試験を組まなければなりません[5]．

[5] 第12講で解説します．

リツキシマブ臨床試験のログランク検定は，p < 0.001でp値がすごく小さいです．臨床試験って，要するにp値が小さければいいんですか？

違います．再発が1/3以下になったとしたら（ハザード比が本当に0.27だったら）リツキシマブの効果は大きいですよね．あるいは無再発期間中央値を見ても，267日と101日の差はかなりのものです．

もしこれが，131日と101日の差だったらどうでしょうか？1カ月の差は大きいとはいえません．しかし，サンプルサイズ（症例数）が大きければp値が小さくなって有意差がつくこともありえます．はたして，このような治療は優れているといえるでしょうか？

また，p値だけに注目すると，かえってミスリードしてしまうこともあります[6]．データを解釈するうえで一番大事なのは，「効果の大きさ」を読み取ることです．

[6] 次の"「解説」3勝1敗のレトロゾール臨床試験 その2"を参照ください．

 3勝1敗のレトロゾール臨床試験 その2：4つのp値

23ページの解説の続きです．

表2は，レトロゾールとタモキシフェンを比較したBIG 1-98試験が公表した論文[1]〜[3]をまとめたものです．この試験では，さまざまな事情があって3本の論文が公表され，4通りの解析結果が報告されました．

p値だけをみると有意水準5%の周辺で上下していて，結論も二転三転しているようにみえます．一方で，ハザード比は0.81〜0.87でそれほど食い違っているわけではありません．もちろん，結果のバラツキはエンドポイント（無病生存期間と全生存期間），追跡期間（2年と5年），解析方法（治療クロスオーバーの取り扱い）の違いによるもので，そのあたりは論文で十分に議論されています．しかし，冷静に振り返ってみると，研究者がp値に踊らされた喜劇のようにも思えます．もちろん，最終的な結論としては，レトロゾールはタモキシフェンに比べて有効ということに行き着くのですが．

表2　レトロゾール臨床試験からの3論文で報告された4通りの解析結果と3つの結論

論文	エンドポイント	解析方法	イベント／人数	ハザード比	p値
NEJM 2005[2]	無病生存期間（主要）	ITT解析	779/8,010（追跡2年）	0.81	$p < 0.05$
【論文の結論】	レトロゾールを用いた補助療法は，タモキシフェンと比べ，再発リスクを減らし，それは特に遠隔部位において顕著だった					
NEJM 2009[1]	全生存期間（副次）	ITT解析	646/4,922（追跡5年）	0.87	0.08
	全生存期間（副次）	PPS解析	641/4,922（追跡5年）	0.81	$p < 0.05$
【論文の結論】	レトロゾール単独療法とタモキシフェン単独療法の全生存の差は，統計学的に有意ではなかった					
JCO 2011[3]	全生存期間（副次）	IPCW解析	641/4,922（追跡5年）	0.82	$p < 0.05$
【論文の結論】	レトロゾールを用いた補助療法は，タモキシフェンと比べ，有意に死亡リスクを減らした					

ITT：Intention-To-Treat　　PP：Per-Protocol set　　IPCW：Inverse Probability of Censoring Weighted
（文献1～3をもとに作成）

理解を深めるための計算2
Wald検定

　ここまで一般論を述べてきましたが，仮説検定にもt検定やログランク検定などさまざまな種類があります❼．ここでは，Cox回帰における**「ハザード比が1かどうか」の検定（Wald検定）**を解説します．Wald検定は，多くの回帰モデルで用いられている汎用的な手法です．

　Wald検定は，推定値が正規分布に従うことを前提にしています．Cox回帰では正規性はサンプルサイズが大きければ成り立つことがわかっています．有意水準5％のとき有意かどうかを判定する手順は，以下のとおりです．

①「ハザード比＝1」という**帰無仮説**（これは「対数ハザード比＝0」と同じ意味ですよね）と**片側か両側か**を決める
②「対数ハザード比／標準誤差」を計算する
③片側検定では，「対数ハザード比／標準誤差」が，**平均0，分数1の正規分布（標準正規分布）の95％点である1.64より大きいかどうか**をみて，大きければ有意と判定する．両側検定では，「対数ハザード比／標準誤差」の絶対値が，**97.5％点である1.96より大きいかどうかをみる**❽

　ちなみに，より一般に有意水準x％のときを考えると，標準正規分布の（$100-x$）％点または（$100-x/2$）％点が，それぞれ片側と両側に対応する判定基準です．

❼第6講でみましたね．

❽このように「推定値／標準誤差」が標準正規分布に従うことを利用する手法がWald検定です．

なぜこれで，αエラーの確率が有意水準よりも小さく保たれるのでしょうか？
わかりやすく有意水準が片側5％のときで説明します．それは，標準正規分布に
従う確率変数が1.64よりも大きくなる確率は，5％だからです[9]．したがって，
「対数ハザード比＝0」が正しいとき，「対数ハザード比／標準誤差＞1.64」にな
る確率[10]は，理論的に5％になるのです．

[9] それがパーセンタイルの定義でした．

[10] これがαエラーの確率でした．

解説 ▶ 推定値が正規分布に従う

Wald検定は，推定値が正規分布に従うと仮定する手法だといいました．これ
は，1人1人の患者で実際に測定された値（リツキシマブ臨床試験の場合は無再発
期間）が，正規分布に従うということではありません．第3講 図4のように，仮
想的反復を想像したときに，推定値が正規分布に従ってばらつく，という意味で
す．臨床研究で用いられている指標（平均，生存曲線，ハザード比など）のほと
んどは，サンプルサイズが大きければ正規分布に従うことが知られています．

ここまでp値は出てきませんでしたが，Wald検定ではp値はどのように計算す
るのでしょうか？ p値を用いる場合には，上の③に代えて以下の手順を用います．

③′ 標準正規分布で，「**対数ハザード比／標準誤差」よりも右の面積（図1右すそ
の青い面積）**を読み取る

④ これが片側p値であり，両側p値は面積を2倍したものになる

つまり，Wald検定のp値の計算では，「対数ハザード比／標準誤差」が，図1の
「データ」に対応しています．

リツキシマブ臨床試験の結果から実際に計算してみましょう．Summary（抄
録）によると，ハザード比は0.27（95％信頼区間0.14〜0.53）でした．そこか
ら，対数ハザード比は「$\log(0.27) = -1.31$」，その標準誤差は「$\{\log(0.53) - \log(0.14)\} / (2 \times 1.96) = 0.34$」と計算されます．その比は3.85ですので，（片側
有意水準2.5％に対応する）1.96よりも大きいですよね．p値を求めるには，標
準正規分布を参照します．図1によると，3.85はずいぶん右すそにあって目盛り
が表示できないほどです．実際，3.85より右の面積は，0.001より小さくなり
ます．

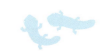

本講のエッセンス

☐ p値と仮説検定は，二者択一の判断において，αエラー（差がないのに差があると判断する誤り）を有意水準以下に制御するための方法です．

☐ 多くの臨床研究では$p<0.05$で有意差を判定しますが，これは有意水準を5％と設定することと同じ意味です．

☐ 見落としがちなのが片側検定と両側検定の違いです．片側有意水準2.5％と両側有意水準5％は，実質，同じ基準で判定していることになります．

☐ また，「有意差がないこと」と「同等」は厳密に区別されています．

文献

1) BIG 1-98 Collaborative Group, et al：Letrozole therapy alone or in sequence with tamoxifen in women with breast cancer. N Engl J Med, 361：766-776, 2009

2) Breast International Group (BIG) 1-98 Collaborative Group, et al：A comparison of letrozole and tamoxifen in postmenopausal women with early breast cancer. N Engl J Med, 353：2747-2757, 2005

3) Colleoni M, et al：Analyses adjusting for selective crossover show improved overall survival with adjuvant letrozole compared with tamoxifen in the BIG 1-98 study. J Clin Oncol, 29：1117-1124, 2011

次は演習問題です

II 臨床試験の統計解析

演習問題

問題1 課題論文4（Cardis E, et al：J Natl Cancer Inst, 2005）のAbstract（抄録）を参照して，p値が両側検定（two-sided）によるものか片側検定（one-sided）によるものかを読み取りなさい．

別冊
33ページ

問題2 以下の問いに答えなさい．いずれも統計用語の意味を確認するためのものです．

1 臨床検査の正常範囲の意味として正しいのはどれでしょうか？

ⓐ ある集団における検査値の平均±1.96×標準偏差
ⓑ ある集団における健常人の検査値の95％が含まれる範囲
ⓒ ある集団における健常人の検査値すべてが含まれる範囲
ⓓ ある集団からのランダムサンプルにおいて95％の値が含まれる範囲

2 試験途中で中間解析をたくさん行うと，治療効果がないのに，治療群間で有意差（$p < 0.05$）がみられやすくなることが知られています．この現象に当てはまるのは次のうちどれでしょうか？

ⓐ αエラー
ⓑ βエラー
ⓒ バイアス
ⓓ ⓐ，ⓑ，ⓒすべて誤り

3 p値の説明として正しいものはどれでしょうか？

ⓐ 帰無仮説が正しい確率である
ⓑ 対立仮説が正しい確率である
ⓒ 0.05よりも小さいと有意差があると判断する
ⓓ ⓐ，ⓑ，ⓒすべて誤りである

4 片側検定のp値から，両側検定によるp値を計算するにはどうすればよいでしょうか？

　　ⓐ 片側検定のp値を2倍する
　　ⓑ 片側検定のp値を2で割る
　　ⓒ 計算できない
　　ⓓ ⓐ，ⓑ，ⓒすべて誤り

5 臨床試験の多くで両側検定が用いられているのはなぜでしょうか？

　　ⓐ 試験治療が優れていたとしても，劣っていたとしても，差があるなら結論を出したいから
　　ⓑ 統計学者の間の決まりごと
　　ⓒ すべての臨床試験で統一すべきであるから
　　ⓓ ランダム誤差は，平均の上方向と下方向の両方のバラツキを生じるから

6 臨床試験で$p = 0.06$だったとき（有意差はみられなかった）の結果の解釈として，正しいものはどれでしょうか？

　　ⓐ 試験治療はコントロール治療より優れていた
　　ⓑ 試験治療はコントロール治療より劣っていた
　　ⓒ 試験治療はコントロール治療と同等
　　ⓓ ⓐ，ⓑ，ⓒすべて誤り

7 末梢B細胞数を測定したのですが，細胞数が一定数より少ない場合には検出限界以下としかわかりませんでした．このようなとき，末梢B細胞数を比較するために適切な検定はどれでしょうか？

　　ⓐ Fisherの正確検定
　　ⓑ 検出限界以下の値を除外して対応のないt検定
　　ⓒ ログランク検定
　　ⓓ χ^2検定

臨床試験のデザイン

リツキシマブ臨床試験と
ダビガトラン非劣性試験を例に

課題論文1　Iijima K, et al：Lancet, 2014［腎疾患］
▶別冊　2〜11ページ

サンプルサイズの計算

本講のテーマ

よく効く薬の有効性を示すことと，あまり効かない薬の有効性を示すこと，どちらがより簡単でしょうか？　きっと前者ですよね．この直感は理論的に正しくて，効果が大きいかどうかによって，研究に必要なサンプルサイズ（症例数）が違うことは統計学的に示すことができます．図1は，効果が大きくなるほど（ハザード比が小さくなるほど），必要なイベント数が（同時にサンプルサイズも）少なくなることを示したものです．論文を読み解くとき，サンプルサイズの計算は最も難しいところなので，しっかり押さえましょう．また，サンプルサイズの計算は，医師が研究計画を立てるときに一番苦労するところです．

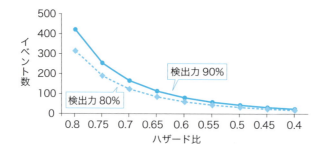

図1　検出したい治療効果（ハザード比）を変化させたときに必要な1群あたりのイベント数

keyword

サンプルサイズ，αエラー，βエラー，有意水準，検出力，検出したい治療効果の大きさ

サンプルサイズはどのような根拠に基づいて計算されるのか

サンプルサイズ計算には，用いる仮説検定の方法に応じてさまざまな公式が使われます．それらは，基本的に次の3つの数字の関係を表すものです．

- 検出力（power）
- 検出したい治療効果の大きさ
- サンプルサイズ

　この3つの数字は，2つの値を設定すれば残りの1つが決まるという関係にあります．

検出力とサンプルサイズ

　臨床試験で避けなければならない失敗の1つは，本当は効果がある治療を「効果がない」と判定して開発中止してしまうことです❶．開発者または臨床試験を行う研究者にとっては，治療が有効であると考えているのですから，このβエラーは極力抑えたいところです．検出力は「$1-\beta$」で定義され，本当は効果がある治療が正しく「効果がある」と判定される確率となります．

　臨床試験のサンプルサイズは，検出力が高くなるように計算されます．一般に，検出力は高くなるほど，サンプルサイズは大きくなります．ただし，検出力を上げたいからといって，倫理的問題と予算の制限のため必要以上に患者を登録することは好ましくありません．通常は，検出力は80〜90％に設定されます．

❶これがβエラーでしたね（第8講参照）．

検出したい治療効果の大きさとサンプルサイズ

　サンプルサイズを計算するためのもう1つの要素は，効果をどのくらいに設定するのか，ということです．効果が大きいほど，有意差を検出しやすくなることから，設定される効果が大きいほど，サンプルサイズは小さくなります．

リツキシマブ臨床試験の場合

　論文によると，

「先行研究に基づいて，リツキシマブ群の患者の40％と，プラセボ群の患者の10％が，登録後6カ月時点で寛解を維持していると仮定した．無再発期間について指数分布（exponential distribution）と比例ハザード性（proportionality of hazards）を仮定したとき，試験治療の有効性を検出力90％，片側有意水準（one-sided significance level）2.5％で示すために，1群30人の患者が必要であった」

ということでした．つまり，この試験の計画は，リツキシマブにより登録後6カ月時点で寛解を維持している患者が4倍になるという治療効果の大きさを見込んだものになっています．

　「効果がない」という仮説のことを**帰無仮説（null hypothesis）**とよぶといいましたが❷，「効果がある」というほうの仮説には，**対立仮説（alternative hypothesis）**という用語を用います．

別冊
5ページ，
Statistical analysis
第1段落

❷第8講を参照ください．

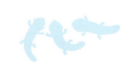

> **知っとこ!** 指数分布と比例ハザード性
>
> 指数分布とは，ハザードが一定のときの生存時間データの確率分布です．比例ハザード性とは，2本の生存曲線全体で（ハザードのスケールで）比例関係があり，ハザード比により生存曲線の違いが1つの数字に要約できることでしたね[3]．

[3] 第7講を参照ください．

サンプルサイズの計算表

表1は，生存時間データをログランク検定で2群比較するときのサンプルサイズの計算結果を示したものです．表1と表2の数字は，有意水準を両側5％，検出力をそれぞれ80％と90％に固定して，検出したい治療効果（試験治療群とコントロール群の生存確率）を動かしたときの，1群あたりに必要なサンプルサイズです．

これらの表から，リツキシマブ臨床試験の条件設定で，何人が必要になるのかを読み取ってみてください（結果は論文のサンプルサイズとは少し異なります）．

表1 ログランク検定による生存曲線の比較に必要な1群あたりのサンプルサイズ
（両側検定，有意水準5％，検出力80％）

		コントロール群の生存確率																
		0.05	0.1	0.15	0.2	0.25	0.3	0.35	0.4	0.45	0.5	0.55	0.6	0.65	0.7	0.75	0.8	0.85	0.9
試験治療群の生存確率	0.1	249	—	—	—	—	—	—	—	—	—	—	—	—	—	—	—	—	—
	0.15	87	483	—	—	—	—	—	—	—	—	—	—	—	—	—	—	—	—
	0.2	51	149	708	—	—	—	—	—	—	—	—	—	—	—	—	—	—	—
	0.25	36	78	204	914	—	—	—	—	—	—	—	—	—	—	—	—	—	—
	0.3	27	51	102	253	1,094	—	—	—	—	—	—	—	—	—	—	—	—	—
	0.35	22	38	64	123	295	1,243	—	—	—	—	—	—	—	—	—	—	—	—
	0.4	19	30	46	76	141	330	1,362	—	—	—	—	—	—	—	—	—	—	—
	0.45	16	24	35	52	85	154	355	1,447	—	—	—	—	—	—	—	—	—	—
	0.5	16	21	29	39	58	92	164	373	1,500	—	—	—	—	—	—	—	—	—
	0.55	13	18	24	31	42	61	97	170	382	1,518	—	—	—	—	—	—	—	—
	0.6	12	16	20	26	34	46	63	99	173	383	1,502	—	—	—	—	—	—	—
	0.65	13	15	17	21	28	35	46	66	98	172	373	1,451	—	—	—	—	—	—
	0.7	12	14	16	19	23	28	36	47	64	98	166	358	1,367	—	—	—	—	—
	0.75	11	13	15	18	20	24	29	36	45	62	92	157	330	1,248	—	—	—	—
	0.8	11	11	14	15	17	21	24	28	35	43	59	87	142	296	1,094	—	—	—
	0.85	10	12	13	13	16	17	21	25	26	34	41	55	80	129	256	909	—	—
	0.9	10	10	11	14	15	15	16	20	22	27	33	40	49	70	109	207	696	—
	0.95	10	11	12	12	13	14	15	16	20	24	27	35	46	60	88	151	440	

10％寛解維持＝生存確率0.1，というように対応します．

ここまでで質問はありますか？

検定ごとに表があるんですか？

まあそうです．表もあるのですが，臨床試験の現場ではサンプルサイズ計算の公式が組み込まれた専用のソフトウェアを用います．最近は，試験計画が複雑になって，公式ではなくコンピューターシミュレーションを行うことも増えてきました．

いずれにしても，サンプルサイズの計算で行っていることは，確率分布を用いた一種のシミュレーションです．「リツキシマブ群40％，プラセボ群10％」といった設定値が正しければ，一定のサンプルサイズで試験を行ったとき有意差が出る確率も予想できるし，逆に治療効果を検出するために必要なサンプルサイズも見積もれるというわけです．

表2 ログランク検定による生存曲線の比較に必要な1群あたりのサンプルサイズ（両側検定，有意水準5％，検出力90％）

		コントロール群の生存確率																
		0.05	0.1	0.15	0.2	0.25	0.3	0.35	0.4	0.45	0.5	0.55	0.6	0.65	0.7	0.75	0.8	0.85	0.9
試験治療群の生存確率	0.1	332	—	—	—	—	—	—	—	—	—	—	—	—	—	—	—	—	—
	0.15	117	645	—	—	—	—	—	—	—	—	—	—	—	—	—	—	—	—
	0.2	67	198	947	—	—	—	—	—	—	—	—	—	—	—	—	—	—	—
	0.25	46	105	273	1,222	—	—	—	—	—	—	—	—	—	—	—	—	—	—
	0.3	36	68	137	338	1,464	—	—	—	—	—	—	—	—	—	—	—	—	—
	0.35	29	50	86	165	395	1,666	—	—	—	—	—	—	—	—	—	—	—	—
	0.4	25	39	61	101	189	441	1,823	—	—	—	—	—	—	—	—	—	—	—
	0.45	22	32	46	70	113	207	475	1,938	—	—	—	—	—	—	—	—	—	—
	0.5	20	28	38	53	77	122	220	499	2,008	—	—	—	—	—	—	—	—	—
	0.55	18	24	31	42	57	82	128	227	510	2,030	—	—	—	—	—	—	—	—
	0.6	17	21	26	34	44	61	86	133	230	512	2,008	—	—	—	—	—	—	—
	0.65	16	20	24	28	35	46	62	87	132	229	500	1,942	—	—	—	—	—	—
	0.7	15	17	21	24	31	36	47	63	85	130	222	478	1,828	—	—	—	—	—
	0.75	14	16	19	21	26	30	38	48	60	83	123	210	444	1,670	—	—	—	—
	0.8	14	15	18	21	24	27	31	38	46	58	81	117	193	400	1,467	—	—	—
	0.85	13	14	17	17	21	24	26	30	35	44	57	73	104	169	341	1,218	—	—
	0.9	14	14	15	16	19	20	22	26	28	34	40	52	67	90	143	274	928	—
	0.95	12	13	14	15	18	19	20	22	24	30	32	36	45	58	74	112	201	600

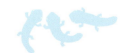

表1から「30」，表2から「39」と読み取れます．では，リツキシマブ臨床試験は，リツキシマブが寛解維持を4倍も増やすほど効くから，1群30人で十分だったということですね

それがサンプルサイズが小さくてすんだ理由の1つです．例えば，かなりよく効く抗がん剤でも，延命効果はハザード比で0.7〜0.8くらいなので，がん臨床試験のサンプルサイズは数百〜数千のオーダーになることがふつうです．

理解を深めるための計算3
サンプルサイズの公式

表1と表2がどのような根拠に基づいているかを理解するために，次の3つの公式を紹介します．なお，生存時間解析の場合，サンプルサイズよりもイベント数のほうが公式が簡単なので，ここではイベント数を計算する式を用います．

$$\text{ハザード} = \frac{-\log(x\text{年生存確率})}{x} \quad \cdots(1)$$

$$1\text{群あたりのイベント数（検出力90％）} = \frac{21}{(\text{対数ハザード比})^2} \quad \cdots(2)$$

$$1\text{群あたりのイベント数（検出力80％）} = \frac{16}{(\text{対数ハザード比})^2} \quad \cdots(3)$$

まず，「効果の大きさ」をハザード比で表します．リツキシマブ群では，登録後6カ月時点で寛解を維持している確率（生存確率）は40％ですから，(1)の公式を用いて1カ月あたりのハザードは

$$-\log(0.4)/6 = 0.153$$

と計算されます❹．プラセボ群では，同じ公式を用いて

$$-\log(0.1)/6 = 0.384$$

と計算されます．したがって，ハザード比は

$$0.153/0.384 ≒ 0.4$$

です．

次に，(2)と(3)の公式を使います．これらの公式は，①**検出力**，②**検出したい治療効果の大きさ**，③**サンプルサイズという3つの数字の関係**を表しています．高い検出力（例えば90％）が必要で，検出したい治療効果が小さいとき（ハザード比が1に近いとき），必要サンプルサイズは大きくなります❺．

ハザード比の対数を計算して，(2)と(3)の公式に代入してみましょう．「log (0.4) = −0.92」ですから，必要イベント数は，検出力90％のときと80％のとき

❹ちなみに，logは高校数学で習う対数のことで，統計学で用いられる対数の底はe = 2.718…です．「log (0.4) = −0.92」，「log (0.1) = −2.30」です．

❺繰り返しになりますが，生存時間解析の場合（ハザード比の解析の場合），サンプルサイズよりもイベント数の公式が簡単なので，ここではイベント数を計算する式を使いました．

で，それぞれ

$$21/(-0.92)^2 = 25$$
$$16/(-0.92)^2 = 19$$

になります．この試験の検出力は90％ですから，25件のイベントを観察するために，打ち切りが5人程度生じると想定して，1群30人の患者が必要と見積もった，というわけです．冒頭の図1は，ハザード比を0.8から0.4まで動かしたときの1群あたりの必要イベント数でした．

質問はありますか？

片側有意水準2.5％という条件は，サンプルサイズの計算に出てきませんでしたが…

説明は省きましたが，先ほどの公式は，片側有意水準2.5％（両側有意水準5％でも同じ）のときのもので，有意水準は分子の21と16に反映されています．**有意水準に応じてこれらの数値が変わります．**

本講のエッセンス

☐ 研究計画を立てるときにはサンプルサイズを計算する必要があります．したがって，ここから研究者が研究実施前にどのような研究結果を予想していたのかを読み取ることができます．

☐ 計算に最低限必要な要素は，有意水準（通常5％），検出力（通常80～90％），検出したい治療効果の大きさ（ハザード比など）の3つです．

☐ サンプルサイズの計算は，βエラーを制御するための方法ともいえます．

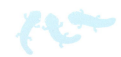

第10講 中間解析

本講のテーマ

第5講で，リツキシマブ臨床試験のStatistical analysis（統計解析）を読み取ったとき，

"We did an interim analysis after 30 patients had relapsed, with a significance level set at 0.25 % (one-sided)."

という記載がありました．片側有意水準 0.25 %は，通常の両側 5 %と比べてずいぶん小さいですが，なぜなのでしょうか？

別冊
5ページ，
Statistical analysis
第2段落

keyword

中間解析，α消費関数，データモニタリング委員会

中間解析の有意水準

臨床試験では，試験の実施途中で群間比較を行う中間解析（interim analysis）を行うことがあります❶．

❶第4講も参照ください．

中間解析で注意すべきことの1つは，最終解析に加えて中間解析を行うと，都合のよい結果が出た時点で結果を公表するという「いいとこどり」ができてしまうことです．そのペナルティとして，**中間解析では有意水準を，通常の5 %よりもずっと小さくします**．

最近のほとんどの試験では，**α消費関数（α spending function）**という統計手法を用いて有意水準を決めています．表1は，4回の中間解析を行ったときの数値例です．

α消費関数による有意水準の決め方

α消費関数による有意水準の決め方は2種類あります．Pocock（ポコック）という統計学者が考えた，有意水準を等間隔に決める**Pocock型**と，最初のほうに行われる中間解析の有意水準を小さく設定する**O'Brien and Fleming（オブライ**

表1　α消費関数により計算した中間解析の有意水準の例

中間解析の回数	等間隔型の有意水準 （Pocock型）	非等間隔型の有意水準 （O'Brien and Fleming型）
第1回（予定症例数の20％）	1.5％	0.0001％
第2回（予定症例数の40％）	1.5％	0.08％
第3回（予定症例数の60％）	1.6％	0.7％
第4回（予定症例数の80％）	1.7％	2.2％
最終解析	1.7％	4.2％

エン・フレミング）型**です．

　いずれも5％よりも小さい基準で有意かどうかを判断することになりますが，O'Brien and Fleming型では，第1回中間解析の基準はp＜0.0001とたいへん厳しくなります．また，中間解析をする場合，最終解析の有意水準も調整する必要があります．表1のケースではPocock型では1.7％，O'Brien and Fleming型では4.2％です．

　いつだったか，中間解析の結果，画期的新薬の有効性が証明されたってニュースを見たことがあります

　それは，**有効性の中止（stopping for efficacy）**のケースですね．中間解析で有意差が判断され，その時点で結果を公表することは，しばしばあります．
　それ以外に中間解析で試験が中止されるケースとしては，有効性を証明する見込みのないことが判明した**無益性の中止（stopping for futility）**，副作用などが理由の**安全性の中止（stopping for safety）**があります．

　研究者だったら，誰でも早く結果を公表したいですよね

　気持ちはよくわかるのですが，中間解析は研究者のためではなくて，患者のために行うものです．
　例えば，中間解析で試験治療の有効性が証明されたのに，劣ることがわかっているコントロール治療を継続したり，さらに患者を登録したりすることは非倫理的ですよね．ですから早期中止の判断では，p値という統計学的な基準だけではなく，患者が早期中止によりどのような利益・不利益を受けるのかが考慮されます．また，第4講 図1Bが示しているように試験途中の解析結果には不確実性が伴いますし，試験途中で結果をオープンにすると試験の実施に影響が出るので，いっそう判断が難しくなります．

そこで，**データモニタリング委員会（または効果安全性評価委員会）**とよばれる第三者的な部門を設けて，研究者に中間解析結果を知らせないまま委員会内だけで結果を検討し，客観的判断ができるようにします．シスプラチン臨床試験の中止を勧告したのもデータモニタリング委員会でしたね．

そういえば，第4講 図1Bでみたシスプラチン臨床試験の生存曲線も中間解析でしたね．あの試験の有意水準はどうだったんですか？

シスプラチン臨床試験では，期待イベント数の1/3，2/3が観察された時点で中間解析が予定されていて，それぞれ片側有意水準0.5％のログランク検定をすると規定されていました．

本講のエッセンス

- ☐ 中間解析では有意水準を，通常の5％よりもずっと小さくします．
- ☐ 最近のほとんどの試験では，α消費関数という統計手法を用いて有意水準を決めています．α消費関数の有意水準の決め方には，有意水準を等間隔に決めるPocock型と，最初のほうに行われる中間解析の有意水準を小さくするO'Brien and Fleming型があります．
- ☐ 中間解析では，データモニタリング委員会を設けて，研究者に中間解析の結果を知らせないまま，委員会内だけで結果を検討し，客観的な判断ができるようにします．

III 臨床試験のデザイン

課題論文1　Iijima K, et al：Lancet, 2014［腎疾患］

第11講　ランダム化

本講のテーマ

　ランダム化の考え方は，1920年頃に統計学者Fisher（図1）により開発された実験計画法までさかのぼります．ここでいう実験とは，誤差を制御できる物理実験や化学実験のことではありません．制御できない誤差の存在下で実施せざるを得ない技術評価のための実験（農事試験や臨床試験など）のことです．Fisherの実験計画法は，以下の3つの原則にまとめられます．

- 反復し，平均をとることにより誤差を相対的に小さくする（**繰り返し：replication**）
- 実験単位内で，均質性を保つようにする（**局所管理：local control**）
- 実験処理や介入は，ランダムに割り付けるべき（**ランダム化：randomization**）

　ランダム化は，交絡（confounding）❶という深刻なバイアスを防ぐための最善の方法です．また，ランダム化は人工的な確率分布を生じさせますので，そこからp値を正確に計算することができます（Fisherの正確検定はその例）．

❶第27講で解説します．

　Fisherは，実験計画法を農事試験に応用し，畑を小区画に分け，列ごとに異なる肥料をランダムに与えるよう指示しました．臨床試験ではランダム化はどのように実践されているのでしょうか？

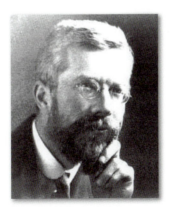

図1　20世紀最大の統計学者R. A. Fisher
　　（1890〜1962年）

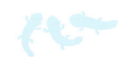

keyword

実験計画法，ランダム化，ランダム化調整因子，最小化法，モデルベースとランダム化ベース

ランダム化の方法

リツキシマブ臨床試験のSummary（抄録）を読んで唐突に感じたのは，

"We used a computer-generated sequence to randomly assign patients（1：1）to…as adjustment factors."

という一文ではないでしょうか？ これはランダム化の方法に関する説明です．すなわち，"computer-generated sequence"はいわゆる（コンピューターで発生させる）乱数のことで，"1：1"はリツキシマブ群とプラセボ群の人数の比のことです．"adjustment factors"とは何でしょう？ これは「ランダム化調整因子」と訳されますが，ここがポイントですので，詳しく解説します．

別冊
3ページ，
Summaryの
Methods
4〜6行目

ランダム化調整因子が偏らない工夫

ランダム化は**比較するグループ間で実験条件をそろえるための手法**ですが，乱数を使うのでまれに患者の特徴が偏ってしまうことがあります．例えば，プラセボ群に特定の施設が偏る（バイアスがかかる）と困りますよね．

これを避けるため，リツキシマブ臨床試験では，**最小化法（minimization）**というアルゴリズムを使って，**4つのランダム化調整因子（adjustment factors）**が偏らないように工夫したと宣言しています．

 ここまでで質問はありますか？

 最小化法以外の方法もあるんですか？

 あります．人数が偏ったら，
- 不均衡が小さくなる方向に割り付け確率を小さくするバイアスコイン法
- ランダム化調整因子で層をつくって，層ごとに割り付ける層別ランダム化
- 2〜6人単位の割り付け結果（ブロック）をランダムに並び替える置換ブロック法

などがあります．

 そういう方法を使って偏りなくランダム化すれば，バイアスがなくなるんですね？

バイアスの可能性が小さくなるのは確かですが，正確には違います．例えば，ランダム化後に生じた計画からの逸脱（例えば治療中止）は，群間で偏っている可能性があります．せっかくランダムに治療を割り付けたのだから，両群で実験条件がそろうように，「ランダム化された全患者を，割り付け群のとおりに解析する」というのがIntention-To-Treat（ITT）の原則[2]でしたね．

[2]第2講を参照ください．

解説 ランダム化の実際

最近の臨床試験では，各医療機関とは別に中央事務局をおき，WEBやFAXで患者登録・ランダム化を行うのが一般的です．臨床試験専用のWEBシステムのアウトソーシングを請け負う企業や団体もあります[3]．

また，ランダム化調整因子には，「比較するグループ間で偏ったら困る変数」を選ぶと考えてください．つまり，疾患の重症度や予後に関係する因子が優先されます．調整因子が多すぎると，患者の数に比べて水準の数が多すぎて，最小化法がうまく機能しません．そのため，試験の規模にもよりますが，10以上の因子をランダム化調整因子として用いることはほとんどありません．

[3]例えば，東京大学はINDICEというシステムを提供しています（http://indice.umin.ac.jp/）．

解説 ランダム化が許容されるとき

研究目的で治療をランダムに割り付けることは，医療行為として倫理的ではない側面があります．ランダム化臨床試験が許容されるのは，試験治療とコントロール治療の間で，均衡（equipoise）が成立しているときだけだといわれています．

理解を深めるための計算4
最小化法

表1が最小化法の数値例です．現時点で，各群15人ずつ登録されており，次の患者をどちらに割り付けるか決めたいとします．

仮に，次の患者の年齢が低かったとしましょう．そのような特徴をもった患者は，すでにリツキシマブ群で10人，プラセボ群で6人登録されています．したがって，偏りを避けるにはプラセボ群に割り付けた方がよさそうですよね．

このアイデアを発展させて，表1における年齢が低く，施設Aで，ステロイド治療歴あり，過去3回の再発の間隔が短い患者の人数を，合計してみましょう．
リツキシマブ群では
$$10+4+5+7=26$$
プラセボ群では
$$6+3+5+10=24$$

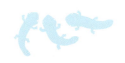

表1　最小化法のアルゴリズム

ランダム化調整因子	水準	次の患者の特徴	リツキシマブ群の人数（現時点で計15人）	プラセボ群の人数（現時点で計15人）
年齢	低	○	10	6
	高		5	9
施設	A	○	4	3
	B		6	7
	C		5	5
治療歴	ステロイド	○	5	5
	免疫抑制薬		7	2
	両方		3	8
過去3回の再発の間隔	短	○	7	10
	長		8	5

です．最小化法では，この数字が小さい群に患者を割り付けます（この場合は26＞24なのでプラセボ群）．

ただし，これは一番単純なアルゴリズムで，最小化法にもいくつかのバリエーションがあります．

理解を深めるための計算5
ランダム化に基づく統計的推測

本講の冒頭で，ランダム化に基づいてp値を正確に計算することができる，と述べました．このことを，6人の患者に試験治療Aとコントロール治療Bを割り付ける臨床試験を例にして，説明しましょう．

＊　　　＊　　　＊

コントロール治療B下の6人の患者のエンドポイントの値は，−5，−3，−1，1，3，5という値をとるとします．また，試験治療Aを行うとコントロール治療Bに比べて＋10されるとします（表2）．これらの治療の比較は，A群のエンドポイントの平均とB群のエンドポイントの平均の差によって行うとします．

治療法を，前から順にA，A，A，B，B，Bという系統的なパターンに従って割り付けたとしましょう．そうすると，

　　平均の差＝(5＋7＋9)/3−(1＋3＋5)/3＝4

です．治療Aの効果は＋10でしたから，10＞4で平均の差を過小評価していることになります．

次に，Aに3人，Bに3人というように，6人から3人を選ぶ20通りの割り付けパターンをランダムに発生させたとしましょう．計算してみると，割り付けパ

表2 ランダム化ベースのアプローチを説明するための数値例

	6人の患者の潜在的なエンドポイントの値					
	①	②	③	④	⑤	⑥
試験治療Aだったとき	5	7	9	11	13	15
コントロール治療Bだったとき	−5	−3	−1	1	3	5

ターンの確率分布は，以下のようになります❹．

平均の差＝ 10 − 18/3　出現確率＝ 1/20
平均の差＝ 10 − 14/3　出現確率＝ 1/20
平均の差＝ 10 − 10/3　出現確率＝ 2/20
平均の差＝ 10 − 6/3　 出現確率＝ 3/20
平均の差＝ 10 − 2/3　 出現確率＝ 3/20
平均の差＝ 10 + 2/3　 出現確率＝ 3/20
平均の差＝ 10 + 6/3　 出現確率＝ 3/20
平均の差＝ 10 + 10/3　出現確率＝ 2/20
平均の差＝ 10 + 14/3　出現確率＝ 1/20
平均の差＝ 10 + 18/3　出現確率＝ 1/20

❹この確率分布は $_6C_3 = 20$ 通りのすべての割り付けパターンを数え上げたものです．

これは，治療Aの効果＋10を中心として対称な確率分布です．つまり，系統的なパターンで割り付けたときに生じたバイアスが，ランダム化を通じて偏りのないランダム誤差に転化されているのです．

＊　　＊　　＊

ランダム化のもう1つの意義は，人工的な確率分布を生じるため確率計算が可能になるということです．ランダム化を行い，A，A，B，A，B，Bという結果が得られたとしましょう．そうすると，

平均の差 − 10 ＝ (5 + 7 + 11)/3 − (−1 + 3 + 5)/3 ＝ 14/3

です．ここで，確率変数は20通りの割り付けパターンであり，エンドポイントの値は定数と考えると，平均の差の分布は，上に示したとおりです．すなわち，平均の差 − 10 の絶対値が 14/3 以上になる割り付けパターンは4通りであり，両側p値は0.2と計算されます．このようにランダム化に基づいて正確にp値を計算する手法を，並び替え検定（permutation test）とよびます．

解説 ▶ 統計的推測 その4：モデルベースとランダム化ベース

統計学は演繹的な学問ですから，どのような根拠に基づいて正しい統計的推測が可能になっているのかは，本質的な問題です．統計的推測の基盤は主に2つあ

り，それぞれモデルベースのアプローチとランダム化ベースのアプローチとよばれています．

● モデルベースのアプローチ

前者は，現実の状況を（確率分布を用いて）数学的に定式化するものです（この定式化を統計学では「モデル」とよびます）．データがどのような確率分布に従うのか正しく特定できれば，その確率分布に適した統計手法を導くことはそれほど難しいことではありません．

ここで重要になるのはモデルが正しいかどうかです．Wald検定[5]は，回帰モデルの回帰係数が0（ハザード比の場合は1）かどうかの検定ですが，Wald検定が妥当であるためには当てはめた回帰モデルが正しいことが前提です．この場合，妥当であるとは，Wald検定によってαエラーが有意水準以下に保たれるという意味です．ところが，当てはめた回帰式が間違っていると（モデルの誤特定）[6]，αエラーがコントロールできるという保証はありません．

[5] 第8講を参照ください．

[6] 第28講で解説します．

● ランダム化ベースのアプローチ

一方，ランダム化ベースのアプローチの代表例は，並び替え検定やFisherの正確検定です．これらは，ランダム化が人工的な確率分布を生じさせることを利用して，p値を正確に計算するものです．

● モデルベースかランダム化ベースか

この異なる2種類の統計的推測の基盤のうち，ランダム化ベースのアプローチはランダム化臨床試験では合理的で頑健です．それに比べ，ランダム化を伴わないコホート研究やケース・コントロール研究では，推測の基盤としてモデルベースに頼らざるを得ません．回帰モデルによる交絡の調整[7]は，モデルベースのアプローチそのものです．

[7] 第28講で解説します．

本講のエッセンス

- ☐ ランダム化は，比較するグループ間で実験条件をそろえるための手法です．
- ☐ ランダム化すれば，ランダム化以前の患者の特徴はグループ間で平均的に等しくなります．
- ☐ 一方で，ランダム化後に生じた計画からの逸脱は，群間で偏っている可能性があります．
- ☐ せっかくランダムに治療を割り付けたのだから，両群で実験条件がそろうように，「ランダム化された全患者を，割り付けの結果どおりに解析する」というのがITTの原則です．

III 臨床試験のデザイン

課題論文1 Iijima K, et al：Lancet, 2014［腎疾患］

第12講 非劣性試験

本講のテーマ

　脳循環改善薬という古い薬をご存知でしょうか？　この薬は脳血管障害の後遺症や認知症などに使われ，累計8,000億円ほどの売り上げがあったようです．脳循環改善薬にはいくつかの類似薬がありましたが，そのほとんどが，最初に承認されたホパンテン酸カルシウム（販売名：ホパテ）と比較した「非劣性試験」を根拠に承認されていました．しかし当時行われていたのは，今回お話しするような正しい解析ではなく，「ホパテと有意差がない」ことに基づいて非劣性を判定していました．1998年にホパテは副作用のため市場から撤退しました．同時期に，厚生省（当時）は製薬企業にプラセボ対照試験による再評価を求めました．その結果が表1です．すべてプラセボに勝てなかったのです．

　この悲劇は，有意差がつかなかったとき，効果が同じと結論するのは間違いであることを明確に示しています．

表1　1998年ホパテ撤退後の脳循環改善薬の再評価の結果

脳循環改善薬	エンドポイント	改善率		有意差
		試験薬群	プラセボ群	
イデベノン	全般改善度	34.2%	32.8%	なし
塩酸インデロキサジン	自発的全般	14.9%	20.9%	なし
塩酸インデロキサジン	情緒改善度	21.6%	24.9%	なし
塩酸ビフェメラン	意欲・情緒全般改善	37.5%	30.8%	なし
プロペントフイリン	全般改善度	25.6%	30.0%	なし

keyword

非劣性試験，優越性試験，非劣性マージン，95％信頼区間，非劣性から優越性への仮説の切り替え

リスクとベネフィットを比較する

第15〜19講では，心房細動患者におけるダビガトランの有効性をワルファリンと比較するメタアナリシスを取り上げるのですが，その事前準備として，今回はそこで解析に含められた臨床試験の1つ，RE-LY試験[1]について解説します．

ダビガトランは新規経口抗凝固薬（Novel Oral Anti Coagulants：NOAC）とよばれる画期的新薬の1つですが，ワルファリンと比べたとき，リスクとベネフィットは複雑です．抗凝固作用はほぼ同等といわれていますが，ダビガトランのほうが出血リスクが低く，臨床上使いやすい薬である一方で，薬剤費は高くなります．このような状況では，「主要エンドポイントに有意差があるか」を調べるだけでは不十分です．ダビガトランとワルファリンを，**リスクとベネフィット両方の観点からうまく比較できるように計画された試験とはどのようなものか**が今回のポイントです．

「劣らない」ことを示す非劣性試験

RE-LY試験のPICO

表2に，RE-LY試験のPICOを示します．

Patientsは心房細動患者18,113人です．この試験は3群比較のランダム化臨床試験で，Interventionはダビガトラン110 mg 1日2回，ダビガトラン150 mg 1日2回であり，コントロール治療はワルファリンです．Outcomesは，主要有効性エンドポイントは脳卒中・全身塞栓症発症，主要安全性エンドポイントは大出血発症です．

非劣性試験の考え方

RE-LY試験では，**非劣性試験（non-inferiority trial）**という臨床試験デザインが用いられています．

RE-LY試験の状況設定で重要なのは，ダビガトランとワルファリンの薬効が同程度だったとしても，データがばらつくため脳卒中・全身塞栓症発生率が全く同

表2　RE-LY試験のPICO

Patients	心房細動患者 18,113人
Intervention	ダビガトラン 110 mg　1日2回 ダビガトラン 150 mg　1日2回
Comparison	ワルファリン
Outcomes	脳卒中・全身塞栓症発症（主要有効性エンドポイント） 大出血発症（主要安全性エンドポイント）

（文献1をもとに作成）

じにはならないだろう，ということです．ワルファリン群に比べ，ダビガトラン群の脳卒中・全身塞栓症予防効果が劣っていたとしても，その度合いがきわめてわずかだったとしたらどうでしょう？許容されませんか？一方で，2群間に臨床的に意味のあるような大きな差があると，非劣性と判定することはできません．

　非劣性試験は，試験治療が標準治療やプラセボに比べ「優れている」ことを示す**優越性試験（superiority trial）**とは異なり，試験治療が標準治療に比べ「劣らない」ことを示すための方法です．

非劣性試験の道具

　優越性試験と非劣性試験では使う道具が違います．優越性試験では有効性を判定する道具はp値と有意水準でしたが，非劣性試験では**信頼区間（confidence interval）**と**非劣性マージン（non-inferiority margin）**を用います．非劣性マージンとは，劣っていることが許容される範囲を表す数字のことで，RE-LY試験では〔Abstract（抄録）には書かれていませんが〕非劣性マージンは相対リスク〔relative risk, 正確にはハザード比（hazard ratio）〕1.46と設定されています．

ここまでで質問はありますか？

前にも出てきましたが，信頼区間って何ですか？

リツキシマブ臨床試験のときは，推定値の誤差を表すのが95％信頼区間だといいましたが，詳しくは説明しませんでした❶．信頼区間の幅は主に，以下の3つの概念により決まります．

- 信頼区間の係数（90％，95％など）
- 両側（two-sided）・片側（one-sided）
- サンプルサイズ

信頼区間の係数は，仮説検定における有意水準に対応する概念です．信頼区間の係数が95％だと有意水準5％（p＜0.05）に対応し，90％だと有意水準10％（p＜0.1）に対応しています．係数が100％に近いほど，信頼区間の幅は広くなります．信頼区間の係数の意味については，仮想的反復❷で説明しましたね．

❶第5講を参照ください．

❷第3講を参照ください．

RE-LY試験の結果

主要有効性エンドポイント

図1は，RE-LY試験の主要有効性エンドポイントに関する結果です．図1には3群の累積発生曲線（生存曲線を上下逆にしたもの）が示されています．

ここで思い出してほしいのは，解析に用いられる統計手法はデータの型によって異なるということです[3]．さらに，3群のアウトカムを比較するための指標として，相対リスクと絶対リスク（absolute risk）の2種類があります．一言でいえば，両者の違いは，「比」か「差」かということです．

RE-LY試験の場合には，2値データ，計数データ，生存時間データの3通りで解析することができ，それぞれに対応して，以下のように4種類の相対リスクが計算できます．

- 2値データ：リスク比（risk ratio），オッズ比（odds ratio）
- 計数データ：発生率比（rate ratio）
- 生存時間データ：ハザード比（hazard ratio）

ここで用語の整理をしましょう．イベント発生割合（リスク）は「一部の数を全体の数で割ったもの」，発生率は「一定時間にイベントが発生するスピードで，人年法（イベントの発生人数/観察人年）で計算したもの」でした[4]．また，オッズとは，

$$リスク/(1-リスク)$$

として計算される指標のことで，あるイベントが起こる確率の，起こらない確率に対する比です．

[3] 第6講を参照ください．

[4] 第7講で述べましたね．

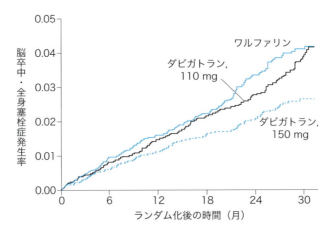

図1　RE-LY試験の脳卒中・全身塞栓症の累積発生曲線
（文献1よりFigure 1を引用）

表3には，3群の解析対象者数と脳卒中・全身塞栓症発生数が示されています．ここから上記の指標を求めてみると，ダビガトラン110 mg群では以下のとおりです．

- リスク＝182/6015＝0.0303
- オッズ＝0.0303/（1－0.0303）＝0.0312
- 発生率＝182/11900＝0.0153

それぞれをワルファリン群の計算結果（表3）で割れば，相対リスクが計算できます．

- リスク比＝0.0303/0.0330＝0.918
- オッズ比＝0.0312/0.0341＝0.915
- 発生率比＝0.0153/0.0169＝0.905

また，図1の生存時間データからCox回帰を用いてハザード比を求めてみると，

- ダビガトラン110 mg群対ワルファリン群のハザード比は0.91（95％信頼区間0.74〜1.11），
- ダビガトラン150 mg群対ワルファリン群のハザード比は0.66（95％信頼区間0.53〜0.82）

です．つまり，いずれの指標であっても，ダビガトラン110 mg群ではワルファリン群に比べ，脳卒中・全身塞栓症の発生は約0.9倍だったということです．ちなみに，絶対リスクとはリスク差（risk difference）のことで，「3.03％－3.30％＝－0.27％」になります．

主要安全性エンドポイント

一方で，主要安全性エンドポイントである大出血発生率は，ワルファリン群では1年あたり3.36％であり，それに比べダビガトラン110 mgを受けたグループでは1年あたり2.71％（p＝0.003），ダビガトラン150 mgを受けたグループで

表3　RE-LY試験の脳卒中・全身塞栓症発生状況

	ダビガトラン群 （110 mg 1日2回）	ダビガトラン群 （150 mg 1日2回）	ワルファリン群
解析対象者数	6,015人	6,076人	6,022人
観察人年	11,900人年	12,070人年	11,780人年
脳卒中・全身塞栓症発生数	182人	134人	199人
イベント発生割合（リスク）	3.03％	2.20％	3.30％
オッズ	0.0312 0.0303/（1－0.0303）	0.0225 0.0220/（1－0.0220）	0.0341 0.0330/（1－0.0330）
発生率	1年あたり0.0153	1年あたり0.0111	1年あたり0.0169

（文献1をもとに作成）

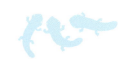

は1年あたり3.11%（p＝0.31）だったということです[1].

非劣性の判定はどう行うか

非劣性が証明されたかどうかの判定は，**非劣性マージンと信頼区間の上限（または下限）の比較**により行われます（図2）.

優越性試験では，p値が0.05より小さいことをもって「優れている」と判定します．このことは，信頼区間が0（相対リスクの場合は1）をまたがないことに対応します．

一方，非劣性を証明するためには，信頼区間が0をまたいでいてもよいのですが，非劣性マージンの値（Δという記号で表します）よりも，信頼区間全体が比較対照の治療よりも優るような位置（図では右）になければなりません．

＊　　＊　　＊

非劣性試験とよく似た**同等性試験（equivalence trial）**という試験デザインがあるのですが，非劣性試験は片側，同等性試験は両側を考える点が主な違いです．つまり，同等性を判定するためには信頼区間全体が−ΔとΔの範囲に入らなければなりません．

何か質問はありますか？

この三角，何ですか？

Δのことですか？これはギリシャ文字でデルタ[5]といいます．統計学では不親切なことに，ギリシャ文字に特別な意味をもたせるというナゾの習慣があ

[5] アルファベットのDに対応しています．

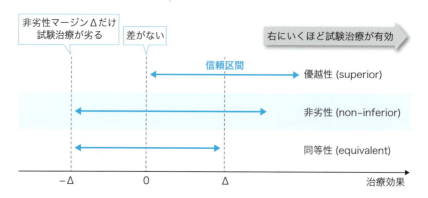

図2　優越性，非劣性，同等性の判定方法の違い

るのです．

　論文でよく用いられるのは，仮説検定で出てきたα（アルファ）とβ（ベータ），非劣性マージンΔ（デルタ），χ^2検定のχ（カイ）くらいでしょうか．

 非劣性マージンをもう少し詳しくお願いします

　ここで考えてほしいのは，非劣性マージンの値が大きいとどうなるか，ということです．非劣性マージンは，統計解析のうえでは一種のハンディキャップとしてはたらいており，**ハンディキャップが大きいほど，非劣性が証明されやすくなります**．また，優越性試験の判断基準は，非劣性マージンがΔ＝0の場合に相当していることにも注意してください．

RE-LY試験結果の解釈

主要有効性エンドポイント

　結果の解釈に戻りましょう．
　脳卒中・全身塞栓症の1年あたりの発生率は，
- ダビガトラン110 mg群　0.0153
- ダビガトラン150 mg群　0.0111
- ワルファリン群　0.0169

でした．この発生率を，ハザード比で比較すると，
- ダビガトラン110 mg群ではワルファリン群に比べ0.91倍（95％信頼区間0.74〜1.11）
- ダビガトラン150 mg群ではワルファリン群に比べ0.66倍（95％信頼区間0.53〜0.82）

となります．この95％信頼区間の上側限界（1.11と0.82）を，非劣性マージン1.46と比べると，いずれも数字が小さい（ダビガトランのほうがよい）ため，ダビガトランの非劣性が判定されます．

主要安全性エンドポイント

　さて，主要エンドポイントについては上のとおりなのですが，リスクとベネフィット両方を評価するためには，これでは不十分です．つまり，主要安全性エンドポイントである大出血に差がないと，ダビガトランがワルファリンに比べて優れているとはいえません．
　その点でいうと，ダビガトラン150 mgの結果は少し微妙です．なぜなら，文献1のAbstract（抄録）を読むと，ワルファリン群の大出血発生率は1年あたり

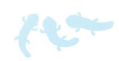

3.36％，ダビガトラン150 mg群では1年あたり3.11％で，有意差がなかったためです（p＝0.31）．もちろん脳出血や死亡率の結果も抄録には示されているのですが．

非劣性試験のなかで優越性の検討？

もう1つ重要な論点は，抄録のResults（結論）によると
「用量150 mgで投与されたダビガトランは，ワルファリンと比べて，脳卒中・全身塞栓症発生率が**低かった（was associated with lower rates）**」
と述べられている点です．優越性試験ではなく非劣性試験なのだから，結論ではそもそもの仮説に従って「劣らない」と述べるべきではないでしょうか？

確認してみると，ダビガトラン150 mg群のハザード比は0.66（95％信頼区間0.53〜0.82）で，95％信頼区間が1をまたいでいませんので，脳卒中・全身塞栓症発生率に（優越性の検定の結果）有意差がついたことがわかります．実際，論文の抄録でも優越性 p＜0.001と報告されています．

このように，非劣性試験で優越性の検定を行うことを，**非劣性から優越性への仮説の切り替え（switching）**といいます．この結果を踏まえると，

①ダビガトラン110 mgはワルファリンに比べ，脳卒中・全身塞栓症予防効果は劣らず，大出血発生率が低い
②ダビガトラン150 mgはワルファリンに比べ，脳卒中・全身塞栓症予防効果が優れており，大出血発生率に有意差はない

という解釈になります．

 非劣性マージンの1.46って誰が決めたんですか？ 数字が大きいと非劣性になりやすいですよね．製薬企業が決めたのなら，自社に都合のよい数字を設定しそうですが…

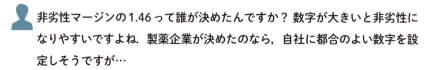 非劣性マージンは，試験実施者（この場合は製薬企業）により設定されることがふつうです．したがって，**非劣性マージンが①事前に，②客観的に設定されたかどうかがきわめて重要**です．

①を補足すると，非劣性マージンをデータを見た後で変更することは一般的に許容されません．ゴルフのハンディキャップをホールアウト後に決めるようなもので，試験治療が勝てる分だけハンディキャップを与えてしまう，ということになりかねないためです．

 ですが，RE-LY試験では，非劣性から優越性への仮説の切り替えをしたんですよね？

そのとおりです．優越性試験の判断基準は，非劣性マージンが Δ ＝ 0 の場合に相当しているのでしたね．ですから，非劣性から優越性への仮説の切り替えは，非劣性マージンを小さくすることを意味します．つまりハンディキャップを小さくするわけなので，アメリカとヨーロッパの規制当局に許容されているのです．一方で，その逆の優越性から非劣性への仮説の切り替えは，明らかにルール違反です．

では，②の客観性についてはどうですか？

論文の Methods（方法）を読んでみると，ワルファリンの有効性に関する過去の臨床試験をメタアナリシスして，「ワルファリンの効果の半分」よりも小さい数字になるように非劣性マージンを設定した，と書かれています．このように，コントロール治療の効果を基準に非劣性マージンを決める方法は，効果維持法（effect retention）とよばれています．効果維持法は，米国食品医薬品局（FDA）に新薬申請をするための試験では標準的に用いられています．

効果維持法のほかには，慣習的に決まった値を用いる疾患領域もあります．例えば，抗菌薬の臨床試験では，有効率が10％（または15％や20％）より劣らなければ非劣性と考えたりします．

疾患領域や研究者の考え方によって非劣性マージンの数字が変わる，ということですか？

そのとおりです．表4は，2010年以前の進行非小細胞肺がん二次治療臨床試験で用いられてきた非劣性マージンをまとめたものです．疾患領域が同じで

表4　2010年以前の進行非小細胞肺がん二次治療臨床試験で用いられてきた非劣性マージン

著者	試験治療	コントロール治療	主要エンドポイント	非劣性マージン（ハザード比）
Hanna et al, 2004	ペメトレキセド	ドセタキセル	全生存期間	1.11 と 1.21
Ramlau et al, 2006	トポテカン	ドセタキセル	全生存期間	ハザード比でない
Kim et al, 2008	ゲフィチニブ	ドセタキセル	全生存期間	1.154
Maruyama et al, 2008	ゲフィチニブ	ドセタキセル	全生存期間	1.25
Krzakowski et al, 2010	ビンフルニン	ドセタキセル	無増悪生存期間	1.325

（文献3をもとに作成）

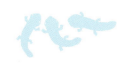

も，非劣性マージンは（ハザード比で）1.11から1.325までバラツキがあることがわかります．

表4の一番上の試験[2]は，アメリカとヨーロッパの規制当局に要求されて2通りの非劣性マージンを設定したことで，一貫性がないと批判をよびました．

論文を取り寄せて詳しく読んでみましたが，ダビガトラン110 mg群，ダビガトラン150 mg群，ワルファリン群では，それぞれ2年後に20.7％，21.2％，16.6％が治療を中止していたと書いてあります．治療をやめたら，効果がないわけだから差がなくなって当たり前です

それは大事なポイントです．**質が悪い試験を行うと2群間の差が薄まってしまい，非劣性が示されやすくなります**．このことを示唆するデータには，以下のようなものがあります．
- 服薬率，治療完遂率，用量，投与スケジュールなどに問題がある
- 治療のクロスオーバーが多い
- 追跡不能例や欠測データが多い
- Intention-To-Treat（ITT）解析とプロトコール逸脱例を除外した解析（Per-Protocol Set解析）の結果が一貫しない

非劣性試験の論文を読むときには，これらのデータは大事なポイントです．ただ，治療中止をゼロにすることは，倫理的観点から難しいのが実際です．RE-LY試験でもやむを得なかったのでしょう．

❻第2講で解説しましたが，大事な内容なのでおさらいです．

ITT，FAS，PPS❻

ITTの原則とは，「ランダム化された全患者を，割り付けの結果どおりに解析すべき」というものです．ただし，これでは厳しすぎるという意見があり，現在最も一般的なルールは，「割り付けられた治療を一度も受けていない患者」と「データが全くない患者」だけは除外してよい，最大の解析対象集団（FAS）を用いるというものです．FASに加えて，プロトコール逸脱や試験治療不遵守の患者を除いた集団をプロトコール遵守集団（PPS）とよんでいます．

本講のエッセンス

- 非劣性試験は，試験治療が標準治療やプラセボに比べ「優れている」ことを示す優越性試験とは異なり，試験治療が標準治療に比べ「劣らない」ことを示すための方法です．
- 非劣性が証明されたかどうかの判定は，非劣性マージンと信頼区間の上限（または下限）の比較により行われます．
- 非劣性マージンは，事前に，客観的に設定されたかどうかがきわめて重要です．
- また，非劣性から優越性への仮説の切り替えが行われることがあります．
- 非劣性試験で気をつけなければならないのは，質が悪い試験を行ったため2群間の差が薄まってしまい，非劣性が示されやすくなっていないかどうかです．

文献

1) Connolly SJ, et al：Dabigatran versus warfarin in patients with atrial fibrillation. N Engl J Med, 361：1139-1151, 2009
2) Hanna N, et al：Randomized phase III trial of pemetrexed versus docetaxel in patients with non-small-cell lung cancer previously treated with chemotherapy. J Clin Oncol, 22：1589-1597, 2004
3) Tanaka S, et al：Statistical issues and recommendations for noninferiority trials in oncology: a systematic review. Clin Cancer Res, 18：1837-1847, 2012

次は演習問題です

III 臨床試験のデザイン

演習問題

問題1 進行非小細胞肺がん患者におけるペメトレキセドのドセタキセルに対する非劣性を検証した論文（Hanna et al, 2004；89ページ参照）では，非劣性マージンは1.11と1.21の2つが用いられ，片側有意水準は2.5％と設定されました．この試験の結果は，全生存期間におけるペメトレキセドのドセタキセルに対するハザード比0.99（95％信頼区間0.82〜1.20）というものでした．おのおのの非劣性マージンについて，非劣性が証明されたかどうか考えてみてください．

問題2 以下の問いに答えなさい．いずれも統計用語の意味を確認するためのものです．

1 2つの集団間で，平均値の差の95％信頼区間が0を含むとき，その意味として正しいのはどれでしょうか？

　ⓐ 平均値の推定精度が低い
　ⓑ どちらかの平均値の推定値が0に近い
　ⓒ 2つの集団間で，平均値に統計学的に有意な差がある
　ⓓ 2つの集団間で，平均値に統計学的に有意な差はない

2 比較する治療が同じとき，優越性試験と非劣性試験のサンプルサイズの違いについて正しいのはどれでしょうか？

　ⓐ 非劣性試験のほうが優越性試験よりも必ずサンプルサイズは大きい
　ⓑ 非劣性試験のほうが優越性試験よりも必ずサンプルサイズは小さい
　ⓒ 非劣性試験と優越性試験でサンプルサイズは同じ
　ⓓ ⓐ，ⓑ，ⓒいずれも誤り

3 非劣性マージンの説明として正しいのはどれでしょうか？

　ⓐ 大きいほど非劣性が示されにくくなる
　ⓑ 大きいほど非劣性の証拠が強くなる

ⓒ 大きいほどサンプルサイズは大きくなる
　　ⓓ ⓐ，ⓑ，ⓒいずれも誤り

4 非劣性試験における統計解析について，正しいものはどれでしょうか？

　　ⓐ データ固定の前であれば，プロトコール改訂により非劣性マージンの値を変更してもよい
　　ⓑ 非劣性が示され，さらに優越性検定を行って有意だった場合，優越性試験として報告してよい
　　ⓒ 非劣性マージンの値は，試験を行う研究者が決定してよい
　　ⓓ 解析対象集団は，Intention-To-Treat（ITT）の原則（第2講参照）に従わなければならない

IV 臨床試験の基礎知識

第13講 臨床試験と規制

本講のテーマ

　華岡青洲は，麻酔薬「通仙散」を開発したことで世界的に有名な，江戸時代の外科医です．青洲は，1804年11月14日に世界初の全身麻酔乳がん手術に成功しますが，その前に，実母，於継と妻，加恵を対象に「臨床試験」を実施しました（図1）．その結果，於継は死亡し加恵は失明したのです．

　これは美談として伝えられていますが，現代ではこのような臨床試験を行うことは考えられません．現代行われている臨床試験の特徴は，①統計学などの科学的方法論が取り入れられ，②同意取得や倫理審査などの被験者保護がなされ，③製薬企業主導でビジネスの一環として行われることがある，という点です．これらはすべて，国による薬事規制と深い関係があります．

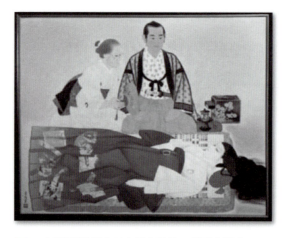

図1　国際外科学会日本部会所蔵の華岡青洲（1760～1835年）の図

keyword

治験，GCP，倫理指針，プロトコール，モニタリング，監査，品質管理・保証

図2 臨床試験の分類

臨床試験の分類

臨床試験にはさまざまな分類があります（図2）.

医薬品が承認され市販される前に，製薬企業は，

- 安全性や臨床薬理を調べる第Ⅰ相試験
- 用量設定をしたり有効性を探索したりする第Ⅱ相試験
- 有効性を検証する第Ⅲ相試験

を行います．これらの試験の目的は，承認申請資料の根拠となるデータを得ることです．このような試験を，薬事法では**治験**とよんでいます．製薬企業には，市販前に行われる治験以外に，市販後も医薬品安全対策の一環として**使用成績調査や製造販売後臨床試験**が義務付けられています．一方で，**医師による自主的な臨床試験**も行われています．

このように臨床試験は，**臨床開発の相・市販前後・医師主導かどうか**によって分類されます．

＊　　＊　　＊

リツキシマブ臨床試験は，医師主導で第Ⅲ相試験（治験）を行った珍しい事例です．リツキシマブには，添付文書上，難治性ネフローゼ症候群への適用がなかったため，この臨床試験が行われ，国の承認審査を経て適用拡大が認められました．

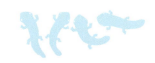

ここまでで質問はありますか？

治験とそれ以外の臨床試験はどこが違うんですか？

用いられている科学的方法論や，被験者保護の考え方について本質的な差はありません．一番の違いは，国による規制の厳しさです．

　実は，治験というのは日本の薬事法上の言葉で，国際的に用いられる用語ではありません．臨床試験には，日米EU医薬品規制調和国際会議（ICH）という会議で国際的に合意されたルール（**Good Clinical Practice：GCP**）があります．例えば，
- 被験者から同意を得ること（インフォームドコンセント）
- 有害事象を国に報告すること
- 試験の内容を試験実施計画書（プロトコール：protocol）として事前に規定すること
- プロトコールは治験審査委員会の審査を受けること
- データの品質管理・保証を行うこと

などが定められています．日本ではGCP省令として運用されています．

　一方で，国内の治験以外の臨床試験には，文部科学省・厚生労働省が定めた**人を対象とする医学系研究に関する倫理指針と臨床研究法**が設けられていますが，内容はGCPとは異なる部分があります．

プロトコールってどんなものなんですか？

あまり目にすることはないかもしれませんので，リツキシマブ臨床試験のプロトコールの章立てを表1に示しておきます．

　プロトコールは，科学性と倫理性を担保して研究を行うために，実施計画と作業内容を示した公式文書です．臨床試験にはさまざまな実施計画がありえますが，科学的または倫理的観点からプロトコールに記載しなければならない必須事項があります．

 医薬品の臨床開発

　医薬品開発は，非臨床開発，臨床開発，市販後という3段階に分かれます（図3）．

　非臨床開発では，薬理，毒性，品質，製品製造などに2〜3年が費やされます．

　臨床開発では，第I相〜第III相までの臨床試験が行われ，有効性・安全性が調べられます（GCPはここで適用されます）．これらのデータは承認申請資料

表1 リツキシマブ臨床試験のプロトコールの章立て

1章	Clinical trial overview（試験の概要）	15章	Data collection（データ収集）
2章	Table of Contents（目次）	16章	Efficacy evaluation（有効性評価）
3章	List of abbreviations and term definitions（略語と用語）	17章	Other evaluation（その他の評価）
4章	RCRNS study group（RCRNS研究グループ）	18章	Safety evaluation（安全性評価）
5章	Introduction（背景）	19章	Statistical Analyses（統計解析）
6章	Purpose（目的）	20章	Direct viewing of source documents and others（原資料の直接閲覧とその他）
7章	Clinical trial design（試験デザイン）	21章	Quality control and quality assurance（品質管理・保証）
8章	Subject inclusion criteria and exclusion criteria（選択基準と除外基準）	22章	Ethical considerations（倫理的配慮）
9章	Investigational drugs（治験薬）	23章	Handling of data and record keeping（データの扱いと保管）
10章	Study plan（実施計画）	24章	Payment of money, other compensations, and insurance（金銭の支払い，その他の補償，保険）
11章	Blinding and key opening（ブラインドとキーオープン）	25章	Arrangements regarding publication（公表に関する協定）
12章	Dosage regimen（用量レジメン）	26章	Clinical trial protocol amendment（プロトコール改訂）
13章	Concomitant drugs, combination therapy and post-treatment（併用薬，併用治療，後治療）	27章	Clinical trial protocol change and clinical trial discontinuation and suspension（プロトコールの変更，試験中止，中断）
14章	Observation, examination and survey（観察，検査，調査）	28章	References（文献）

（Common Technical Document：CTD）にまとめられて国に申請がなされます．そして1〜2年の審査を経て市販されるわけです．

市販後には，幅広い患者に使用したときの適正使用や安全性を確保するため，使用成績調査や製造販売後臨床試験が行われます．これらの結果は，国により承認後4〜10年後に行われる再審査の資料として用いられます．

解説 ▶ 倫理指針改訂のポイント

「人を対象とする医学系研究に関する倫理指針」は，臨床研究にかかわるいくつかの不祥事の影響で，2014年に旧倫理指針を改訂して作成されました．最も大きく変わったところは，臨床試験を行う研究責任者に以下の3つが義務付けられたことです．

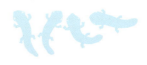

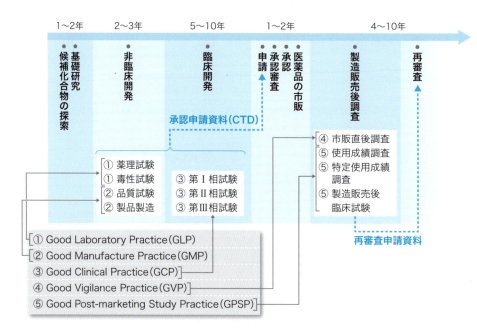

図3 医薬品の臨床開発と薬剤規制（GCPなど）

- モニタリングを行うこと
- 必要に応じて監査を行うこと
- 研究に用いられる情報および資料の保管

モニタリングとは，試験依頼者側（例えば製薬企業）の立場で，被験者保護，データの質，実施手順を中心に医療機関での試験実施状況を確認し，記録する業務のことです．例えば施設訪問モニタリングでは，医療機関に行って同意説明文書があるか，データとカルテの内容が一致しているか，プロトコールどおり治療がなされているか，などが確認されます．

一方，監査とは，プロトコールやGCPなどに従って実施されているかについて，臨床試験にかかわる業務および文書を体系的かつ独立に検証することです．

解説 臨床統計家（生物統計家：biostatistician）とは

臨床統計学（Clinical Biostatistics）は，臨床試験でどのようにデータを集めるか（研究計画），どのように解析するか（統計解析）といった方法論を提供する生物統計家の一分野です．アカデミアや製薬メーカーは医薬品などさまざまな医療技術を開発していますが，実用化するためには人を対象とした臨床試験を行い，有効性・安全性を評価する必要があります．科学的に厳密な評価を行うために統計学が活用され，臨床試験と数理の両方に強い臨床統計家の参画が不可欠です．

臨床統計家の仕事は，臨床試験の実務と臨床試験方法論の研究とに大きく分かれます．臨床試験の実務では，試験実施計画書（プロトコール）の作成，中間解

析，統計解析（プログラミング・報告書作成），データの解釈を行います．これらは医師との共同作業で行われるため，医療一般に関する知識とコミュニケーション能力が求められます．方法論の研究では，数学的な証明・導出，コンピューターシミュレーション，実データへの適用を通じて新しい統計手法を開発し，その性能を評価します．

本講のエッセンス

- ☐ 臨床試験を実施する際には，治験であればGCP，国内の治験以外の臨床試験では「人を対象とする医学系研究に関する倫理指針」を遵守しなければなりません．
- ☐ 具体的には，被験者から同意を得ること，有害事象を国に報告すること，試験実施計画をプロトコールとして事前に規定すること，プロトコールは治験審査委員会の審査を受けること，データの品質管理・保証を行うことなどが求められています．

IV 臨床試験の基礎知識

第14講 データの流れと品質管理・品質保証

Good Clinical Practice（GCP）で求められているデータの品質管理・保証を理解するには，臨床試験のデータの流れを知る必要があります．図1に沿って，具体的にどのような作業が発生し，どのようなエラーが起こりうるのかをみていきましょう．

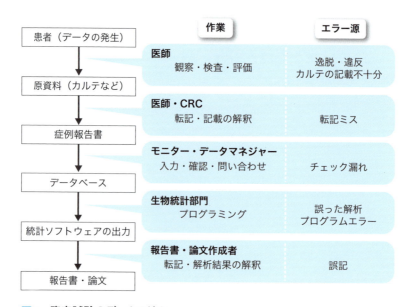

図1 臨床試験のデータの流れ

keyword

GCP，品質管理・保証，原資料，データ固定，モニタリング，監査

データの流れ

データの多くは患者から発生するものであり，カルテ，臨床検査伝票，患者日

誌などさまざまな媒体に記録されます．このような，臨床試験の事実経過の再現と評価に必要な記録のことを**原資料**とよびます．

原資料に含まれる情報の一部は，医師またはClinical Research Coordinator (CRC) とよばれる専門のスタッフによって，データ収集用の質問票〔**症例報告書（Case Report Form：CRF）**〕に転記され，医療機関からデータセンターに送られます．最近では，紙ベースの症例報告書ではなく，専用のWEBシステム（**Electric Data Capture：EDC**）を用いることが一般的です．データセンターに送られた臨床データは，電子的にデータベースに格納されます．

データ固定

データ収集はこの手順の繰り返しであり，患者の来院や別の患者の登録があるごとに，データベースは更新されます．そのため，データ管理部門から生物統計部門に統計解析用データセットを渡す前に，特定の日付で**データ固定（data lock）**を行うことになります．生物統計部門はSASなどの統計解析ソフトウェアを用いて解析を行い，ソフトウェアの出力に基づいて統計解析報告書や論文を作成します．

なお，がんなどの長期追跡が行われる疾患領域では，一部の統計解析が行われた後もデータベースが更新されることがあります．したがって，統計解析用データセットは，データベースのスナップショットのようなものであり，**どのタイミングのものかを特定するためデータ固定日を記録することが重要**です．

品質管理の目標

この流れの背後には，人間が行う作業があることはいうまでもありません．すなわち，どれほど真剣に作業に取り組んだとしても，人為的なエラーがつきものです（図1）．例えば，医師によるエラーとして，プロトコール逸脱，カルテの記載不十分や症例報告書の転記ミスなどがあります．

すなわち，品質管理の目標とは，**これらのエラー源をできるだけ早期に特定し，現場にフィードバックすることにより，作業を改善しデータのエラーを減らすこと**です．

事前準備も重要

さらに，図1には示されていませんが，**エラーの原因は臨床試験の準備段階にもあります**．典型的なのは，プロトコールの記載があいまいだったり，症例報告書のデザインがまずかったり，EDCシステムに不具合があったり，医師への手順の説明が不足していたり，といったケースです．

データ管理部門と生物統計部門のはたらきどころは試験開始以降だと思われがちですが，事前の準備に十分なエフォートを割くことも重要です．

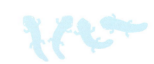

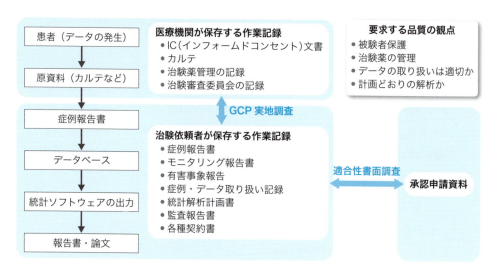

図2 GCP実地調査と適合性書面調査で照合される作業記録

 品質管理についてはわかってきました．では，品質保証とは何ですか？

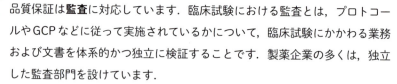 品質保証は**監査**に対応しています．臨床試験における監査とは，プロトコールやGCPなどに従って実施されているかについて，臨床試験にかかわる業務および文書を体系的かつ独立に検証することです．製薬企業の多くは，独立した監査部門を設けています．

また，医薬品の承認後には，**承認申請書類の信頼性を保証するために，規制当局からの査察（GCP実地調査や適合性書面調査）**が入ります（図2）．図の左側に示しているのは図1のデータ処理の流れですが，おのおのの段階で，医療機関側が保存する作業記録と治験依頼者（データセンターや製薬企業）が保存する作業記録が生じます．医療機関側の記録と治験依頼者側の記録を照らし合わせるのがGCP実地調査，治験依頼者側の記録と承認申請資料を照らし合わせるのが適合性書面調査です．

なお，英語では規制当局による査察のことをinspection，監査のことをaudit とよんでいます．

 記録がなかったら品質保証できないですね

 そのとおりです．そこで重要になるのが，作業記録，プロトコール，手順書，データベースやシステムに関する書類などの事前に準備した文書や，データ修正履歴といったデータ以外の情報（メタデータ）です．われわれ生物統計

家は，臨床試験にかかわる際には「作業記録を残す」ことを心掛けなければならないと，口をすっぱくして教わるものです．

 データ固定ってどういう意味があるんですか？

統計解析して都合が悪い結果だったからといって，データを修正するのは明らかにおかしいですよね．解析の公正性を保つうえで，
①事前に解析計画を規定し，
②データ固定を行うこと
はきわめて重要です．データ固定の前には，症例・データの取り扱いに関するデータレビューを通じて，**対象者1人1人の解析対象集団への採否，エンドポイントの評価結果，プロトコール逸脱**などを確定することがふつうです．

本講のエッセンス

☐ 医療機関で発生したデータは，カルテなどの媒体に記録され，症例報告書としてデータセンターに送付されます．データベースに格納された後に，統計解析が行われ，その結果が論文として公表される，というのが一連のデータの流れです．

☐ このプロセスで生じるエラー源をできるだけ早期に特定し，現場にフィードバックすることにより，作業を改善しデータのエラーを減らすことが，品質管理の目標です．

☐ 一方で，品質保証は，審査のことを意味します．

☐ また，解析の公正性を保つうえで，①事前に解析計画を規定し，②データ固定を行うことはきわめて重要です．

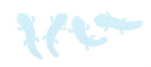

メタアナリシス
抗凝固薬に関するエビデンスの統合

課題論文2 Ruff CT, et al：Lancet, 2014［循環器疾患］
▶別冊　12〜20ページ

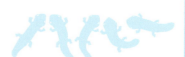

メタアナリシスの大前提
― 偏りのない試験選択

皆さんは**公表バイアス（publication bias）**という言葉を聞いたことがあるでしょうか？公表バイアスをめぐる社会問題として有名なのが、グラクソ・スミスクライン社の抗うつ薬パロキセチンに関する一連の事件です。

きっかけは、パロキセチン中断による離脱症状や自殺企図について、2001年に患者団体が起こした訴訟でした。その後2004年には、未成年者を対象とした臨床試験データを隠匿したとして、ニューヨーク州検事が訴訟を起こしました。ある研究者は、1987～2004年に米国食品医薬品局（FDA）に承認された12種類の抗うつ薬の第Ⅱ相および第Ⅲ相試験（全74試験）の審査報告書を入手し、論文として公表されたかどうかを検討しました[1]。これによると、FDAが主要エンドポイントにおける有効性についてポジティブと判断した38試験のうち、37試験が公表されていた一方で、FDAがポジティブとはいえないと判断した36試験では、報告書と一貫した結論で公表されたものは3試験にすぎなかったそうです。

このような研究結果の隠匿の背景には、**臨床試験の結果の公表・報道が、マーケッティング上の広告の役割を果たしている**という、社会的・経済的構造があります。これから解説するメタアナリシスでは、公表バイアスは深刻なテーマです。

keyword
メタアナリシス，公表バイアス，ファンネルプロット，臨床試験登録データベース

メタアナリシスとは

メタアナリシス（meta-analysis）とは、過去に行われた複数の研究結果を統合し、定量的な結果を得るための統計手法のことです。

ワルファリンと比べた新規経口抗凝固薬（NOAC）の心房細動患者における効果は、患者の特徴やワルファリンコントロールの質によって異なる可能性がありますが、1つ1つの試験では、サブグループ解析を行うために十分な症例数があ

りません．そのため，今回の論文では，すでに公表されたRE-LY試験，ROCKET AF試験，ARISTOTLE試験，ENGAGE AF-TIMI 48試験の結果を統合したメタアナリシスを行っています．

論文の集め方は適切か

さて，最初の疑問は「なぜこの4試験なのか？」ということです．意地悪な見方をすれば，NOACの効果が大きかった論文ばかりを集めれば，NOACに有利な（偏った）メタアナリシスができてしまいます．意図的に論文を選ばなくても，ネガティブな結果が出た研究は，ポジティブな結果が出た研究に比べて論文公表されにくいという公表バイアスはよく知られている現象です．

公表バイアスを防ぐために，専門家の間では，次のような手順が勧められています．
① 臨床試験を行うときには，「臨床試験登録データベース」に登録し，すべての臨床試験の概要を誰でも把握できるようにする．
② メタアナリシスを行うときには，研究実施計画書（プロトコール）を「系統的レビュー登録データベース」に登録し，試験選択ルールを事前に宣言する．
③ 事前に決めたルールに従い，PubMedなどの文献データベースを検索し，該当するすべての臨床試験を解析に含める．

この論文では，NOACの有効性と安全性をワルファリンと比べたすべての第Ⅲ相試験を選択しています．

ここまでで質問はありますか？

臨床試験登録データベースや系統的レビュー登録データベースって何ですか？ 聞いたことありません

いくつかの公的機関がHPを設けていますので，臨床試験や系統的メタアナリシスを行うときには，それらのHPに登録することになります．

前者で有名なのは，世界保健機関（WHO）の臨床試験登録国際プラットフォーム（ICTRP；http://www.who.int/ictrp/en/），大学病院医療情報ネットワーク（UMIN）のUMIN臨床試験登録システム（UMIN-CTR；http://www.umin.ac.jp/ctr/index-j.htm）の2つです．

臨床試験のメタアナリシスでは，PROSPERO（http://www.crd.york.ac.uk/PROSPERO/）というデータベースが利用できます．事前に登録しないと論文が採択されないこともあります．

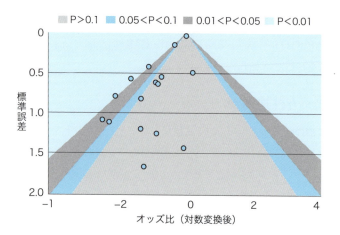

図1 心筋梗塞後のマグネシウム静注と死亡率に関するファンネルプロット
(文献2より引用)

解説 公表バイアスを見つける手がかりは？

　公表バイアスがあるかどうかを，公表されたデータだけから調べることは簡単ではありません．ただ，その手がかりとしてよく用いられるのが，図1のような**ファンネルプロット（funnel plot）**です[2]．ファンネルプロットは，縦軸に試験の規模（人数や標準誤差など）を，横軸に効果の推定値（相対リスクの対数など）をとった図で，漏斗（funnel）を逆さにした形をしていることが名前の由来です．

　仮に，試験はその規模によらず必ず公表されるとすると，ファンネルプロットは平均を中心に左右対称にばらつくと考えられます．一方，大規模な試験は必ず公表され，小規模で，有意差がなかった試験は公表されにくいとすると，**ファンネルプロットは左右非対称**になるはずです．

　図1は，あるメタアナリシスでみられたファンネルプロットの例ですが，標準誤差が大きい小規模な試験は，明らかに左側（試験治療に有利な側）に偏っており，公表バイアスがあることを示唆しています．

本講のエッセンス

- 臨床試験登録データベースができた理由は，「ネガティブな結果が出た研究は，ポジティブな結果が出た研究に比べて公表されにくい」という公表バイアスを防止するためです．
- メタアナリシスを行うときには，ファンネルプロットが左右対称かどうかに基づいて，公表バイアスがあるかどうかを調べることが一般的です．

文献

1) Turner EH, et al：Selective publication of antidepressant trials and its influence on apparent efficacy. N Engl J Med, 358：252-260, 2008
2) Sterne JA, et al：Recommendations for examining and interpreting funnel plot asymmetry in meta-analyses of randomised controlled trials. BMJ, 343：d4002, 2011

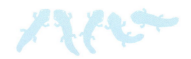

| V メタアナリシス | 課題論文2 Ruff CT, et al：Lancet, 2014［循環器疾患］|

第16講 メタアナリシスの本質は「平均値」

本講のテーマ

別冊
15ページ

第12講では，ダビガトランの非劣性試験であるRE-LY試験を取り上げました．抗凝固薬メタアナリシスでは，RE-LY試験を含めFigure 1（図1）の4試験のデータが用いられました．図1の右側をみると，RE-LY試験の行には，ちゃんとAbstract（抄録）と同じ相対リスクが示されていることがわかります．また，ほかの試験で報告された相対リスクも，図1に示されているとおりでした．これらの結果を統合して，新規経口抗凝固薬（NOAC）の効果（相対リスク）を推定するにはどうすればよいでしょうか？

実は，一番素朴な方法が正解です．メタアナリシスの本質は，「1つ1つの試験から得られた推定値（ここでは0.66，0.88，0.80，0.88）の平均をとること」です．メタアナリシスで用いられる統計手法は2つあり，**変量効果モデル（random-effects model）と固定効果モデル（fixed-effects model）**というものなのですが，いずれも一種の平均値を計算します．ただし，計算にはちょっとした工夫があるのですが❶．

❶詳しくは第17講で解説します．

	NOAC （イベント）	ワルファリン （イベント）		相対リスク （95％信頼区間）	p
RE-LY	134/6,076	199/6,022		0.66（0.53-0.82）	0.0001
ROCKET AF	269/7,081	306/7,090		0.88（0.75-1.03）	0.12
ARISTOTLE	212/9,120	265/9,081		0.80（0.67-0.95）	0.012
ENGAGE AF-TIMI 48	296/7,035	337/7,036		0.88（0.75-1.02）	0.10
全体（ランダム）	911/29,312	1,107/29,229		0.81（0.73-0.91）	<0.0001

図1　NOACとワルファリンの脳卒中・全身塞栓症発生率を比較したメタアナリシス
（課題論文2よりFigure 1を転載）

keyword

メタアナリシス，変量効果モデルと固定効果モデル

理解を深めるための計算6
メタアナリシス

「平均をとること」を素朴に実行すると，

$$(0.66 + 0.88 + 0.80 + 0.88)/4 = 0.805$$

となります．これでも悪くありませんが[2]，メタアナリシスでは，さらに2つの工夫をしています．

● **第1の工夫：対数をとる**

第1の工夫は，**対数をとること**です．相対リスク[3]では，比較する治療を逆にする（NOACを基準にする）ためには，逆数をとります．ところが，相対リスクの単純平均だと，ワルファリンを基準にしたとき

$$(0.66 + 0.88 + 0.80 + 0.88)/4 = 0.81$$

とNOACを基準にしたとき

$$(1.52 + 1.14 + 1.25 + 1.14)/4 = 1.26$$

とで，結果が逆数の関係にならないことがあるのです（0.81 と 1/1.26 = 0.79）．これでは困りますよね？ そこで，相対リスクでは，対数[4]をとってから平均を計算します．

● **第2の工夫：試験ごとに重みを付ける**

第2の工夫は，**試験ごとに重みを付けること**です．

図1の"NOAC（イベント）"や"ワルファリン（イベント）"には，試験ごとの人数とイベント数が示されており，試験の規模がまちまちであることがわかります．また，図1の中央には，相対リスクの推定値が四角（■）で，95％信頼区間が横線で表されています．これによると，RE-LY試験の95％信頼区間はほかの試験よりも広く，相対リスクの推定精度が低いことがわかります．これらを単純平均するのは違和感がありますよね．そこで，このメタアナリシスでは，上から順に，0.19，0.28，0.25，0.28 という重みを付けて，平均を求めています．

● **メタアナリシスの結果の再現**

これで，図1の数字からメタアナリシスの結果を再現できます．計算式は，

$$\exp(-0.42 \times 0.19 - 0.13 \times 0.28 - 0.22 \times 0.25 - 0.13 \times 0.28) = 0.81$$

です[5]．ここで，-0.42，-0.13，-0.22，-0.13 は，試験ごとの相対リスクの対数をとったものです．

❷図1の"全体"の結果 0.81 と比べてみてください．

❸第12講で，相対リスクには，ハザード比，発生率比，リスク比，オッズ比などがあると解説しましたね．

❹例えば，「log (0.66) = -0.42」

❺expとは exponential（指数）の略で，「$\exp(x) = e^x = 2.718\cdots^x$」のことです．

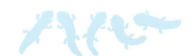

解説 メタアナリシスでもPICOは重要

　クリニカルクエスチョンの基本形は,「どんな患者に(Patient),どんな介入を行うと(Intervention),何と比べて(Comparison),どうなるか(Outcomes)が知りたい」だと解説しました.これはメタアナリシスでも同じです.
　この研究では,
- Patients：心房細動患者
- Intervention：NOAC
- Comparison：ワルファリン
- Outcomes：脳卒中と全身塞栓症,虚血性脳卒中,脳出血,総死亡,心筋梗塞,大出血,頭蓋内出血と消化管出血

です.

本講のエッセンス

☐ メタアナリシスでは,個々の試験の結果を統合するための統計手法として,変量効果モデルと固定効果モデルが用いられますが,どちらも計算は本質的に「平均値」です.

第17講 固定効果モデルと変量効果モデルの使い分け

V メタアナリシス　　　課題論文2　Ruff CT, et al：Lancet, 2014［循環器疾患］

本講のテーマ

メタアナリシスのMethods（方法）のStatistical analysis（統計解析）は，どのような記載になっているのでしょうか？ 図1は，その第2段落です．第5講 図1の臨床試験のものとはかなり違いますね．特に大切なのが，

「アウトカムは変量効果モデル（random-effects model）を用いて併合し，比較した」

という一文です．

別冊 15ページ

> We calculated relative risks (RRs) and corresponding 95% CIs for each outcome and trial separately and checked findings against published data for accuracy. When necessary, we calculated numbers of outcome events on the basis of event rates, sample size, and duration of follow-up. Outcomes were then pooled and compared with a random-effects model.[24] We assessed the appropriateness of pooling data across studies with use of the Cochran Q statistic and I^2 test for heterogeneity.[25]

図1　抗凝固薬メタアナリシスのStatistical analysis（統計解析）第2段落の記述
（課題論文2より転載，ハイライトは著者追記）

keyword

メタアナリシス，変量効果モデルと固定効果モデル，試験内分散と試験間分散，不均一性の検定

別冊 15ページ，Figure 1

❶読み飛ばされた方は，これから述べる試験ごとの重みの違いが，モデルの違いに対応していることだけでも押さえてください．

試験ごとの重みの付け方

第16講では，第16講 図1の4試験のデータからメタアナリシスの結果を再現しました❶．対数変換を行って，上から順に0.19，0.28，0.25，0.28という重みを付けて，平均を求めることで，第16講 図1の"全体"の結果0.81が計算できました．さて，この重みはどこからきたのでしょうか？

基本的な考え方は，**推定値の精度が高いものには大きい重みを，低いものには小さい重みを与える**，ということです．実際，統計学の理論によると，「推定値の分散」の逆数で重みを付けることが最適ということがわかっています．「推定値の分散」は，誤差にどのような確率分布（モデル）を考えるかで違ってきます．メタアナリシスでは，**固定効果モデル（fixed-effects model）** と変量効果モデルとよばれる2種類のモデルが用いられます．

固定効果モデルと変量効果モデル

　第16講 図1をみると，相対リスクの推定値には明らかなバラツキがあります．固定効果モデルと変量効果モデルの違いは，**推定値のバラツキを，「試験内分散」だけによるものだと考えるか，「試験内分散」と「試験間分散」の2つがあると考えるか**，です．ここで，「推定値の分散」は，試験ごとに報告された標準誤差の2乗のことです．

固定効果モデル

　固定効果モデルは，すべての試験を通じて，真の効果は1つ（固定値）と考えます．「試験間分散」はゼロと考えるので，「推定値の分散」は，「試験ごとに報告された標準誤差の2乗」そのものになります（その逆数が重み）．

変量効果モデル

　一方で，変量効果モデルは，試験ごとの真の効果がランダムに分布する，というものです．「試験ごとに報告された標準誤差の2乗」に，「試験間分散」（これはデータから推定する必要があります）を加えたものが「推定値の分散」になります．

抗凝固薬メタアナリシスではどうか

　このメタアナリシスでは，変量効果モデルが用いられています．すなわち，先ほどの0.19，0.28，0.25，0.28という重みは，変量効果モデルのものです．固定効果モデルを用いると，重みは0.16，0.29，0.24，0.31というように変わってきます．

　一般的に，**固定効果モデルは，変量効果モデルに比べ，推定値の精度が低い試験に小さな重みを付ける性質**があります（例えばRE-LY試験では0.19＞0.16）．

ここまでで質問はありますか？

すみません，よくわからないんですが，固定効果モデルと変量効果モデルのどちらを使えばいいんですか？

変量効果モデルの「試験ごとの真の効果がランダムに分布する」というのは，簡単にいうと「試験ごとに効果が違う」ということです．人によっては，そもそも試験ごとにデザインや状況設定が異なるのだから，すべての試験を通じて真の効果は固定値と考えるのは間違いで，常に変量効果モデルを使うべきだ，という意見もあります．

しかし，より一般的な意見は，「試験間分散」がゼロかどうかを調べて，ゼロのときには固定効果モデルを，試験間分散があるときには変量効果モデルを用いる，というものです．

 試験間分散って何ですか？ もう少し具体的にお願いします

試験間分散がゼロとは，今回の例でいうと，**NOACの効果の大きさが4試験の間で同じ**，ということを意味します．試験間分散がゼロかどうかの検定を**不均一性の検定（test for heterogeneity）**，バラツキ全体のうち試験間分散が占める割合を**不均一性（heterogeneity）のI^2統計量**とよんでいます．第16講 図1のデータでは$I^2 = 47％$です❷．$I^2 = 0$でないということは，言い換えると，「RE-LY試験，ROCKET AF試験，ARISTOTLE試験，ENGAGE AF-TIMI 48試験の間で，NOACの効果の大きさが不均一である」ということを示唆しています．

❷詳しい計算法は知らなくても大丈夫です．

試験間の不均一性の原因は，さまざまなものが考えられます．試験ごとに患者の臨床的特徴（脳卒中既往の有無など）がばらついていたためかもしれませんし（試験ごとに脳卒中リスクの異なる患者を対象にしていた），NOAC（ダビガトラン，リバーロキサバン，アピキサバン，エドキサバン）の間で薬効が異なる可能性もあります．

 結果の解釈はなんとなくわかりました．では，Methods（方法）のStatistical analysis（統計解析）にはどう書かれているんですか？

これまで解説した内容に対応するのは，第2段落です（図1）．

最初に，アウトカム・試験ごとに，相対リスク（relative risk）と信頼区間（95％ CI）を計算し，公表されたデータの正確性をチェックしたと書かれています．次に書かれているのは，変量効果モデル（random-effects model）を用いてアウトカムを併合し，比較したという部分でしたね．最後に，不均一性を調べるために，Cochran（コクラン）のQ統計量（Cochran Q statistic）とI^2統計量に関する検定（I^2 test）を用いたと書かれています．ただ，Cochran

のQ統計量はI^2統計量を計算する途中に出てくるだけで,この論文で報告はされていないようです.

本講のエッセンス

- ☐ 固定効果モデルと変量効果モデルの実質的な違いは,重み付き平均を計算するときの重みに表れます(固定効果モデルのほうが,推定値の精度が低い試験により小さな重みを付けます).
- ☐ モデル間で重み付けに違いが生じる理由は,前者は推定値のバラツキを「試験内分散」だけによるものだと仮定しており,後者は「試験内分散」と「試験間分散」の2つがあると考えているためです.
- ☐ 試験間分散がゼロかどうかの検定を,不均一性の検定とよんでいます.

| V メタアナリシス | 課題論文2 Ruff CT, et al：Lancet, 2014 ［循環器疾患］|

サブグループ解析と交互作用の検定

このメタアナリシスの目的の1つは，新規経口抗凝固薬（NOAC）の効果が患者の特徴やワルファリンコントロールの質によって異なるかどうかを調べることでした．Figure 4A（図1）は，年齢，性別，糖尿病の有無，脳卒中または一過性脳虚血発作（TIA）既往の有無，クレアチニンクリアランス，$CHADS_2$ スコア，ビタミンK拮抗薬（VKA）使用状況，治療域内時間（TTR）によって患者を2グループに分けたときの，脳卒中と全身塞栓症の相対リスクを示したものです．この

17ページ

	NOAC 全体 （イベント）	ワルファリン全体 （イベント）		相対リスク （95% 信頼区間）	$p_{interaction}$
年齢					
<75	496/18,073	578/18,004		0.85 (0.73–0.99)	0.38
≧75	415/11,188	532/11,095		0.78 (0.68–0.88)	
性別					
女性	382/10,941	478/10,839		0.78 (0.65–0.94)	0.52
男性	531/18,371	634/18,390		0.84 (0.75–0.94)	
糖尿病					
なし	622/20,216	755/20,238		0.83 (0.74–0.93)	0.73
あり	287/9,096	356/8,990		0.80 (0.69–0.93)	
脳卒中 or TIA					
なし	483/20,699	615/20,637		0.78 (0.66–0.91)	0.30
あり	428/8,663	495/8,635		0.86 (0.76–0.98)	
クレアチニンクリアランス(mL/分)					
<50	249/5,539	311/5,503		0.79 (0.65–0.96)	
50〜80	405/13,055	546/13,155		0.75 (0.66–0.85)	0.12
>80	256/10,626	255/10,533		0.98 (0.79–1.22)	
$CHADS_2$スコア					
0〜1	69/5,058	90/4,942		0.75 (0.54–1.04)	
2	247/9,563	290/9,757		0.86 (0.70–1.05)	0.76
3〜6	596/14,690	733/14,528		0.80 (0.72–0.89)	
VKA 使用状況					
経験なし	386/13,789	513/13,834		0.75 (0.66–0.86)	0.31
経験あり	522/15,514	597/15,395		0.85 (0.70–1.03)	
TTR で分けた相対リスク					
<66%	509/16,219	653/16,297		0.77 (0.65–0.92)	0.60
≧66%	313/12,642	392/12,904		0.82 (0.71–0.95)	

0.5　　　1　　　2
←NOAC 有利　　ワルファリン有利→

図1　抗凝固薬メタアナリシスにおけるサブグループ解析
（課題論文2より Figure 4A を転載）

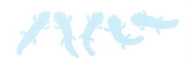

種の検討をサブグループ解析といいます．この図はどのように読み取るべきなのでしょうか？

> **keyword**
>
> メタアナリシス，サブグループ解析，交互作用の検定

サブグループ解析のポイント

図1で最初に気づくのは，多くのサブグループでNOACに好ましい結果であり，一方でクレアチニンクリアランスが80 mL/分より高いサブグループでは，相対リスク0.98（95％信頼区間0.79〜1.22）と，ワルファリンとNOACの差があまり大きくないということです．クレアチニンクリアランス高値のサブグループでは，NOACの効果がないと結論すべきでしょうか？

＊　　　＊　　　＊

15ページ,
Figure 1

第16講 図1別冊の結果を思い出してください．この結果は，（クレアチニンクリアランスの値を問わず）心房細動患者全体で，NOACに効果があることを意味しています．それと，クレアチニンクリアランス高値のサブグループ解析の結果は，矛盾しませんか？

ここがサブグループ解析のポイントです．サブグループ解析は，**全患者を対象とした解析で有意な場合とそうでない場合**で，解釈が変わります．

ケース1：全体で有意な場合

全体の結果に基づいて考えると，「相対リスク≠1」ということ（この場合だとNOACに効果があること）がわかっているわけです❶．それなのに，サブグループごとに「相対リスク＝1」かどうかの検定を行うのは論理が一貫しません．そこで，サブグループ解析では，「相対リスク＝1」かどうかの検定ではなく，後述する**交互作用の検定（test for interaction）**を用います．

❶この場合は，相対リスクが1より小さいと，NOAC群のリスクが低いのでしたね．

ケース2：全体で有意ではない場合

サブグループ解析で有意差が出ても，何回も検定を行ったことによる偶然の結果かもしれません．したがって，サブグループ解析の結果から，治療が有効とは結論できないのです．

サブグループ間の効果の違いを検定する

交互作用（interaction）とは，どこかの**サブグループで効果の向き（相対リス

クが＞1と＜1など）や大きさが異なることを意味します．メタアナリシスの例では，比較しているNOACの効果のことを主効果（main effect）とよび，サブグループとNOACの組み合わせによる効果を交互作用（interaction effect）といいます．

＊　　　＊　　　＊

図1では，クレアチニンクリアランス＜50 mL/分のサブグループでは相対リスク0.79，50〜80 mL/分では相対リスク0.75，＞80 mL/分では相対リスク0.98と3つの相対リスクがありますよね．これらを仮に，相対リスクA，相対リスクB，相対リスクCとよびましょう．

主効果の検定と交互作用の検定は，それぞれ以下の仮説を調べるものです．
- 主効果の検定：相対リスクA＝1（特定の相対リスクが1かどうか．相対リスクB，Cでもよい）
- 交互作用の検定：相対リスクA＝相対リスクB＝相対リスクC（3つの相対リスクが同じかどうか）

図1の交互作用p値（$p_{interaction}$）を見ると，交互作用のp値は0.12で，クレアチニンクリアランスに関する交互作用は有意ではありません．それ以外のサブグループも同じですので，著者は「NOACの相対的な有効性と安全性は，多様な患者層を通じて一致している」と結論したわけです．

別冊 13ページ，Summary（抄録）のInterpretation（解析）

質的交互作用と量的交互作用

交互作用は，効果の向きの違いによって，**量的交互作用**と**質的交互作用**に分類されます．量的交互作用とは，「どのサブグループでも一貫して因果的（または予防的）な効果があるが，効果の大きさは一定していない」ことであり，質的交互作用とは「あるサブグループでは因果的な効果があり，別のサブグループでは予防的な効果があるように，効果の方向が逆転してしまう」ことを示します．

今回の例では，サブグループの群間で相対リスクの向きが違うことはないので，量的交互作用の関係がみられていると考えます．

ここまでで質問はありますか？

交互作用の検定は，相対リスクと相対リスクの違いを調べているってことですか？

そうです．交互作用の検定は，差の差（difference in differences）をみているのだといわれます．

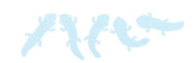

なお、図1の相対リスクの95％信頼区間が1をまたいでいるもの（主効果が有意でないもの）と、またいでいないもの（有意なもの）がありますが、これを根拠に**サブグループ間で効果の大きさが異なると結論することはできません**。これでは主効果をみているにすぎず、差（相対リスク）の差を調べたことになっていませんから。

サブグループをみると、どれも医学的に重要なものばかりで、交互作用はいかにもありそうです。全体で有意かどうかは気にせず、いきなり交互作用を調べたらいいのでは？

その考え方が用いられない理由は2つあります。第1に、交互作用の検定は、全患者を対象とした主効果の検定に比べて、検出力が低いという問題があります。第2に、NOACの適応症は心房細動患者全体なので、そこで有効かどうかを検証しないと、議論が先に進まないのです。

交互作用の検定が有意になることもあるかもしれないけど、たくさん検定するわけだから、いいとこどりの一種なんじゃないですか？

それはサブグループ解析の重要な側面です。たくさんのサブグループを検討して有意なものだけを報告する、ということができないように、解析するサブグループは、プロトコールに事前に規定しておくことが勧められています[1]。

解説　交互作用を検討するほかの状況

　複数の国をまたいで行われる国際共同臨床試験では、国ごとに治療効果が異ならないかどうかが論点の1つです。その場合の考え方も、サブグループ解析・交互作用の検定と同じで、"global first"です（全体の結果より先に日本だけの結果を見る"local first"ではだめ）。また、観察研究でも交互作用を調べることはあります。チェルノブイリのケース・コントロール研究のTable 4がその例です。

本講のエッセンス

- □ サブグループ解析は，全患者を対象とした解析で有意な場合とそうでない場合で，解釈が変わります．
- □ 全体で有意な場合，交互作用の検定を用いて，サブグループ間で効果の大きさが異なるかどうかを調べます．
- □ 一方で，全体で有意でない場合，サブグループで有意差が出ても，何回も検定を行ったことによる偶然の結果かもしれません．したがって，サブグループ解析の結果から，治療が有効と結論することはできません．
- □ 解析するサブグループは，プロトコールに事前に規定しておくことが勧められています．

文献

1) Wang R, et al：Statistics in medicine-reporting of subgroup analyses in clinical trials. N Engl J Med, 357：2189-2194, 2007

第19講 試験ごとのバイアスの評価

V メタアナリシス　　課題論文2　Ruff CT, et al：Lancet, 2014［循環器疾患］

本講のテーマ

臨床試験にも，適切に実施されたものもあれば，質の低いものもあります．個々の臨床試験の結果にバイアスがあると，メタアナリシスの結果も偏ってしまいます．

図1は封筒を使ってランダム化を行った悲惨な事例です．この試験では，好みの治療が割り付けられるまで，医師が封筒を開けてしまいました．その結果，施設によってAばかりまたはBばかりが割り付けられる，という偏りが生じています．これは**選択バイアス（selection bias）**の例です．

今回のテーマは，メタアナリシス論文において，1つ1つの試験に生じたバイアスはどのように調べられているかということです．

消化器がんを主体とする化療122例/12施設
　非治癒切除適格例　A：化療対照　　41例
　　　　　　　　　　B：化療＋SSM　40例
年齢，性，部位，ステージ，検査値などに群間差は認められない

封筒法割り付けのA，Bの分布

	施設番号	
	6	BBBBBBBB
	5	B
AAAA	10	BBBBBBBBBBBB
AAA	9	BBBB
AAAAA	3	BBBBB
AA	1	BB
A	12	B
	7*	
AAAAAAA	8	BBBBB
AAAAAAA	2*	B
AAAAAAAAAA	11	B
AA	4*	
41	計	40

＊世話人施設

図1　封筒法によるランダム化を用いて施設によって偏ってしまった例
化療：化学療法，SSM：Specific Substance MARUYAMA（丸山ワクチン）

keyword

リスクオブバイアス評価ツール，選択バイアス，パフォーマンスバイアス，検出バイアス，脱落バイアス，報告バイアス

バイアスを見抜くポイント

個々の臨床試験の結果にバイアスの可能性があるかどうかを論文から読み取るために，表1のリスクオブバイアス評価ツールを用いることが推奨されています[1]．表1は，バイアスの種類❶ごとに，論文のどこを読むべきなのかを示しています．具体的には，以下の5点が主なポイントです．

- 割り付け結果が患者や医師に漏れていないか
- 二重盲検試験かどうか
- アウトカムの評価は偏っていないか
- 脱落などによりアウトカムは不完全でないか
- 都合のよいアウトカムばかり公表されていないか

解説 ランダム誤差とバイアス

相対リスクなどの推定値が真の値から系統的にずれていること（過大評価や過小評価）をバイアスといい，系統的でない（過大評価や過小評価でない）バラツキのことをランダム誤差といいます（図2）．

生存時間解析では脱落バイアスに注意すべきだと述べました❷．研究を実施するときには，バイアスを可能なかぎりゼロに近づけることが第1の目標です．それができなかったとしても，バイアスの可能性をチェックし，どちらの方向に偏りが生じているのかを考察することは不可欠です．

❶脱落バイアス（attrition bias）については第4講，実際の研究でバイアスについてどのような議論がなされているかについては第30講で解説しています．

❷第4講，第7講を参照ください．

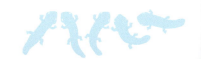

表1 Cochrane（コクラン）共同計画のリスクオブバイアス評価ツール

バイアスのドメイン	バイアスの原因	判断の手がかり	レビュワーの判断の基準（低，不明，高リスク）
選択バイアス	乱数列の発生	割り付け乱数列の発生方法の記載（群間の比較可能性を判断できる程度に詳細に）	割り付け乱数列の発生が不適切であることによる選択バイアス（介入割り付けの偏り）
	割り付け情報の管理	管理方法の記載（登録前や途中に割り付け結果が予見できたかどうかを判断できる程度に詳細に）	割り付け前に割り付けが秘匿されないことによる選択バイアス（介入割り付けの偏り）
パフォーマンスバイアス	参加者と医師のブラインディング	参加者と研究者に介入結果を知らせないためのすべての手段の記載，その手段が効果的だったかに関する情報も	参加者と医師が割り付けられた介入を知ることが治療成績に影響するというバイアス
検出バイアス	アウトカム評価のブラインディング	アウトカム評価者に介入結果を知らせないためのすべての手段の記載，その手段が効果的だったかに関する情報も	アウトカム評価者が割り付けられた介入を知ることにより生じる検出バイアス
脱落バイアス	不完全アウトカムデータ	脱落や解析からの除外など主なアウトカムごとにデータの完全性の記載〔脱落と除外が報告されていたか，群ごとの人数（ランダム化された人数と比べて），脱落や除外の理由が報告されていたか，レビューで異なる扱いをしたかどうか〕	不完全なアウトカムデータの量，特性，扱いにより生じる脱落バイアス
報告バイアス	選択的な報告	選ばれたアウトカムのみ報告されていないかを，どのように調べ，その結果どうだったかの記載	選ばれたアウトカムのみ報告されることによる報告バイアス
その他のバイアス	どのようなものでもよいが，事前に特定されていることが望ましい	このツールのほかのドメインに含まれない重要なバイアスの懸念の記載	ほかに含まれていない問題によるバイアス

（文献1より引用）

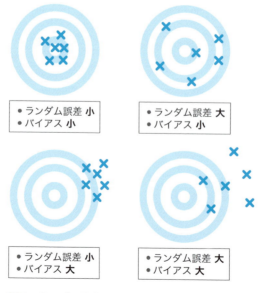

図2 ランダム誤差とバイアスのイメージ

本講のエッセンス

☐ メタアナリシスで個々の試験をレビューするときには，リスクオブバイアス評価ツールを用いて，選択バイアス，パフォーマンスバイアス，検出バイアス，脱落バイアス，報告バイアスがあるかどうかが調べられます．

☐ 割り付け結果が患者や医師に漏れていないか，二重盲検試験かどうか，アウトカムの評価は偏っていないか，脱落などアウトカムは不完全でないか，都合のよいアウトカムばかり公表されていないか，などがポイントです．

文献

1) Higgins JP, et al：The Cochrane Collaboration's tool for assessing risk of bias in randomised trials. BMJ, 343：d5928, 2011

次は演習問題です

V　メタアナリシス

 演習問題

問題1　課題論文3（Miura T, et al：Lancet Psychiatry, 2014）を読んで，以下の問いに答えなさい．

22〜31ページ

1 文献データベースから見つかったのは何件の臨床試験で，解析に用いられたのはそのうち何件でしょうか？

2 解析に用いられたのは，固定効果モデルと変量効果モデルのどちらでしょうか？

3 公表バイアス，選択バイアス，パフォーマンスバイアス，検出バイアス，脱落バイアス，報告バイアスに関する記述を調べなさい．著者は，どのようなバイアスを最も懸念していたでしょうか？

ネットワークメタアナリシス

17通りの双極性障害治療レジメンを比較するには

課題論文3 Miura T, et al：Lancet Psychiatry, 2014 ［精神疾患］
▶別冊　22〜31ページ

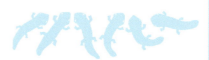

VI ネットワークメタアナリシス

課題論文3　Miura T, et al：Lancet Psychiatry, 2014 ［精神疾患］

第20講　大流行のネットワークメタアナリシス

本講のテーマ

第15〜19講に取り上げたメタアナリシスでは，4つの臨床試験の結果を統合し，新規経口抗凝固薬（NOAC）はワルファリンに比べ，脳卒中または全身塞栓症を減らす❶ことが示されました．しかし，論文をよく読むと，ダビガトラン，リバーロキサバン，アピキサバン，エドキサバンをまとめてNOAC群として解析しています．この点について疑問が生じませんでしたか？医師として本当に知りたいのは，NOAC同士の比較（ダビガトラン対リバーロキサバンなど）や，4剤のうち一番優れているのはどれか，といったことではないでしょうか？

今回は，より高度な手法であるネットワークメタアナリシス（network meta-analysis）について解説します．ネットワークメタアナリシスは，**3つ以上の治療を比較するための強力な手法**で，このところLancetやBMJなどトップジャーナルで大流行しています．

❶相対リスク0.81, 95％信頼区間 0.73〜0.91, $p < 0.0001$

keyword

ネットワークメタアナリシス，直接比較と間接比較

ネットワークメタアナリシスの原理

22〜31ページ：課題論文3

27ページ

ケーススタディとして，双極性障害の長期治療に関するネットワークメタアナリシスを取り上げます．双極性障害の長期治療ではリチウムなどさまざまな薬剤が用いられており，臨床試験も数多く行われています．

Figure 2（図1）は，今回の論文で解析に用いられた個々の試験で，どのような比較がなされたのかを表しています．図に示されている18の円は，17レジメンの実薬群とプラセボ群を意味しており，線が結ばれている治療間ではランダム化臨床試験がなされています．円の大きさは患者数に，線の太さは試験の数に比例しています．例えば，線の太さから，一番線の太いリチウム（LIT）とプラセボ（PLB）を比較した臨床試験が一番多く行われていることや，線の接続関係か

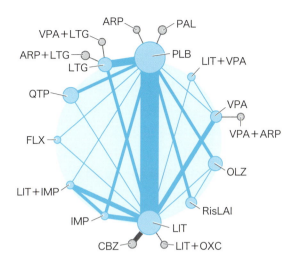

図1　双極性障害メタアナリシスの治療ネットワーク
略語は次のとおりです．ARP：アリピプラゾール，CBZ：カルバマゼピン，FLX：フルオキセチン，IMP：イミプラミン，LIT：リチウム，LTG：ラモトリギン，OLZ：オランザピン，QTP：クエチアピン，OXC：オクスカルバゼピン，PAL：パリペリドン，PLB：プラセボ，RisLAI：リスペリドン特効性注射剤，VPA：バルプロ酸（課題論文3よりFigure 2を転載）

らは，それ以外の薬剤はリチウムまたはプラセボと比較されることが多かったことがわかります．これだけデータがあれば，いろいろなことが調べられそうです．

直接比較と間接比較

仮に，カルバマゼピン（CBZ）がプラセボより有効かどうかが知りたいとしましょう．ところが，カルバマゼピンとプラセボを**直接比較**（direct comparison）した臨床試験はありません．そこで用いるのが，**間接比較**（indirect comparison）という手法です．

カルバマゼピンとリチウムの臨床試験で推定された再発リスク比が1.10（CBZ群のリスク/LIT群のリスク）だとしましょう．また，リチウムとプラセボの臨床試験で推定された再発リスク比が0.62（LIT群のリスク/PLB群のリスク）だとしましょう．そうすると，CBZ群のリスク/PLB群のリスクが知りたければ，

$$1.10 \times 0.62 = 0.68$$

と計算できますよね．これが間接比較です．

ネットワークメタアナリシスは，**このような直接比較と間接比較を統合解析することによって，一度に多くの治療を比較する手法**です．

ここまでで質問はありますか？

よくわからないんですが，メタアナリシスは平均値を計算するんでしたよね？

第16講の内容ですね．NOACのメタアナリシスでは，4試験から報告された相対リスクを統合するために，試験ごとに重みを付けて対数相対リスクの平均値を計算していました（直接比較）❷．つまり，従来型のメタアナリシスの本質は「平均値」です．

　しかし，**ネットワークメタアナリシスでは直接比較だけでなく間接比較も考慮してリスク比を求めるため，単純な平均値にはなりません**．ただ，直感的な理解としては，直接比較の推定値と間接比較の推定値の重み付き平均を求めている，と考えて差し支えありません．今回の講義では詳細は割愛しますが，この論文ではマルコフ連鎖モンテカルロ法（Markov chain Monte Carlo）という数値積分の手法を用いてリスク比を計算しています．

❷読み飛ばされた方は，気にせずこの結果だけ押さえてください．

本講のエッセンス

☐ ネットワークメタアナリシスは，直接比較と間接比較を統合解析することによって，一度に多くの治療を比較する手法です．

☐ 直感的な理解としては，直接比較の推定値と間接比較の推定値の重み付き平均を求めている，と考えて差し支えありません．

VI ネットワークメタアナリシス

課題論文3　Miura T, et al：Lancet Psychiatry, 2014 ［精神疾患］

第21講　273通りのリスク比

図1に論文のFigure 3を示します．この図は，17の実薬とプラセボの273通りの組み合わせについて，リスク比と95％信頼区間（正確にはcredible interval）をまとめたものです．このたくさんのリスク比はどのように求められた

別冊 28ページ

図1　双極性障害メタアナリシスで推定されたリスク比
（課題論文3よりFigure 3を転載）

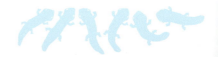

ものなのでしょうか？

> **keyword**
> ネットワークメタアナリシス，変量効果モデルと固定効果モデル

ネットワークメタアナリシスの解析結果

23ページ

Summary（抄録）を読んでみましょう．

まず，PICOを確認すると，Patientsは「双極性障害患者6,846人」，InterventionとComparisonは「17の双極性障害のための治療・プラセボ」です．Outcomesについては，主要アウトカムは気分障害を再発（または再燃）した患者数と有害事象により試験を中止した患者数と述べられています．

抄録からすべてを読み取るのは，正直言って難しいのですが，33試験6,846人の患者のデータを解析したところ，再燃リスクについては，「アリピプラゾール，カルバマゼピン，イミプラミン，パリペリドンはプラセボと有意差がなく，それ以外の治療は再燃リスクが有意に低かった」，と述べられています．直接比較だけでなく間接比較の結果をもとにして，プラセボ対照試験がない薬剤でも，リスク比が推定できた，というわけです．

結果の読み取り方

図1は，17の実薬とプラセボを273通りの組み合わせで比較したもので，左下の白色部分が再燃（recurrence of any mood episode）のリスク比，右上の薄青部分が有害事象による中止（忍容性：tolerability）のリスク比です．リスク比の方向は，右下にある治療がリスク比の基準（分母）になるようにしてあります（つまり数字が1より小さいと，左上にある治療のほうが，リスクが小さい）．

リチウム（LIT）対プラセボ（PLB）のリスク比を調べてみると，LITとPLBが交差する数字から，再燃のリスク比は0.62（95％信頼区間0.53〜0.72，リチウムが有意によい），有害事象による中止のリスク比は2.58（95％信頼区間1.33〜5.39，リチウムが有意に悪い）と読めます．

 ここまでで質問はありますか？

 つまり，図1は，17の実薬とプラセボについて有効性と忍容性を比べた結果で，リスク比が1より小さいということは，左上にある薬剤で有効性が高

い（再燃リスクが低い）ということですね．

結果の読み方まではわかりましたが，統計手法がまだイマイチです．ここまでのことを一度整理していただけるとありがたいです

抄録に登場する統計用語は，
① Bayes（ベイズ）統計学の枠組みでの変量効果ネットワークメタアナリシス
　（a random-effects network meta-analysis within a Bayesian framework）
② リスク比（risk ratio）
③ 95％信頼区間（95％ credible interval）
の3つです．いずれもこれまでの講義で近い内容が出てきましたので，まずはここを押さえてください．

まず，①については，固定効果モデル（fixed-effects model）と変量効果モデル（random-effects model）を復習しましょう❶．この2つのモデルの違いはなんだったでしょうか？固定効果モデルでは，**推定値のバラツキを，「試験内分散」だけによるもの**だと考えます．一方で変量効果モデルでは，**「試験内分散」と「試験間分散」の2つがある**と考えます．今回のメタアナリシスでは，試験間分散を考慮した（不均一性を仮定した）変量効果モデルを用いています．

②のリスク比は，**相対リスクの一種で，イベント発生割合の比をとったもの**でしたね❷．

最後に，③の"credible interval"は，第3講で解説した"confidence interval"とほぼ同じ意味の指標だと思ってください❸．先ほどは，95％信頼区間が1をまたいでいなかったので，リチウムが有意によい（悪い）ことが読み取れたのですね．

別冊
23ページ，下線
❺❼❽

❶ 第17講に解説しましたね．

❷ リスク比については，第12講で詳しく説明しました．

❸ これはBayes統計学の用語です．簡単のため日本語では用語を「信頼区間」に統一しました．

そうですか．ではメタアナリシスとの違いは，①直接比較と間接比較の結果を統合すること，②リスク比の計算にマルコフ連鎖モンテカルロ法を用いていること，③ Bayes統計学のモデルを用いていること，くらいでしょうか？Bayes統計学なんて初めて聞きました

そうですね．Bayes統計学については後述の「解説」を読んでみてください．でも実用上は，②，③はあまり気にしなくても構いません．

リスク比や95％信頼区間の意味については，前回やった従来型のメタアナリシスと大きく違わないと思っていいってことですね．ふつうのメタアナリシスより，ネットワークメタアナリシスのほうがよい手法なんですか？

表1　メタアナリシスとネットワークメタアナリシスの比較

	メタアナリシス	ネットワークメタアナリシス
統計解析の考え方	・直接比較	・直接比較＋間接比較
統計モデル	・固定効果モデル ・変量効果モデル	・ほとんどの場合，変量効果モデル
特長	・プラセボや無治療と比べた有効性を示しやすい ・バイアスが生じる余地が少ない	・複数の治療を比較可能
エビデンスの質を評価するためのポイント[1]	・公表バイアスは？ ・個々の試験にバイアスはないか？ ・不均一性はないか？ ・信頼区間は十分に狭いか？	・公表バイアスは？ ・個々の試験にバイアスはないか？ ・不均一性はないか？ ・信頼区間は十分に狭いか？ ・**間接比較への依存度は？** ・**一貫性は成立しているか？**

そうでもありません．従来型のメタアナリシスは，基本的にランダム化臨床試験で得られた推定値を平均したものですから，バイアスが生じる余地が少ない点がメリットです．

　ところが，ネットワークメタアナリシスのように，間接比較の考え方を用いるには，「直接比較と間接比較の結果が一貫している」という仮定をおく必要があるのです❹．表1に，両者の違いをまとめておきました．従来型のメタアナリシスのほうが偏りが小さいのか，それともネットワークメタアナリシスのほうが優れているのかについては，まだ議論が分かれています．言い換えると，ネットワークメタアナリシスにも落とし穴があります．

　これまで，メタアナリシスで必ず検討すべき問題には以下の2つがあるといいました❺．

● 公表バイアス（publication bias）
● 不均一性（heterogeneity）

ネットワークメタアナリシスではこの2つに加えて，次の3つのポイントがあります❻．

● 間接比較への依存度
● 直接比較と間接比較の一貫性（consistency）
● ランキングの解釈

❹第23講で解説します．

❺第15～19講を参照ください．

❻これらについては第22～24講で解説します．

解説　公表バイアスとネットワークメタアナリシス

　公表バイアスとは，特定の治療の効果が大きかった試験ばかりを集めれば，その治療に有利な（偏った）メタアナリシスができてしまう，という問題のことで

す．ネットワークメタアナリシスでは，**直接比較だけではなくて間接比較も考慮されているため，公表バイアスが入りにくいのではないか**，という意見もあります．

いずれにしても，ネットワークメタアナリシスが行われる前に試験選択ルールを事前に宣言して，PubMedなどの文献データベースを検索し，該当するすべての臨床試験を解析に含める，という手続きが重要なことに変わりはありません．

解説 統計的推測 その5：Bayes統計学と主観確率

第3講では95％信頼区間について，第8講ではp値について，「仮想的反復」という考え方を用いて説明しました．いずれも，**確率とは同じ研究を仮想的に反復したときの相対頻度**である，という解釈です．

一方でBayes統計学では，95％は**主観的な確信の度合い**（主観確率）を表しています．例えば，図1のリチウム（LIT）対プラセボ（PLB）の再燃リスク比（0.62, 95％信頼区間 0.53〜0.72）だと，再燃リスク比は95％の確率で0.53〜0.72の範囲にあると確信しているという意味になります．信頼区間に相当する用語として，英語ではconfidence intervalとcredible intervalを使い分けるのは，そのためです．

ただし実用上は，Bayes統計学でも，95％といった信頼区間の係数を仮説検定の有意水準に対応させて，結果を読み取ることがあります．Bayes統計学の信頼区間（credible interval）でも，信頼区間の係数が95％だと有意水準5％（p＜0.05）に対応し，90％だと有意水準10％（p＜0.1）に対応します．

統計学の流派間の違いについて，統計学者の竹内 啓先生が講義でおもしろいことをおっしゃっていましたので紹介します．

「具体的データをどう扱うかというときには，BayesianとNon-Bayesian，Fisher流とNeyman-Pearson流というのは，そう差は出てこないものです．あるいは差がやたら出てくるような手段で解析をする人のほうがトンチンカンなのでして，そういう人は"基礎"ばかりに凝っていて現実の統計はできないのです」

本講のエッセンス

☐ 公表バイアスと不均一性が，メタアナリシスで必ず検討されるべき問題でした．

☐ ネットワークメタアナリシスではこの2つに加えて，間接比較への依存度，直接比較と間接比較の一貫性，ランキングの解釈の3つがポイントです．

文献

1) Salanti G, et al：Evaluating the quality of evidence from a network meta-analysis. PLoS One, 9：e99682, 2014

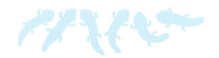

第22講 間接比較への依存度

本講のテーマ

第20講では間接比較の例として，カルバマゼピン対リチウムのリスク比1.10（CBZ群/LIT群）と，リチウム対プラセボのリスク比が0.62（LIT群/PLB群）から，カルバマゼピン対プラセボのリスク比を1.10×0.62＝0.68（CBZ群/PLB群）と計算しました．しかし，間接比較によるリスク比の推定では，全く異なる試験の結果を組み合わせています．そんなことをして本当によいのでしょうか？

keyword

ネットワークメタアナリシス，治療ネットワーク，直接比較と間接比較の一貫性

間接比較することは適切か？

別冊 27ページ，Figure 2

「本講のテーマ」であげた疑問はもっともです．第20講 図1の，プラセボ（PLB），ラモトリギン（LTG），リチウム（LIT）の三角形に注目してください．ラモトリギン対プラセボのリスク比が知りたいとしましょう．ネットワークがつながっていることから，ラモトリギン対プラセボを直接比較した試験結果が得られていることがわかります．

そうすると，一貫性の検定（test for consistency）を用いて直接比較と間接比較の結果が食い違っているかどうかを調べることによって，間接比較することは適切かどうかを確認することができそうです．

確認が可能な場合，不十分な場合

このような確認が可能なのは，**ネットワークが，ループ（例えば三角形）の形をしているときだけ（ネットワークがループ状に閉じているときだけ）**です（第20講 図1の青色の部分）．ループになっていない治療に関するリスク比は，直接比較による検証がなされていません．さらに，直接比較した試験がきわめて少ないときも，似たようなことがいえます．

❶第20講 図1の灰色で示されたARP＋LTG，VPA＋LTG，ARP，PAL，VPA＋ARP，LIT＋OXC，CBZ．

＊　　＊　　＊

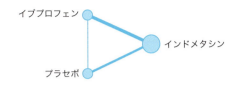
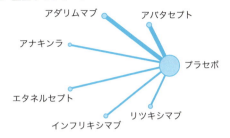
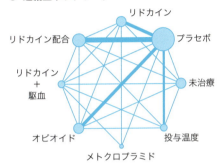
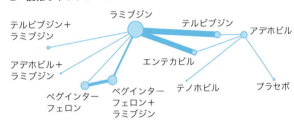

図1　さまざまな治療ネットワークの例
A) 1つの閉じたループで構成され，直接比較と間接比較ができるもの
B) プラセボを中心とする「星型」で，実薬間は間接比較しかできないもの
C) 相互によく連結したもの
D) 1つのループからなる複雑でまばらなもの
（文献1より引用）

図1に，典型的な治療ネットワークを4つ示します[1]．図1A, Cでは直接比較と間接比較の両方ができるので，相互に検証が可能です．

ところが，図1Bでは，実薬同士を比較しようとしても，プラセボを介した間接比較しかできないので，それが妥当かどうかデータから判断ができません．**治療ネットワークが偏っているときには，間接比較に過度に依存してしまう**ことがあり，確認が不十分になるので注意が必要です．

ここまでで質問はありますか？

確認が不十分だったらどうすればいいんですか？

例えばこの論文のDiscussion（考察）では，第2段落でループの閉じているメインのネットワーク（the main network consisting of closed loops）に

29ページ

含まれる薬剤を議論していて，それ以外の独立した薬剤（the single-standing nodes）は第3段落で分けて扱っています．

 どの薬剤のことです？

 第20講 図1でいうと，ループの外にある薬剤はARP + LTG，VPA + LTG，ARP，PAL，VPA + ARP，LIT + OXC，CBZですよね．

 ループってどんな形でもいいんですか？

どんな形でもよいです．試験の数が増えてくると，三角形だけでなくてさまざまな形が出てきますよね．ただし，ループの形が複雑になると，直接比較と間接比較の一貫性を調べるときはややこしくなります．

本講のエッセンス

- ☐ 治療ネットワークがループになっていなかったり，直接比較した試験がきわめて少なかったりすると，間接比較に過度に依存してしまうことがあります．
- ☐ ネットワークメタアナリシスでは，治療ネットワークの偏りを見抜くことが重要です．

文献

1) Cipriani A, et al：Conceptual and technical challenges in network meta-analysis. Ann Intern Med, 159：130-137, 2013

| Ⅵ ネットワークメタアナリシス | 課題論文3　Miura T, et al：Lancet Psychiatry, 2014 ［精神疾患］|

第23講　直接比較と間接比較の一貫性

本講のテーマ

　第22講に引き続いて，直接比較と間接比較を統合解析してよいかどうかがテーマです．今回は，直接比較と間接比較の一貫性とはどのような概念なのかを学びます．

keyword

ネットワークメタアナリシス，治療ネットワーク，直接比較と間接比較の一貫性

直接比較と間接比較の結果は一致するのか

　プラセボ（PLB），オランザピン（OLZ），リスペリドン特効性注射剤（RisLAI；以下，リスペリドン）の三角形に注目して，直接比較と間接比較の結果（オランザピン対リスペリドンのリスク比）が食い違っているかどうか調べてみましょう（図1）．

　オランザピン対リスペリドンを比較した試験は1件しかなく，そのリスク比は0.61でした．これが直接比較です．

　オランザピン対プラセボ，リスペリドン対プラセボの組み合わせは複数試験がありますから，従来型のメタアナリシスを用いてリスク比を推定してみると，おのおの0.52と0.61です．間接比較によるリスク比は，この比をとれば計算でき，

　　0.52/0.61 = 0.85

となります．

　直接比較の0.61と間接比較の0.85では，オランザピンのほうがリスクが低いという方向性は同じであるものの，全く同じ結果ではありません．これが，一貫性がないといわれる状況です．

一貫性についての記載は？

　論文のResults（結果）では，どのように直接比較と間接比較の一貫性について述べられているのでしょうか？　具体的な記載を抜き出すと，

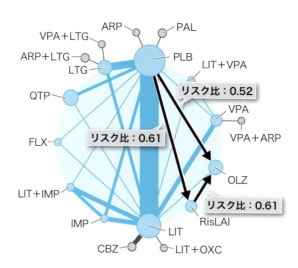

図1 プラセボ，オランザピン，リスペリドンを直接比較した試験から得られたリスク比

「局所的に一貫性の仮定が満たされているかどうかについて検定したところ，（中略）有効性の主要アウトカムについては10のループのうち一貫性が成り立っていないものは1つだけであり，忍容性については7のループで一貫性が成り立っていないものはみられなかった」

28ページ左段，4〜8行目

と書かれています．したがって，一貫していない結果が一部でみられたものの，全体としては，直接比較と間接比較の結果は一貫していたと考えられます．このあたりが，（目立たないですが）ネットワークメタアナリシス特有の論点です．

ここまでで質問はありますか？

どういうときに，一貫性が成り立たないんですか？

例えば，重症な患者には治療がよく効いて，軽症な患者にはあまり効かないとしましょう．試験ごとに，対象患者の重症度が大きく異なっていると，一貫しないことがありえますよね．例えば，直接比較の試験には重症患者が多くて，間接比較の試験には軽症患者ばかりだと，おのおののリスク比が異なるかもしれません．

　対象患者以外にも，さまざまな試験デザインの違いが一貫性を妨げる要因になります．

では，ネットワークがループになっていて，直接比較と間接比較の結果が一貫していることが確認できたとき，ネットワークメタアナリシスの結果が信頼できるってことですか？

平たく言うとそのとおりです．ループになっていないと，一貫性の確認すらできませんよね．

本講のエッセンス

☐ 直接比較によるメタアナリシスは，ランダム化臨床試験で得られた推定値を平均したものなので，バイアスが生じる余地が少ない点がメリットです．

☐ 一方，ネットワークメタアナリシスでは，「直接比較と間接比較の結果が一貫している」という仮定が必要です．

第24講 ランキングの解釈

本講のテーマ

別冊 28ページ, Figure 3

第21講 図1 は，左上から有効性が高い順に並んでいますから，一種のランキングと考えることもできます．ランキング第1位は，アリピプラゾールとバルプロ酸の併用（ARP＋VPA）です．しかし，ランキングの解釈には注意が必要といわれています．

keyword

ネットワークメタアナリシス，ランキングの解釈

ランキング第1位の落とし穴

ランキング第1位はARP＋VPAですが，ARP＋VPAが有意に優っているかどうか，についてはどうでしょうか？

第21講 図1のARP＋VPAの再燃のリスク比と95％信頼区間をもう一度みてみると，有意に優っている（95％信頼区間が0をまたがない）比較対照は，パリペリドン（PAL），イミプラミン（IMP），プラセボ（PLB）だけです．つまり，ARP＋VPAは試験の数が少ないので，リスク比の数字は一見よくても，エビデンスは十分ではないのです．実際，Summary（抄録）でもARP＋VPAのことを強調していませんよね．

別冊 23ページ

もう1つ注意しなければならないのは，ARP＋VPAは閉じたループの外にあるため，間接比較に依存していることです（第20講 図1）．

＊　＊　＊

このように，ランキングに惑わされず，リスク比の95％信頼区間の幅が十分に狭いか，プラセボに有意に優っているか，全体ではなく特定の薬剤について試験数・対象者数は十分か，一貫性の仮定は成り立っているか，といったことを踏まえ，総合的に判断することが重要です．

ここまでで質問はありますか？

やっぱりよくわかりません．ランキング第1位がベストなんじゃないですか？

やっぱりそうなっちゃいますよね．臨床試験では，最初に仮説を立てて「試験治療群はコントロール群に比べて差がある」と「差がない」の二者択一の判断を行います．抗凝固薬メタアナリシスでも，考え方は同じです．

　ところが，一度に多くの治療を比較するネットワークメタアナリシスでは，よくも悪くも仮説があいまいなのです．ランキングだけではなく，双極性障害メタアナリシスのFigure 4もきちんと確認してください．これは，一貫性が確認された薬剤について，プラセボとの比較を示したものです．個々の薬剤がどれくらい優れていたのか，ランダム誤差はどの程度なのか，有効性・忍容性・治療継続のバランスが一目瞭然です．

別冊 29ページ

本講のエッセンス

- ☐ ネットワークメタアナリシスではランキングが強調されがちですが，よくみるとプラセボと比べて有意差がついていないことがあります．
- ☐ ランキングに惑わされず，総合的に判断することが重要です．

次は演習問題です

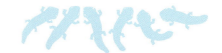

VI ネットワークメタアナリシス

演習問題

問題1 以下の問いに答えなさい．

1 ネットワークメタアナリシスは，従来型のメタアナリシスに比べてどのような利点があるでしょうか？ 正しいものを選びなさい．

ⓐ 公表バイアスが生じない
ⓑ サブグループ解析が可能になる
ⓒ 直接比較だけでなく間接比較の結果を利用するため，信頼区間が狭くなる
ⓓ 直接比較した臨床試験がない薬剤同士でも，リスク比を推定できる

2 不均一性の原因として，最も適切なものは，次のうちどれでしょうか？

ⓐ 海外の試験に比べ日本の試験では，全体として高齢者が多かった
ⓑ 海外の試験に比べ日本の試験では，重篤な副作用が多かった
ⓒ 試験薬の投与量が欧米人の体格に合わせて設定されており，海外に比べ日本の試験では試験薬群の成績が悪かった
ⓓ 固定効果モデルを用いて解析を行った

3 第22講 図1の4つの治療ネットワークのうち，直接比較と間接比較の一貫性を確認できないものは，次のうちどれでしょうか？

ⓐ 1つの閉じたループで構成されたもの（図1A）
ⓑ プラセボを中心とする「星型」のもの（図1B）
ⓒ 相互によく連結したもの（図1C）
ⓓ 1つのループからなる複雑でまばらなもの（図1D）

解答▼ 別冊 52ページ

コホート研究と
ケース・コントロール研究

放射線被曝問題でみる疫学研究の実際

課題論文4　Cardis E, et al：J Natl Cancer Inst, 2005［がん］
▶別冊　32〜41ページ

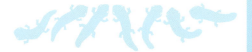

VII コホート研究とケース・コントロール研究

課題論文4 Cardis E, et al：J Natl Cancer Inst, 2005〔がん〕

第25講 長年の議論に決着をつけたケース・コントロール研究

1992年，Nature誌に「チェルノブイリ後の甲状腺がん」という記事が掲載されました（図1）[1]．この記事に示されているのは，1986年4月のチェルノブイリ原発事故から1992年までのベラルーシ共和国における小児甲状腺がん発生数です．1986～1989年には年間数人だったのが，1990年以降は小児甲状腺がん発生数が30人前後まで増えています．これは，放射線被曝が甲状腺がんを生じる可能性を示唆する初めてのまとまった臨床データで，世界中で論争を巻き起こしました．

当時の結論は，「このデータだけでは因果関係を示す証拠と考えてはならない」というものです．その主な理由は，以下のとおりです．

- 発生数は人口規模に依存するので，甲状腺がん発生数が多いのか少ないのかわからない
- 1990年にがん検診が導入されたため，見過ごされてきた甲状腺がんが見つかっただけかもしれない
- 被曝線量が不明で，線量が低い集団と高い集団を比較したものではない

今回は，この議論に一定の決着をつけた論文 を取り上げます．

32～41ページ：
課題論文4

図1　1992年にNature誌に載った記事
（文献1より引用）

keyword

コホート研究，ケース・コントロール研究，スクリーニング効果，交絡

コホート研究，ケース・コントロール研究というアプローチ

　これまでの講義は，臨床試験とメタアナリシスについてのものでした．臨床医学にはもう1つ別のアプローチがあります．それは**コホート研究（cohort study）**や**ケース・コントロール研究（case-control study）**です．

　コホート研究やケース・コントロール研究などのランダム化や介入を伴わない研究は，観察研究とよばれ，**環境因子，生活習慣，遺伝子**などの介入が難しい要因と疾患との関連を調べるときに威力を発揮します．

ケース・コントロール研究の抄録

　いつものようにAbstract（抄録）を読むところから始めましょう．介入がないので代わりに曝露（Exposure）という言葉を用いて，PICOではなくPopulation, Exposure, Comparison, Outcomes（PECO）で整理します．この論文では，

- Population：ベラルーシ共和国・ロシア連邦の一般住民
- Exposure・Comparison：甲状腺被曝線量と安定ヨウ素摂取状況
- Outcomes：甲状腺がん発生

です．PECOをよく読むと，Nature誌の記事との違いがわかります．前者は「チェルノブイリ原発事故後に甲状腺がん発生数が増えた」ことを報じたものですが，この論文は「甲状腺被曝線量と甲状腺がん発生リスクに関連はあるか」を調べたものです．

別冊 33ページ

ここまでで質問はありますか？

「本講のテーマ」で出てきた因果関係ですが，難しい言葉ですよね

　因果（causality）とは，原因と結果の関係のことで，さまざまな学問分野で用いられる言葉ですが，その正確な意味や考え方はさまざまです（表1）．
　同じ医学でも，基礎医学の例〔Koch（コッホ）の原則〕では，
①ある一定の病気には一定の微生物が見出されること

表1 さまざまな因果論

	仏教	Descartesの機械論	Humeの因果論	法律	基礎医学	臨床医学（有害事象）	臨床医学（疫学）
分野	宗教	自然科学	哲学	実学	自然科学	実学	実学
対象	宇宙	宇宙	科学的方法論	訴訟	人体	個人	人間集団
因果の表現	因果律	物理法則や解剖学	原因と結果の認識	特定の原因と結果	生命システムとしての理解	診断	特定の原因と結果
証明	非経験的	経験的	経験的	経験的	経験的	経験的	経験的

②その微生物を分離できること
③分離した微生物を感受性のある動物に感染させて同じ病気を起こせること
④その病巣部から同じ微生物が分離されること
が病原体と感染症の因果関係を判断する基準として提唱されました．

また，有害事象を分類するときには，医薬品と事象の発生との因果関係があるかどうかが重要ですが❶，その判断は主に診断によるものです．

人間集団を対象とする疫学ではどうでしょうか？ その場合，統計学的な意味での相関から，因果関係を推測することになりますよね．しかしながら，チェルノブイリの事例は，**相関関係（correlation）は必ずしも因果関係（causal relationship）ではない**ということを示しています．疫学研究では，スクリーニング効果や交絡などのバイアス❷の影響がないかどうかについて，因果関係を述べる前に慎重な議論が必要です．

❶第1講を参照ください．

❷スクリーニング効果については後述，交絡については第27講で解説します．

がん検診が導入されたため，見過ごされてきた甲状腺がんが見つかっただけだっていうのはどういうことですか？

それまで検査をしていなかった健常者に一斉にスクリーニング検査を行ったり，検査機器の検出精度が向上したりすると，無症状で今までは見つからなかった疾患が高い頻度で見つかることが知られています．これを疫学では，**スクリーニング効果（screening effect）**とよんでいます．

図2は，1973～2002年にかけて，米国のコネチカット州，ハワイ州，アイオワ州，ニューメキシコ州，ユタ州，アトランタ市，デトロイト市，サンフランシスコ市，シアトル市における甲状腺がん発生率と甲状腺がん死亡率の年次推移を，米国がん登録により調べた結果です[2]．発生率が1970年前半から目立った増加傾向を示していますが，死亡率はほぼ一定ですよね．ちなみに超音波を用いたがん検診は，1980年代に普及しました．

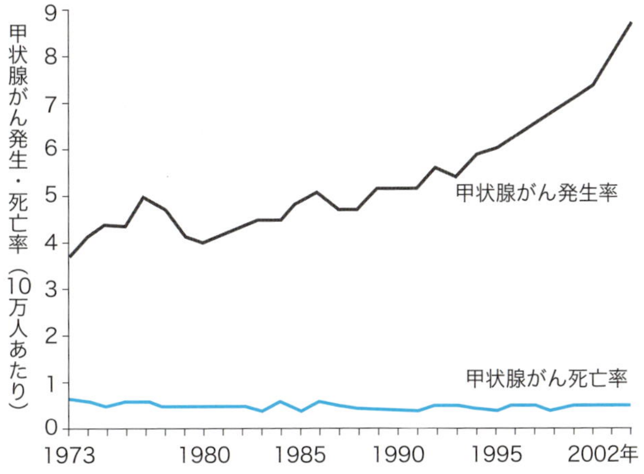

図2　米国における甲状腺がん発生率・死亡率
（文献2より引用）

　つまり，このような現象が知られていたため，チェルノブイリでもスクリーニング効果により，見かけ上，甲状腺がん発生数が増加したにすぎないのではないか，という批判があったのです．

本講のエッセンス

- □ コホート研究とケース・コントロール研究で代表される観察研究は，環境因子，生活習慣，遺伝子などの介入が難しい要因と疾患との関連を調べるときに威力を発揮します．
- □ ただし，相関関係（correlation）は必ずしも因果関係（causal relationship）ではありません．
- □ 疫学研究では，スクリーニング効果や交絡などのバイアスの影響がないかどうかについて，因果関係を述べる前に慎重な議論が必要です．

文献

1) Baverstock K, et al：Thyroid cancer after Chernobyl. Nature, 359：21-22, 1992
2) Davies L & Welch HG：Increasing incidence of thyroid cancer in the United States, 1973-2002. JAMA, 295：2164-2167, 2006

VII コホート研究とケース・コントロール研究　　課題論文4　Cardis E, et al：J Natl Cancer Inst, 2005［がん］

第26講　ケースとコントロールの選択と調査

本講のテーマ

　第25講に引き続いて，放射線被曝・甲状腺がんケース・コントロール研究をみていきます．コホート研究は，特定の集団（コホート：cohort）を追跡して，疾患の発生を調べる研究です（図1A）．ケース・コントロール研究は，潜在的なコホートのなかから疾患を発生したケースを特定し，疾患を発生しなかったもののなかからコントロールを選択し，ケースとコントロールの曝露状況を比較する研究です（図1B）．

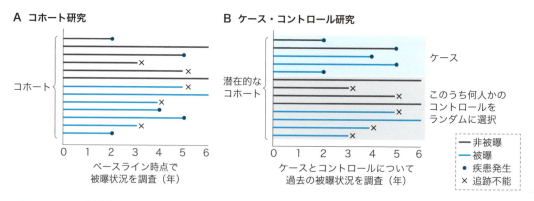

図1　コホート研究とケース・コントロール研究のイメージ

keyword

コホート研究，ケース・コントロール研究，マッチング，条件付きロジスティック回帰，思い出しバイアス，リスク比，オッズ比，ハザード比，発生率比，誤分類

ケース・コントロール研究の方法

ケースとコントロールの選択

　このケース・コントロール研究は，276人の甲状腺がん（ケース）と1,300人のコントロールを対象としたものです．

　まず，ベラルーシ共和国とロシア連邦の住民のうち事故当時15歳未満の人について，1992年1月1日〜1998年12月31日までの間に，276人の甲状腺がんが特定されました．甲状腺がんの診断は，病理組織スライドを用いて病理学者により行われており，11人を除いて甲状腺乳頭がんでした．その後，276人の患者と年齢，性，居住地がマッチした1,300人の健常者（コントロール）がランダムに選択されました．

調査方法

　甲状腺への被曝線量は，アンケートを用いた面接を通じて，食事とヨウ素剤服用情報および居住地を調べ，そのデータを数式に代入することにより計算されました．線量推定のための数式は，事故直後一部の対象者でのどに放射線測定器を当てる直接測定を行うことで構築されました．

結果：被曝線量とがん発生の関係

　Figure 2（図2）は，甲状腺被曝線量（横軸）と甲状腺がん発生〔縦軸，正確にはケースかコントロールかに関するオッズ比（odds ratio）〕との関連を調べたものです．曲線は，全データに二次関数を当てはめた結果です．2本の直線は，2Gy未満までのデータに一次関数を当てはめたものと，1Gy未満までのデータに一次関数を当てはめたものです❶．

　いずれも強い量・反応関係がみられています．線量1Gyにおけるオッズ比は，順に4.9（95％信頼区間2.2〜7.5），5.5（95％信頼区間2.2〜8.8），6.6（95％信頼区間2.0〜11.4）です．すなわち，さまざまなモデルを仮定しても，一貫して放射線により甲状腺がんリスクが増えるという結果です．図2の曲線を推定したモデル（excess relative risk model）は，**条件付きロジスティック回帰（conditional logistic regression）**とよばれる回帰モデルの一種です❷．

ここまでで質問はありますか？

線量1Gyにおけるオッズ比が4.9ということは，被曝するとリスクが4.9倍になるってことですか？

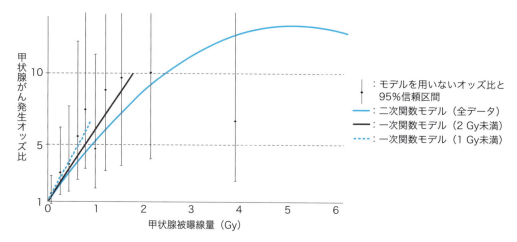

図2　放射線被曝・甲状腺がんケース・コントロール研究で3種類の回帰モデルから推定された甲状腺がんオッズ比と甲状腺被曝線量の関連
〔課題論文4より転載．Figure 2のうち excess relative risk（ERR）model の結果のみを抜粋〕

　オッズ比を読み取るときには，**グループ間の比較なのか（非被曝群対被曝群），量・反応関係を調べているのか（被曝線量が増えるとリスクが上昇するのか）**に気をつけましょう．前者では，どちらのグループを基準に比較しているのかが，後者では，回帰係数やオッズ比の「単位」が重要です．

　この研究の「線量1Gyにおけるオッズ比が4.9」とは，0Gyと1Gyという2つのグループ間を比較すると，リスクが4.9倍になる，という意味です

　相対リスクには，リスク比，オッズ比，ハザード比，発生率比があるんでしたっけ？

　それは第12講で解説しましたね．そもそもリスク（risk）とは，集団全体の人数に対する疾患発生人数の割合を意味します．オッズは，「リスク／（1－リスク）」のことです．つまり，あるイベントが起こる確率の，起こらない確率に対する比です．オッズ比が小さいほど，イベントが起こる確率は小さくなります．

　リスクはケース・コントロール研究からは計算できません[❸]．ただしケース・コントロール研究は，ケースとコントロールしかデータが得られない状況でも，コホート研究と同じように「疾患リスクが何倍になるか（相対リスク）」が推定できるように設計されています．

❸ ケースもコントロールもコホートから選ばれた一部の集団なので，全体の人数はわからないですよね．

> どういうことですか？

それでは図1に戻って確認してみましょう．典型的なコホート研究の手順は以下のとおりです．
① コホートを設定し，時間原点（ベースライン時点）を決める
② ベースライン時点の曝露情報（例えば被曝線量）などを調査する
③ 対象者を追跡し，疾患発生状況を調査する
④ 曝露群と非曝露群を比較する
復習のため，図1Aのようなデータからリスク比を計算してみてください．●は疾患発生を表しています[4]．

一方でケース・コントロール研究は，先ほど述べたように一部の集団のみ（ケースとコントロール）について過去の曝露状況を調査します（図1B）．そうすると，曝露群・非曝露群のリスクの分母がわかりませんよね．そこで代わりにオッズ比を求めます．図1Bで，仮に疾患を発生しなかった全員をコントロールとしたとき，ケース内の被曝オッズ，コントロール内の被曝オッズ，オッズの比を計算してみてください．ただし，被曝オッズとは「被曝確率/(1－被曝確率)」のことです[5]．

> つまり，リスク比1.3とオッズ比1.5が近い値だってことですか？

そうです．この計算のポイントは，このように疾患リスクが低いときには**オッズ比がリスク比の近似になる**という点です．

コホート研究とケース・コントロール研究は，「特定の集団における疾患発生」という同じ現象を，別のアプローチにより調べたものです．適切に計画すれば結果はほぼ同じになる（正確には，疾患リスクが低い[6]か，密度サンプリングという方法でコントロールを選んだとき，正確に同じになる）ということが，理論的に知られています．

> ですが，図1Aには途中で追跡不能になった対象者がいるのが気になります

図1Aは，正確には人口の流入のない**閉じたコホート（closed cohort）**です．しかし，現実のコホート研究では，人口が流入したり（**開いたコホート：open cohort**），途中で転出，追跡拒否，死亡などにより追跡が妨げられたりすることがありますよね．このように，**追跡期間の長さが対象者により異なるときは割合ではなく率（発生率）**が用いられます．

発生率とは，追跡期間の合計（人年）を計算し，疾患発生人数をこれで

[4] 答えは，非曝群のリスク：2/6＝0.33，被曝群のリスク：3/7＝0.43，リスク比1.3

[5] 答えは，ケース内の被曝オッズ：0.6/0.4＝1.5，コントロール内の被曝オッズ：0.5/0.5＝1，オッズ比1.5

[6] 「オッズ＝リスク/(1－リスク)」ですから，リスクが低いほどオッズはリスクに近づきますね．

割ったものです．図1Aの非被曝群6人の直線の長さを合計すると，27人年です．したがって，非被曝群の発生率は，2/27 = 0.074，つまり1,000人年あたり74人です．同様に，被曝群の発生率は3/29 = 0.103，つまり1,000人年あたり103人で，発生率比は1.39です．

今回の被曝調査では，食事とヨウ素剤服用情報および居住地を，面接で思い出してもらったんですか？甲状腺がんを発症したケースのほうが，コントロールよりも事故当時のことを思い出しやすいですよね

そのとおりです．被曝線量の根拠になった情報の一部は，事故から数年後の対象者の記憶によるものなので，**思い出しバイアス（recall bias）** が生じている可能性は否定できません．これがケース・コントロール研究の最大の弱点です．論文を読むときには，その研究で用いられた測定方法が適切かどうか（信頼性と妥当性）にも気を配りましょう．

解説 回帰モデルの誤特定

図2では，二次関数（全データ），一次関数（2 Gy未満までのデータに当てはめ），一次関数（1 Gy未満までのデータに当てはめ）という3通りの回帰モデルを当てはめています．ほとんどの疫学研究では，データがどのような関数形に従うのかについて事前の知識は乏しいので，いくつか異なる回帰式を当てはめて，データへの当てはまりを確認するということが行われます．

間違った回帰式を当てはめてしまうことを回帰モデルの誤特定といいます．回帰モデルの誤特定は，推定値にバイアスが生じる原因の1つです．

解説 測定の信頼性と妥当性

放射線疫学研究では，過去にさかのぼって被曝線量を推定せざるをえないことが多いのですが，直接測定したときに比べ誤差が大きい（特に内部被曝）ことが指摘されています．

一般に，測定誤差を評価するときには，**信頼性（reliability）** と **妥当性（validity）** を区別することが必要です．信頼性とは，同じ条件で繰り返し測定したとき，どのくらい近い結果が得られるか，ということです．妥当性とは，測定したいものをどのくらい正しく測れているか，ということです．妥当性は，妥当性が確認されている別の測定方法（ゴールドスタンダード）との相関を調べることで，評価することができます．

理解を深めるための計算7
誤分類によるバイアス

思い出しバイアスは解析結果にどのような影響を与えるのでしょうか？

それは，**誤分類（misclassification）**が生じる確率を用いた数値例で説明できます（表1）．簡単のため，被曝群と非被曝群の2群を比較するとしましょう．そうすると，この場合の誤分類には，

①被曝者が誤って非被曝群として扱われること
②非被曝者が誤って被曝群として扱われること

の2通りがあります．ここでは①が生じない確率（被曝者を正しく被曝群に分類できる確率）を感度，②が生じない確率（非被曝者を正しく非被曝群に分類できる確率）を特異度とよびましょう．

＊　　　＊　　　＊

表1によると，誤分類が生じていない真のデータでは，オッズ比は3です．

仮に，真に被曝した520人のうち20％が誤って非被曝群に誤分類されたとしましょう（感度0.8，特異度1.0）．被曝群のうち，ケース30人，コントロール74人が非曝露群として扱われることになります．そうすると，オッズ比は2.6と真のオッズ比よりも小さくなります．

同様に，真に被曝した520人のうち60％が非被曝群に，真に被曝しなかった1,056人のうち40％が被曝群に誤分類されたとしましょう（感度0.4，特異度0.6）．計算してみると，オッズ比は1です．もちろんこれは，測定が極端にまずいケースです．

表1　ケース・コントロール研究における被曝状況の誤分類によるバイアスの数値例

	被曝群	非被曝群	オッズ比
真のデータ			
ケース（276人）	150人	126人	3倍
コントロール（1,300人）	370人	930人	$(150/126) \div (370 \times 930) = 3$
真に被曝した520人のうち，20%が非被曝群に誤分類されたとき（感度0.8，特異度1.0）			
ケース（276人）	120人	156人	2.6倍
コントロール（1,300人）	296人	1,004人	$(120/156) \div (296/1004) = 2.6$
被曝・非被曝の両方で誤分類が起きたとき（感度0.4，特異度0.6）			
ケース（276人）	110人	166人	1倍
コントロール（1,300人）	520人	780人	$(110/166) \div (520/780) = 1$

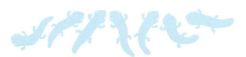

＊　　＊　　＊

このように，**誤分類が生じるとオッズ比の推定値に系統的な偏りを生じます**．数値例のように，ケースとコントロール間で感度・特異度が同じであれば，オッズ比は1に近づく方向にバイアスが生じることが知られています．ただし，ケースとコントロール間で感度・特異度が同じであるかどうかは，多くの場合わかりません．

本講のエッセンス

☐ コホート研究，ケース・コントロール研究，リスク比，オッズ比，ハザード比，発生率比といった疫学用語を整理しましょう．

☐ ケース・コントロール研究は，単にケースとコントロールを比較すればよいというわけではなく，コホート研究と同じように相対リスクが推定できるように設計されています．

☐ 過去にさかのぼって曝露状況を調べるときには，思い出しバイアスが問題になります．

VII コホート研究とケース・コントロール研究

課題論文4　Cardis E, et al：J Natl Cancer Inst, 2005［がん］

第27講　交絡とはリンゴとバナナを比較すること

　第11講で登場した統計学者Fisherは，1950年代に相次いで報告された喫煙と肺がんに関するケース・コントロール研究を，激しく批判したことで知られています．Fisherは，Nature誌に投稿したレターで，「いかなる直接的因果関係がなかったとしても，両方の特徴（注：喫煙と肺がん）は，共通の原因により，大きく影響されることがある」と述べています（図1）[1]．

　共通の原因（**交絡因子：confounder**）としてFisherは遺伝子を指摘していますが，このレターは単に喫煙と肺がんの因果関係を否定することを意図したものではありません．Fisherが提唱するランダム化試験（喫煙の場合は倫理的に不可能ですが）でなければ因果関係は証明できないため，結論を保留すべきである，という統計学的視点からの主張なのです．これが，今回のテーマである**交絡（confounding）** に関する最も有名な論争です．

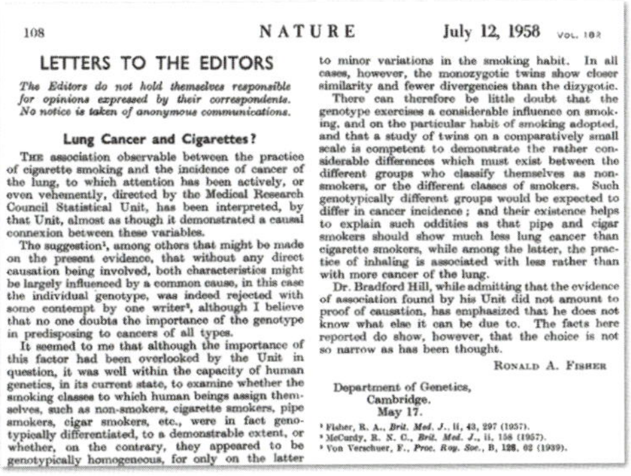

図1　Fisherによる喫煙と肺がんの因果関係に反論するレター
（文献1より引用）

> **keyword**
> 交絡

バイアスとの戦い

　第26講で述べたように，コホート研究やケース・コントロール研究で相対リスクを計算することは，難しいことではありません．しかし，計算された相対リスクは，本当に「疾患リスクが何倍になるか」を表しているのでしょうか？ バイアス❶はないと考えてよいのでしょうか？

　そこがまさにこの論文を読み解くうえでの最重要ポイントです．**コホート研究やケース・コントロール研究はバイアスとの戦い**といわれています．

❶第19講では臨床試験におけるバイアスを解説しました．

関係をゆがめる第3の因子

　図2は，仮想的なコホート研究のデータを示しています．

　下の表は，被曝群と非被曝群の疾患発生数と集団の人数（分母）です．合計の

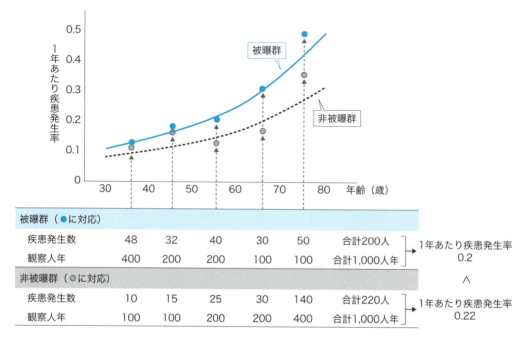

図2　コホート研究における年齢による交絡の数値例

欄によると，1年あたり疾患発生率は，被曝群では200/1,000 ＝ 0.2，非被曝群では220/1,000 ＝ 0.22 と非被曝群のほうが高くなります．

ところが，10歳きざみで年齢をグループ化して発生率を計算し，グラフにすると，疾患発生率を表す点は，被曝群のほうが明らかに上にあります．

この現象が生じた理由は，年齢分布の違いです．被曝群では30歳代が多く，非被曝群では70歳代が多いことに注目してください．非被曝群では高齢者が多く，年齢が高くなるほど疾患発生率が高いため，非被曝群では被曝群より見かけの疾患発生率が高くなったのです．

＊　　　＊　　　＊

このように，**原因（放射線被曝）と結果（疾患発生率）の関係を第3の因子（年齢）がゆがめる現象**を，交絡とよんでいます．そもそも被曝群・非被曝群の間で年齢分布が違う場合には，同じ年齢グループ内で比較するべきですよね．

交絡とリンゴとバナナ

交絡とはあまり耳慣れない言葉ですが，疫学の教科書では**しばしばリンゴとバナナを比べること**と説明されます．

例えば，日本全国の喫煙者と非喫煙者の乳がん発生率を比較しようとしているとしましょう．しかし，よく考えると日本全国を対象にするのは広すぎて比較可能性がありません．というのは，喫煙者には（乳がんリスクがきわめて低い）男性が多く含まれていますよね．したがって，日本全国の喫煙者と非喫煙者は，男女比の違いを考えると「リンゴとバナナ」なわけです．せめて女性に限定して調べないとまずいですよね．

ここまでで質問はありますか？

すみません，よくわかりません．ほかの例はありませんか？

たくさんあります．花粉症の季節にはマスクをする人が増えますよね．マスクによる花粉症予防効果を調べるため，これを集計して，マスク群と非マスク群で，花粉症の有病率❷を比較したらどうでしょう？マスク群のほうが花粉症有病率が高いでしょうが，マスク着用によって花粉症が増えたわけではなく，花粉症だからマスクをしているのです．これも交絡の例で，マスク群と非マスク群で（そもそも花粉症かどうかが偏っているわけだから）比較することが妥当でないのです．

また，昔，コーヒーを飲むと膵がんになる，という論文が出ました．そこ

❷有病率とリスク・発生率は違う指標です．有病率は，ある時点で疾患を有しているものの割合のことで，疾患の発生をみているわけではありません．

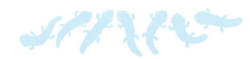

で議論になったのが，コーヒーと一緒にたばこを吸う習慣があるので，コーヒーではなくたばこが膵がんのリスクを上げているのではないか，ということでした．

どちらも，見かけの関連がゆがめられて，解析結果が因果関係を反映していなかったのです．このように交絡は，比較対照群の設定がまずかったり，統計解析で交絡因子を調整し忘れたりするときに生じます．

 どういう現象なのかはわかりましたが，いまいちすっきりしません．定義はあるんですか？

疫学の文脈では，交絡は昔から議論されてきた問題で，定義はいくつかあるのですが，広く受け入れられているのは比較対照の妥当性に基づく定義です．

ある線量の甲状腺被曝を受けたとき，「被曝していないときに比べて甲状腺がんリスクが何倍になるか」を調べるときに，理想的な比較対照は何なのかを想像してみましょう．実際には不可能ですが，ある個人が，被曝したときと被曝しなかったときを比較するのが最も理想的です．これを**事実と反事実の比較**（counter-factual comparison）といいます．

ランダム化臨床試験は，この理想にかなり近い状況です．同一個人の比較ではありませんが，2つのグループに治療をランダムに割り付ければ，おのおののグループには似たような特徴をもつ対象者が含まれているはずです．このような**ランダム化した比較**（randomized comparison）では，交絡によるバイアスは生じません❸．

しかし，放射線被曝の研究では，仮に被曝しなかったときに甲状腺がんが生じたかどうかを知ることや，ランダム化を行うことは不可能です．そのため，コホート研究やケース・コントロール研究が行われているわけです．ところが，ランダム化を伴わない研究では，（図2の年齢のように）グループ間で対象者の特徴が異なることがほとんどで，理想的な比較対照を見つけられないことがほとんどです．言い換えると，**異なる人間集団を観察したときの比較**（observational comparison）では，ランダム化臨床試験のように実験条件がそろっていないので，バイアスが生じてしまうわけです．

次の「理解を深めるための計算」では，オッズ比の値の違いを通じて交絡を説明しています（これをコラプシビリティに基づく交絡の定義といいます）．

❸たまたま特徴が偏る可能性はゼロではありませんが，ある程度人数がいれば無視できます．

理解を深めるための計算8
交絡と層別解析

　表1は，仮想的なケース・コントロール研究の数値例です．ここで示されているのは，男女合計と男女別の集計結果です．男女を合わせて解析するとオッズ比は3で，被曝群のほうが非被曝群に比べて，疾患リスクが高いことがわかります．ところが，男女で層に分けて計算すると，オッズ比は男女ともに1になります．これが正しいとすると，被曝と疾患リスクの間に関係はないことになります．

　なぜこのような計算結果になったのでしょうか？ それは，
① 被曝群には女性が，非被曝群には男性が多いという偏りがあり，
② 女性では男性に比べて疾患リスクが高かった（ケースが多かった）
ためです❹．このように，原因と結果の両方に関係する第3の因子があると，層別する場合としない場合で，オッズ比の計算結果が大きく異なることがあります．

❹計算して確かめてください！

　この仮想例では，被曝群と非被曝群の比較を行っているわけですが，そもそも2群間で性の分布が違うことが問題です．この場合は，性別が交絡因子と考えて，男女で層別した解析結果のほうを信じるべきです．

表1　ケース・コントロール研究における性別による交絡の数値例

	被曝群	非被曝群	オッズ比
男女合計			
ケース（276人）	150人	126人	3倍
コントロール（1,300人）	370人	930人	(150/126)÷(370/930)＝3
女			
ケース（187人）	143人	44人	1倍
コントロール（389人）	296人	93人	(143/44)÷(296/93)＝1
男			
ケース（89人）	7人	82人	1倍
コントロール（911人）	74人	837人	(7/82)÷(74/837)＝1

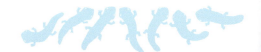

本講のエッセンス

- ☐ コホート研究やケース・コントロール研究では，ランダム化臨床試験のように実験条件がそろえられず，グループ間で対象者の特徴が異なることがほとんどです．
- ☐ このように比較対照が妥当でないため，原因と結果の関係がゆがめられてしまう現象を，疫学では交絡とよんでいます．
- ☐ したがって疫学研究では，年齢や健康状態などの原因と結果以外の第3の因子に注意が必要です．

文献

1) Fisher RA. Lung cancer and cigarettes. Nature, 182：108, 1958

第28講 回帰モデルを用いた交絡の調整

本講のテーマ

回帰モデル（regression model）は，簡単にいうと結果変数（PECOのOutcomeに対応）と説明変数（ExposureとComparisonに対応）の関係に数式を当てはめる統計手法です（図1）．回帰モデルは，交絡を調整するために必須の道具です．

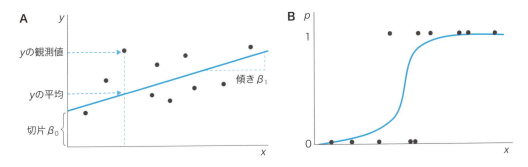

図1　連続データ（A）と2値データ（B）への回帰モデルの当てはめ

keyword

交絡，線型モデル，ロジスティック回帰，Poisson回帰，Cox回帰，変量効果モデル

回帰モデルの例

連続データの場合

図1Aは単回帰〔最近では**線型モデル（linear model）**とよばれます〕の例です．結果変数yと説明変数xの関係に，$y = \beta_0 + \beta_1 x$という一次関数を当てはめています．

両者の関連は傾きが大きいほど強いことになりますから，傾きβ_1を**回帰係数**

❶回帰モデルでは，結果変数を確率変数と考えて，その確率分布をモデル化します．

(regression coefficient) は関連の強さを表しているといえます．この回帰直線は，y を確率変数❶と考えたときの平均を表したものです．

2値データの場合

2値データの場合はどうでしょうか？ y は0または1の値しかとりません．その場合，直線は不自然ですよね．そこで，y が1になる確率 p に，S字型の曲線を当てはめることになります．これが**ロジスティック回帰（logistic regression）**です（図1B）．ここでも回帰係数とは，x が大きくなるにつれ，曲線の変化が急になるかどうかを表す係数のことです．

ここまでで質問はありますか？

ロジスティック回帰はオッズ比を推定するってどこかで聞いたことがあるような気がするんですが…

そのとおりです．ちょっと補足しましょう．よく用いられる回帰モデルを表1にまとめました．

この5つのモデルを押さえておいてください．これらは，オッズ比，発生率比，ハザード比などの指標と結びつけると覚えやすいものです．例えば，ロジスティック回帰からはオッズ比が計算されます．ロジスティック回帰の数式をみてみると，指数変換（exp）が用いられています．指数変換すると足し算が掛け算になるので，「比のモデル」になります．

まとめると，線型モデルは回帰係数がそのまま指標として用いられますが，**ロジスティック回帰，Poisson回帰，Cox回帰は，数式に指数変換があり，回帰係数の指数をとることで，それぞれオッズ比，発生率比，ハザード比が計算されます**．

表1 データの型と回帰モデル

データの型	モデル	数式	指標
連続データ	線型モデル	平均＝$\beta_0+\beta_1 x$	回帰係数＝β_1
2値データ	ロジスティック回帰	オッズ＝$\exp(\beta_0+\beta_1 x)$	オッズ比＝$\exp(\beta_1)$
計数データ	Poisson回帰	発生率＝$\exp(\beta_0+\beta_1 x)$	発生率比＝$\exp(\beta_1)$
生存時間データ	Cox回帰	ハザード＝ベースラインハザード×$\exp(\beta_1 x)$	ハザード比＝$\exp(\beta_1)$
反復測定データ	変量効果モデル	平均＝$\beta_0+\beta_1 x$＋変量効果	回帰係数＝β_1

回帰モデルを用いた交絡の調整

第27講 図2 に戻って，回帰モデルを用いた交絡調整の原理を説明しましょう．

この図の曲線は，点で示されている1つ1つのデータへの距離が最も近くなるように引いたものです．年齢を無視した表の合計の欄とは違い，被曝群の曲線のほうが上にあります．すなわち，回帰モデル（曲線）を当てはめることによって，年齢によるバイアスが調整されたわけです．

これは，実際の統計解析でいうと，疾患発生率を結果変数，被曝の有無と年齢を説明変数とするPoisson回帰を用いて，被曝群と非被曝群の発生率比を推定することに相当します．

被曝群と非被曝群のようなグループの比較だと，図1 みたいに曲線の傾きを調べられませんよね．よい方法はあるんですか？

グループを比較するときには，グループを指定する0または1の説明変数（ダミー変数）を用います．

例えば，非被曝群の対象者だと $x = 0$，被曝群の対象者だと $x = 1$ とコーディングして，$y = \beta_0 + \beta_1 x$ という線型モデルを当てはめることはできますよね．各グループの y の平均を求めるには，回帰式に，ダミー変数の値を代入すればよいのです．例えば，非被曝群だとダミー変数は0ですので，y の平均は β_0 そのものです．被曝群だとダミー変数は1ですので，y の平均は $\beta_0 + \beta_1$ です．

3グループだったらどうしますか？

その場合，まず比較の基準となるグループを決めます．それを仮にグループ1，それ以外をグループ2とグループ3としましょう．次に，ダミー変数を2つ使って，グループ1だと $x_1 = 0$，$x_2 = 0$，グループ2だと $x_1 = 1$，$x_2 = 0$，グループ3だと $x_1 = 0$，$x_2 = 1$ とコーディングして，$y = \beta_0 + \beta_1 x_1 + \beta_2 x_2$ という線型モデルを当てはめます．

ここで重要なのが回帰係数の解釈です．
① β_0 はグループ1の y の平均
② β_1 はグループ2とグループ1の y の平均の差
③ β_2 はグループ3とグループ1の y の平均の差
④ $\beta_0 + \beta_1$ はグループ2の y の平均
⑤ $\beta_0 + \beta_2$ はグループ3の y の平均

回帰モデルが使われているときには，とにかく回帰式と回帰係数の意味を

理解することが第一歩です．

マッチングを考慮した回帰モデル

38ページ，
Figure 2

　第26講 図2の3本の曲線を推定した回帰モデル（excess relative risk model）は，どのような数式だったのでしょうか？ 被曝線量と疾患の定量的な関係を調べるには，どうしても数学的な表現を使わざるを得ませんので，数式アレルギーの方も少しだけ我慢してお付き合いください．
　一次関数モデル（linear model）は，
　　甲状腺がん発生オッズ比＝$\alpha_i(1+\beta x)$
と表されます．二次関数モデル（linear-quadratic model）は，
　　甲状腺がん発生オッズ比＝$\alpha_i(1+\beta x+\gamma x^2)$
です．左辺の甲状腺がん発生オッズは「リスク/(1−リスク)」のことでしたね．右辺のxは甲状腺被曝線量です．α_i，β，γは回帰係数で，特にβとγは，被曝線量と甲状腺がん発生リスクの関係性の強さを表しています．

　α_iは，マッチング因子とよばれる部分です．この研究では，1,300人のコントロールは，甲状腺がんを生じたケースにマッチした住民から選ばれていました．これは，年齢・性別・居住地が一致するように選ばれた，という意味です．数式にα_iがあることで，実は276組のケースとコントロールのマッチングが考慮されているのです．マッチング因子を含む回帰モデルのことを，**条件付きロジスティック回帰（conditional logistic regression）**とよびます．

　交絡の調整という観点では，マッチング因子は重要です．なぜなら，**年齢・性別・居住地による交絡が生じていたとしても，条件付きロジスティック回帰を用いてマッチングを考慮して解析することで，バイアスを排除できているはず**だからです．

33ページ，
Abstract

❷添え字のiは，$i=1, 2, \ldots$ 276という意味です．

　調整する交絡因子は，年齢・性別・居住地だけでいいんですか？

　そこがこの研究の弱点です．このケース・コントロール研究では，年齢・性別・居住地くらいしか対象者の背景情報が得られていません．したがって，それ以外の要因が交絡を生じていたとしても，調整することができないのです．
　一般に，がんのコホート研究では，人種，体重，感染症，既往歴，喫煙歴，食事・運動習慣など，がんの主なリスク因子を調査項目に含めておくことがふつうです．

　ほかに注意すべきところはありませんか？

私たち，生物統計家が実際に解析するときにうっかりしがちなのは，説明変数に1つでも欠測データがあると，その対象者はソフトウェアの仕様で自動的に除外されてしまうということです．

回帰モデルによる解析結果を読むときには，**解析対象となった人数や欠測データの扱いがちゃんと説明されているかどうか**に注意しましょう．論文に書かれていないときには，問題があることが意外と多いです．

解説 ▶ 95％信頼区間は必ず対称か？

回帰係数の95％信頼区間は，

　回帰係数±1.96×標準誤差

で計算することが一般的です．これは，回帰係数が正規分布に近似できることを利用したものです．そうするとしかし，オッズ比，発生率比，ハザード比の95％信頼区間は，

　exp（回帰係数±1.96×標準誤差）

という計算になり，上下対称になりません．論文を読んでいて，これらの指標の95％信頼区間が上下対称だったら，間違いを疑うべきかもしれません．

解説 ▶ 回帰モデルでも95％信頼区間とp値を報告すべき

回帰モデルによるp値として，回帰係数がゼロかどうかの検定（Wald検定）[3]のものを報告することが一般的です．ロジスティック回帰では，このp値はオッズ比が1かどうかの検定結果として用いられることがあります（同じ意味ですよね）．回帰モデルを用いた解析でも，どのくらい誤差があるのかを示すために95％信頼区間とp値を報告することは必須です．

[3] 第8講を参照ください．そこでは回帰係数ではなくて対数ハザード比でした．表1によると，$\beta_1 = \log$（ハザード比）ですよね．

解説 ▶ 交互作用は回帰モデルの用語

抗凝固薬メタアナリシス[4]では，治療とクレアチニンクリアランスの**交互作用（interaction）**の検定について解説しました．一般に，説明変数x_1とx_2の交互作用とは，$y = \beta_0 + \beta_1 x_1 + \beta_2 x_2 + \beta_3 x_1 x_2$のような，掛け算の項（$\beta_3 x_1 x_2$）のことです．**$\beta_3 = 0$の検定が交互作用の検定**です．一方，$\beta_1 x_1$や$\beta_2 x_2$は主効果とよばれます．

[4] 第18講を参照ください．

解説 ▶ 統計的推測 その6：モデルの誤特定と感度解析

統計的推測の基盤として，モデルベースのアプローチ（確率分布を仮定）とランダム化ベースのアプローチ（ランダム化に基づいて確率計算）の2つがあると述べました[5]．前者では，誤った確率分布を仮定してしまう「モデルの誤特定」が問題になります．モデルの誤特定が生じるのは，これまでの講義でいうと以下のような状況があります．

- 正規分布に従わないとき（第3講）

[5] 第11講を参照ください．

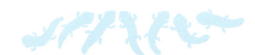

- 増悪や副作用など，疾患の悪化に関係して打ち切り（脱落バイアス）が生じているとき（第4・7講）
- 比例ハザード性が成り立たないとき（第7講）
- 公表バイアスがあり，偏った試験ばかり選ばれているとき（第15講）
- 直接比較と間接比較の一貫性が成り立たないとき（第23講）
- 誤分類が生じているとき（第26講）
- 回帰モデルを誤特定したとき（第26講）
- 未測定の交絡因子があるとき（第27講）

これらは，モデルの誤特定を通じて推定値のバイアスを生じさせます．真のモデルが誰にもわからないため，モデルの誤特定を完全に防ぐことは不可能です．実践的な対処法の1つは，異なるモデルを用いて同じような結果が得られるかを調べることです．これを**感度解析**（sensitivity analysis）とよびます．

本講のエッセンス

☐ よく用いられる回帰モデルは，線型モデル（連続データ），ロジスティック回帰（2値データ），Poisson回帰（計数データ），Cox回帰（生存時間データ），変量効果モデル（反復測定データ）の5つです．

☐ これらの回帰モデルは，データの型と「比のモデルかどうか」が主な違いです．

☐ ロジスティック回帰，Poisson回帰，Cox回帰は比のモデルで，回帰係数の指数をとることで，それぞれオッズ比，発生率比，ハザード比が計算されます．

☐ 解析結果を読むときには，調整された交絡因子は何か，解析対象となった人数や欠測データの扱いがきちんと説明されているかに注意しましょう．

次は演習問題です

VII コホート研究とケース・コントロール研究

演習問題

問題1 課題論文4 (Cardis E, et al：J Natl Cancer Inst, 2005) を読んで，測定されていない交絡因子を3つ指摘しなさい．

別冊 32〜41ページ

問題2 膵がんの画期的な診断が開発され，一般集団を対象としたマススクリーニングが導入されたとします．がん登録のデータによると導入前と導入後で，3年生存率が5％増えました．さて，マススクリーニングに効果はあったといえるでしょうか？

問題3 以下の問いに答えなさい．

1 野球選手の打率は次のうちどれに分類されるでしょうか？

ⓐ 割合
ⓑ 率
ⓒ ⓐとⓑどちらにも分類できる
ⓓ ⓐとⓑどちらにも分類できない

2 1年あたりの自殺件数は次のうちどれに分類されるでしょうか？

ⓐ 割合
ⓑ 率
ⓒ ⓐとⓑどちらにも分類できる
ⓓ ⓐとⓑどちらにも分類できない

3 生存曲線（Kaplan-Meier曲線；第4講 図1，図2参照）の縦軸は次のうちどれに分類されるでしょうか？

　　ⓐ 割合
　　ⓑ 率
　　ⓒ ⓐとⓑどちらにも分類できる
　　ⓓ ⓐとⓑどちらにも分類できない

4 ある疾患について，これまでの検査法よりも1年早く診断可能な検査法が導入されました．ただし，有効な治療はないため，早期発見してもこの疾患の自然経過に変化はありません．今後10年間で，この疾患について起こる可能性が最も高いものは次のうちどれでしょうか？

　　ⓐ 発生率が低下する
　　ⓑ 年齢調整死亡率が低下する
　　ⓒ 有病率が低下する
　　ⓓ 見かけの生存率が上昇する

5 ケース・コントロール研究の特徴として，正しくないものは次のうちどれでしょうか？

　　ⓐ ほかの研究デザインに比べてコストが低い
　　ⓑ 発生率を直接推定できる
　　ⓒ ケースとコントロールの曝露状況を比較する
　　ⓓ ケースより，コントロールの定義が難しい

6 血圧を結果変数，LDL-Cを説明変数として線型モデルを当てはめたとします．LDL-Cの単位を，mg/dLからmmol/Lに変換したとき，回帰係数は何倍になるでしょうか？
ただし，LDL-C(mmol/L) = LDL-C(mg/dL) × 0.02586 です．

7 脳卒中発症を結果変数，LDL-Cを説明変数としてロジスティック回帰を当てはめたとします．LDL-Cの単位を，mg/dLからmmol/Lに変換したとき，オッズ比はどう変化するでしょうか？

プロペンシティスコア
受動喫煙の影響を正しく推定するには

課題論文5　Tanaka S, et al：BMJ, 2015［歯科疾患］
▶別冊　42〜50ページ

| VIII プロペンシティスコア | 課題論文5　Tanaka S, et al：BMJ, 2015［歯科疾患］|

プロペンシティスコアを用いた交絡の調整

本講のテーマ

別冊
42〜50ページ：
課題論文5

❶ 7万人を超えるデータを解析した結果，家庭内の受動喫煙により，子どもが虫歯（う蝕）になる可能性が2倍になったという研究です．

図1は，受動喫煙と乳歯う蝕の関連を報告した研究❶に関するネットの書き込みです．「タバコを吸う親だと低学歴・低所得の割合が多くて，食生活とか生活習慣が乱れてるのが理由なんじゃないか」は，まさに**交絡（confounding）**に関する指摘です．果たしてこの書き込みを論破することができるのでしょうか？

```
1：受動喫煙より，家庭環境の悪影響のほうが大きいのでは？

2：昔に比べたら受動喫煙は減っているのでは？
　以前ならいろいろな場所で受動喫煙のリスクがあったが…
　家庭に限った話ってことでありえるんですかね．

3：直接の因果関係にはならないように思います．
　むしろ，低所得者層は歯みがき粉の使用を控えてしまう，とか，
　そういった話につながっていくのでは？

4：やっぱり，タバコを吸う親だと低学歴・低所得の割合が多くて，
　食生活とか生活習慣が乱れてるのが理由なんじゃないか．
```

図1　受動喫煙・う蝕コホート研究に関する匿名掲示板への書き込み
（匿名掲示板を一部変更して掲載）

 keyword

コホート研究，交絡，プロペンシティスコア，プロペンシティスコアのオーバーラップ，測定されていない交絡因子はないという仮定，VanderWeele-Shpitserの基準，中間因子，合流点因子

受動喫煙・う蝕コホート研究の概要

いよいよ最後の論文です．この受動喫煙・う蝕コホート研究のPECOは

- Population：2004〜2010年の神戸市内出生児
- Exposure：「家庭内喫煙あり・タバコ煙曝露なし群」と「タバコ煙曝露あり群」
- Comparison：家庭内喫煙なし群
- Outcomes：3歳児健診の乳歯う蝕の発生

です．この論文は，神戸市による母子健診を受けた76,920人の出生児を対象にしたコホート研究で，家庭内喫煙なし群と比べて，2つの曝露群におけるう蝕のプロペンシティスコア調整ハザード比（propensity score adjusted hazard ratios）はそれぞれ1.46（95％信頼区間，1.40〜1.52）と2.14（1.99〜2.29）だったということです（表1）．

別冊 47ページ, Table 3

表1　受動喫煙・う蝕コホート研究における4カ月健診時のタバコ煙曝露とう蝕リスクとの関連（プロペンシティスコア解析）

変数	家庭内喫煙なし (n=34,395)	家庭内喫煙のみあり (n=37,257)		タバコ煙曝露あり (n=5,268)	
		ハザード比 (95％信頼区間)	p値	ハザード比 (95％信頼区間)	p値
すべてのう蝕発生（調整なし）(%)	4,453 (14.0*)	6,925 (22.0*)		1,351 (27.6*)	
調整なし	基準	1.54 (1.48〜1.61)	<0.01	2.35 (2.19〜2.52)	<0.01
プロペンシティスコア調整*1	基準	1.46 (1.40〜1.52)	<0.01	2.14 (1.99〜2.29)	<0.01
感度解析*2	基準	1.71 (1.56〜1.87)	<0.01	2.29 (2.48〜3.43)	<0.01
感度解析*3	基準	1.46 (1.40〜1.52)	<0.01	2.13 (1.99〜2.29)	<0.01
感度解析*4	基準	1.32 (1.24〜1.40)	<0.01	1.77 (1.58〜1.98)	<0.01
感度解析*5	基準	1.40 (1.35〜1.46)	<0.01	1.94 (1.83〜2.07)	<0.01

*　Kaplan–Meier法により推定．
*1　児の出生年，母親年齢，妊娠時アルコール摂取，妊娠時喫煙，性別，第一出生児，多胎，妊娠中毒症，貧血，切迫流産，在胎週数，帝王切開，吸引分娩，臍帯纏絡，仮死，黄疸光線輸血，けいれん，保育器，酸素吸入，出生時の体重・身長・頭位・胸囲，4カ月時体重，4カ月時の人工乳，4カ月時の保育者，4カ月時の家族・友人・隣人のサポート，4カ月時の母親の精神状態で調整．
*2　多胎でない第一出生児に限定．
*3　プロペンシティスコアが1％点以下と99％点以上の児を除外．
*4　追加で，9カ月時の歯数，18カ月時と3年時のフッ素塗布，18カ月時と3年時の歯みがき，18カ月時と3年時の仕上げみがき，4カ月時と9カ月時の人工乳，9カ月時の離乳食，離乳食開始年齢，18カ月時と3年時のおやつ頻度，18カ月時と3年時のおやつ摂取時間が決まっているか，18カ月時と3年時のジュース摂取が毎日か，で調整．
*5　生存時間データを区間打ち切りと扱った指数回帰分析．
（課題論文5より転載．Table 3を一部抜粋）

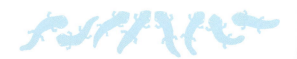

背景因子の比較

交絡があるのかどうか検討するためには，まずは**比較するグループ間の背景因子の違い**を調べることになります．

論文を読むと，受動喫煙に曝露した子どもは，非曝露に比べて母親の平均年齢が2歳ほど若く，歯みがきをしていた割合が低く，人工乳，ジュースをよく飲んでいて，保育所やベビーシッターをよく利用していた（すべて有意）と報告されています．つまり，これらは交絡因子である可能性が高く，その影響を調整していない解析は正しいかどうか疑問が生じます．

別冊
46ページ，
Table 1, 2

 そういえば，リツキシマブ臨床試験も，放射線被曝・甲状腺がんケース・コントロール研究も，Table 1か2は対象者の背景を記述してたように思います

最初に対象者のことをていねいに説明して，グループ間で比較することが妥当かどうかを示すことは，臨床研究の基本ですね．

プロペンシティスコアによる交絡の調整

プロペンシティスコアとは

Abstract（抄録）に書かれているとおり，この研究ではプロペンシティスコアを用いて交絡を調整しています．プロペンシティスコアとは，「個人が治療や曝露を受ける確率」のことです．

ランダム化臨床試験では，治療が50％など決まった確率に従って割り付けられます．そうすると，比較群間で実験条件がそろうため，バイアスは生じないと解説しました．

ところがランダム化していないコホート研究では，プロペンシティスコアは未知です．受動喫煙・う蝕コホート研究では，母親の特性や家庭環境によって曝露するかどうかが変わってくると予想されます．そこで**ロジスティック回帰（logistic regression）**を用いて対象者1人1人のプロペンシティスコアを推定してやり，その数値を用いて交絡を調整します．具体的な解析手順は，以下のとおりです．

ステップ1：変数選択

まず，測定しておいた数ある変数のなかから，どれを交絡因子として調整するのか選択します．

ステップ2：プロペンシティスコアの計算

次に，交絡因子を説明変数，曝露の有無（ここでは受動喫煙）を結果変数とし

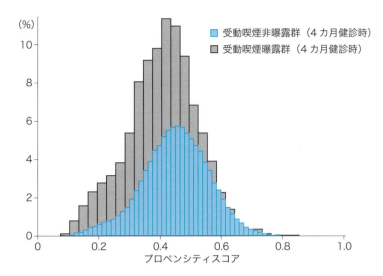

図2 受動喫煙・う蝕コホート研究における曝露群と非曝露群のプロペンシティスコアの分布
(課題論文5よりSupplementary figure 2を引用)

たロジスティック回帰を当てはめ，1人1人のプロペンシティスコアを計算します．

ステップ3：回帰モデル

曝露の有無とプロペンシティスコアを説明変数，関心のあるアウトカム（ここではう蝕）を結果変数とした回帰モデルを用いて，ハザード比などの指標を推定します．

*　　　　*　　　　*

表1の注釈に注目してください．プロペンシティスコア調整ハザード比では，注釈（＊1）に示されている30の因子（出生年，母親年齢，妊娠時の飲酒など）の影響が取り除かれています．

プロペンシティスコアの妥当性

なぜこのような方法で交絡が調整できるのでしょうか？ その理由は，プロペンシティスコアが同じ値の対象者内では，曝露群と非曝露群の間で，交絡因子の分布が等しくなるという性質があるからです．

ただし，プロペンシティスコア解析は必ずしもバイアスを排除できているとは限りません．妥当であるための必要条件が2つあります．

①プロペンシティスコアの分布が曝露群と非曝露群でオーバーラップしていること
②測定されていない交絡因子はないこと

図2は，受動喫煙に曝露していた子どもと非曝露の子どものプロペンシティスコ

アのヒストグラムを描いたものです．2つの分布は重なり合っているので，①の条件を満たしていることがわかります．

重なってなかったらどうなるんですか？

プロペンシティスコアが同じ値の対象者同士を比べる，というのがプロペンシティスコア解析の考え方です．分布が全く重なっていない場合，プロペンシティスコアが近い値をもつ対象者が見つけられないということになり，解析は妥当ではありません．

　分布の一部は重なっていて一部は重なりがないような場合，**重なりがない範囲にプロペンシティスコアの値が含まれる対象者を除外**して，全体がオーバーラップするようにします．もちろん，除外の結果，対象者が少なすぎて困ることもありますが．

プロペンシティスコアが同じ値の対象者同士を比べる，ということは，第26講で学んだ放射線被曝・甲状腺がんケース・コントロール研究（年齢，性，居住地が同じコントロールを選んだ）みたいにマッチングしてもよさそうですが…

それでもいいです．プロペンシティスコア解析にもいろいろあって，以下のようなものが用いられています．
- プロペンシティスコアでマッチング
- プロペンシティスコアで層別解析
- プロペンシティスコアに基づいて重み付け
- 今回のように回帰モデルの説明変数に利用

どれを用いるかは本質ではなくて，とにかく2つの必要条件が満たされているかどうかが，結果を読み取るときのポイントです．

交絡因子の選ばれ方

　2つの必要条件のうち，②の測定されていない交絡因子はない，という条件について考えてみましょう．

　これは結局，ロジスティック回帰を用いてプロペンシティスコアを推定したときの説明変数が適切だったか，ということに帰着します．まず，臨床的に重要な因子（例えば歯みがきの有無）を測定し忘れていた場合には，明らかに必要条件を満たしていません．

また，測定された変数はたくさんあるでしょうから，そのなかでロジスティック回帰の説明変数はどのように選ばれたのでしょうか？ 解析に用いる交絡因子を選ぶ際には，VanderWeele-Shpitser（ヴァンダーウィル・シュピツァー）の基準を用いるのが便利です．それは，①曝露前の因子で，②曝露に影響するか，③**またはアウトカムに影響する因子は，すべて交絡因子として選ぶべき**，というものです．

 臨床的に重要な因子を測定し忘れたらどうなるんですか？

 残念ながら，統計学を駆使したとしても救ってあげることはできません．

 なぜ，曝露後（この場合，4カ月以降）の因子（例えば，1歳6カ月健診時の歯みがきの有無）を交絡因子として調整したらいけないんですか？

 それは，曝露がアウトカムに影響を与える過程の**中間因子（intermeidate variable）**かもしれないからです．例えば，降圧薬による脳卒中予防効果を調べるとき，投与後の血圧の影響を排除してしまうと，降圧薬の効果を純粋に評価できないですよね．

 では，歯みがきの有無，人工乳，ジュース，保育所・ベビーシッターの利用について，4カ月以降のデータは調整できないですね

 そのとおりです．それらを調整していたのは，（メインの解析ではなく）**感度解析（sensitivity analysis）**だったのは，そういう理由からです（表1の下から2行目）．

 逆に，基準を満たすものはすべて交絡因子として選ぶのはなぜですか？ 回帰モデルの説明変数が多すぎだと思います

 理由は2つあります．第1に，交絡因子がもれているとバイアスがあるかもしれないということ．第2に，アウトカムについて解析するときに用いる説明変数は，結局のところ曝露の有無とプロペンシティスコアの2つだけだということです．交絡因子（プロペンシティスコアを求めるためにロジスティック回帰に含める説明変数）の数が多くても，それほど問題にはならないのです．

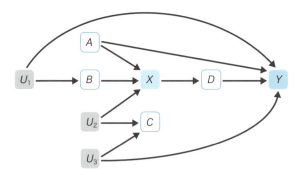

図3 VanderWeele-Shpitserの基準を確認するための因果ダイアグラム

曝露X, アウトカムY, 測定されたそれ以外の変数A, B, C, D, 未測定の変数U_1, U_2, U_3の因果関係を表す.

解説 VanderWeele-Shpitserの基準と因果ダイアグラム

図3は, 曝露XのアウトカムYへの効果を調べる研究において, 変数間の因果関係を表しているとします.「→」は, 矢印の前の変数が後の変数に, 直接影響していることを意味します. 変数A, B, C, Dは測定されており, U_1, U_2, U_3は測定されていません. この因果関係に関係する変数はこれ以外にはないとします. 変数A, B, C, Dのうち, VanderWeele-Shpitserの基準を満たすものはどれでしょうか？

答えはAとBです. なぜなら, 基準②または③を満たすものはA, B, Dですが, Dは曝露後の因子で基準①を満たさないからです. Dのように, 曝露XとアウトカムYの経路の途中にある変数が**中間因子**です. また, Cのように, 矢印が合流している変数を**合流点因子（collider）**とよぶことがあります.

解説 回帰モデルの説明変数の選択

回帰モデルの変数選択にはさまざまな考え方があります.「交絡因子」を選ぶときに私が勧めているのはVanderWeele-Shpitserの基準です. 予後因子研究では, 死亡率などの予後と相関する「予測因子」が選ばれることがありますが, その場合には**p値に基づいた変数選択の方法（p値が小さいものを優先）**が用いられます.

本講のエッセンス

☐ プロペンシティスコア解析は交絡を調整するためによく用いられる手法ですが，それが妥当であるためには，①プロペンシティスコアの分布が曝露群と非曝露群でオーバーラップしており，②測定されていない交絡因子はない，という2つの必要条件を満たす必要があります．

☐ 解析に用いる交絡因子を選ぶときには，①曝露前の因子で，②曝露に影響するか，③またはアウトカムに影響する因子は，すべて交絡因子として選ぶべき，というVanderWeele-Shpitserの基準を用いるのが便利です．

☐ 回帰モデルやプロペンシティスコアによる解析では，中間因子を交絡因子として調整することはできません．

第30講 バイアスと感度解析

本講のテーマ

バイアスとは，統計学では「得られた推定値が真の値から系統的にずれていること」を意味します．バイアスは，対象者の選択から研究結果の報告にいたるまで，研究実施のあらゆるプロセスで生じます（表1）．

表1 研究デザインごと・プロセスごとに注意すべきバイアス

	ランダム化臨床試験	メタアナリシス	ケース・コントロール研究	コホート研究
例	対象者を2群にランダムに分け，異なる介入を行う	ランダム化臨床試験の文献データを集め，研究結果を統合	甲状腺がんの有無に基づきケースとコントロールを特定し，線量を比較	被曝者を登録し，甲状腺がん発生まで追跡
対象の選択	・選択バイアス	・公表バイアス	・選択バイアス	・選択バイアス
比較対照群の設定	―	＊	・思い出しバイアス ・交絡	・交絡
介入	・パフォーマンスバイアス	＊	―	―
アウトカムの評価	・脱落バイアス ・検出バイアス	＊	・脱落バイアス ・検出バイアス	・脱落バイアス ・検出バイアス
統計解析と結果の報告	・報告バイアス	・報告バイアス	・交絡 ・報告バイアス	・交絡 ・報告バイアス

＊ 個々の試験の質による．

keyword

感度解析，選択バイアス，脱落バイアス，検出バイアス，交絡，プロペンシティスコアのオーバーラップ，中間因子，区間打ち切り

コホート研究の典型的なバイアス

第27～29講に解説した交絡（confounding）もバイアスの一種ですが，それ

以外にどのようなバイアスが問題になるのでしょうか？コホート研究の典型的なバイアスについて，受動喫煙・う蝕コホート研究で影響はあったのか，どのような対応がなされたのかみてみましょう．

42〜50ページ：
課題論文5

選択バイアス (selection bias)

選択バイアスは，対象者を選択するプロセスで生じるバイアスのことです．例えば，チェルノブイリのケース・コントロール研究では，ケースはベラルーシ共和国・ロシア連邦住民に発生したすべての甲状腺がん，コントロールは健常人からランダムに選択されたと書かれています．完全にランダムなら選択バイアスは生じませんが，実際には，同意が得られなかったりもしますよね．

選択バイアスについて論文から読み取るときには，

- 解析対象集団に組み入れられたのは母集団の何割か（組み入れ率）
- 選択プロセスで懸念される要因はあるか

が重要です．受動喫煙・う蝕コホート研究では，組み入れ率は93.2％と報告されています．

脱落バイアス (attrition bias)

疾患の悪化に関係して打ち切りが生じた場合，Kaplan–Meier法を用いたとしても正しく生存曲線を推定することはできないといいました❶．これは，ハザード比をCox回帰を用いて推定するときも同じです．脱落バイアスを読み取るときには，

❶第4講で述べましたね．

- 予定追跡期間が完遂されたのは何割か
- 追跡プロセスで懸念される要因はあるか

の2点を押さえておきましょう．

この研究の3年追跡率は91.9％です．ただし，健康状態や生活習慣の悪い子どもが健診未受診になっている可能性はあります．その場合，**見かけ上予後がよくなる方向に**バイアスが入ると考えられます．

同一家族の影響に伴うバイアス

小児を対象としたコホート研究では，遺伝子・環境因子が近い双子や兄弟を特別に扱うことがあります．この研究では，双子・兄弟を特定できるような情報は得られていないのですが，出生順位・多胎かどうかはわかっています．

そこで，同一家族の影響があるかどうかを確認するために，第29講 表1では，双子でない第一子のみに対象を限定して，それ以外の条件は同じCox回帰を用いた解析（感度解析：sensitivity analysis）を行っています．

47ページ，
Table 3

プロペンシティスコアのオーバーラップ

第29講 図2によると，プロペンシティスコアがあまり重なっていない部分がわずかにあります．そこで，2つ目の感度解析として，プロペンシティスコアの

値が1％点より高い対象者と99％点より低い対象者を除外して，主たる解析結果が変わるかどうか確かめています．

中間因子であるため調整しなかった交絡因子によるバイアス

第29講で述べたVanderWeele-Shpitserの基準によると，**曝露後（この場合，4カ月以降）の因子は，中間因子（intermediate variable）かもしれないので，交絡因子として選択しない**，ということでした．さらに，「個人が治療や曝露を受ける確率」というプロペンシティスコアの定義に戻ると，曝露後の因子が曝露確率を決めるとは考えられません．しかし，4カ月以降の生活習慣による交絡があるかどうかは気になるところです．

そこで，3つ目の感度解析では，歯数，フッ化物塗布の有無，歯みがきの有無，仕上げみがきの有無，人工乳の有無，離乳食開始時期，おやつ摂取頻度，おやつ摂取が定期的かどうか，毎日ジュースを飲むかどうかという9個の因子を，**（プロペンシティスコアの推定ではなく）Cox回帰の説明変数に追加した解析**を行っています．

検出バイアス（detection bias）

健康診断に基づくコホート研究では，数カ月の健診間隔が生じるので，疾患発生日が正確に特定できないことがあります〔このようなデータを**区間打ち切りデータ（interval censored data）**とよびます〕．これは診断の遅れの一種ですので，**生存曲線が右方向に（遅れる方向に）シフトするといったバイアス**を生じます．

う蝕発生日の場合も同じ懸念があります．そこで，4つ目の感度解析として，区間打ち切りデータを扱うことができる**回帰モデル〔指数分布（exponential disbribution）を仮定した回帰モデル〕**を用いた結果が報告されています．

これまでの論文のバイアスを確認しよう

さて，これまでの総決算として，双極性障害メタアナリシス，放射線被曝・甲状腺がんケース・コントロール研究の，研究の限界（study limitation）に関する記述を読み，バイアスについてどのような議論がなされたのかを確認してみましょう．

双極性障害メタアナリシス

● Discussion（考察），第5段落，2文目

"First, the evidence network in our network meta-analyses was well connected overall, but had a relatively small number of trials and participants in comparison with the other network meta-analyses previously undertaken in psychiatry."

双極性障害メタアナリシスでは，"This study is not without limitations."か

ら始まる段落全体をみてみてください．研究の限界が3つあげられています．これは，「治療ネットワークは十分な接続があったが，試験数や対象者数が少ない部分があった」という意味なので，**間接比較への依存度**が高いことを述べているようです．

- **Discussion（考察），第5段落，3文目**

"Second, we were unable to do separate analyses for bipolar II disorder or for rapid-cycling bipolar disorder, and different drugs might have different efficacy profiles for different subtypes."

「双極II型障害や急速交代型双極性障害などを区別して解析することができなかった」というコメントで，必ずしもバイアスとはいえないかもしれません．

- **Discussion（考察），第5段落，5文目**

"Third, many of the studies of maintenance treatment for bipolar disorder were funded by pharmaceutical companies and used the enrichment design to select patients who responded to treatment in the acute phase (tables 1, 2), which might give clear advantage to the investigational drug and cause a sponsorship bias."

この問題は医薬品のメタアナリシスではつきものなのですが，**製薬企業が自社製品の試験を行ったものが含まれている**ので，そこから生じるバイアス（スポンサーシップバイアス：sponsorship bias）を指摘しています．エンリッチメントデザイン（enrichment design）とは，治療反応性のよい患者だけを対象に試験を行うことです．バイアスの方向としては，**プラセボに比べて実薬に有利に偏っているかもしれない**と著者は述べています．

先ほどのコホート研究とメタアナリシスでは，全然バイアスに関する視点が違いますよね．

放射線被曝・甲状腺がんケース・コントロール研究

- **Discussion（考察），第7段落，1文目**

"Uncertainties in thyroid dose estimates and possible biases resulting from selection, recall, confounding, or effect modifiers need to be considered carefully when interpreting the results of this study."

この論文では，第7～9段落の冒頭の文章をみてみましょう．これは，甲状腺被曝線量の推定値は不確実なので，**選択バイアス，思い出しバイアス（recall bias），交絡，交互作用（interaction❷）**などが生じている可能性を述べたものです．

- **Discussion（考察），第8段落，1文目**

"The low participation rate among control subjects, particularly in the Russian Federation, is of concern because it may have introduced a selec-

30ページ：
課題論文3

30ページ：
課題論文3

39ページ：
課題論文4

❷原文では effect modifiersですが，同じ意味です．

40ページ：
課題論文4

tion bias."

「特にロシアでは，コントロール群への組み入れ率が低かった」ので，**選択バイアス**があるかもしれないようです．

● Discussion（考察），第9段落，1文目

"Interviews were carried out with case patients and control subjects (or their mothers) years after the Chernobyl accident, and the possibility that recall bias may have played a role in the magnitude of the observed risk estimate cannot be excluded."

これは，「対象者への面接が事故後数年経ってから行われた」ことにより，**思い出しバイアス**の影響は否定できないというコメントですね．甲状腺がんを発症したケースとコントロールで，思い出しの程度に差があるでしょうから，思い出しの差が被曝線量の差を生じさせた可能性は否定できません．

ケース・コントロール研究の著者は，ほかの研究に比べて，かなり深刻にバイアスの影響があるのではないかと気にしているようにみえます．

本講のエッセンス

☐ バイアスとは，統計学では「得られた推定値が真の値から系統的にずれていること」を意味します．

☐ バイアスは，対象者の選択から研究結果の報告に至るまで，研究実施のあらゆるプロセスで生じます．

☐ さらに，ランダム化臨床試験，メタアナリシス，ケース・コントロール研究，コホート研究といった研究デザインごとに注意すべきバイアスが異なります．

次は演習問題です

VIII プロペンシティスコア

演習問題

問題1　以下の問いに答えなさい．

1 プロペンシティスコアのオーバーラップがないときの解釈として正しいものは次のうちどれでしょうか？

　　ⓐ どちらの曝露を受けるのかが，対象者の特徴によってほとんど決まっている
　　ⓑ 測定されていない交絡因子があることを意味する
　　ⓒ マッチングを用いれば対処できる
　　ⓓ ⓐ，ⓑ，ⓒすべて誤り

2 回帰モデルとプロペンシティスコア法の違いについて正しいものは次のうちどれでしょうか？

　　ⓐ サンプルサイズがかなり大きいときは，プロペンシティスコア法のほうがバイアスが小さい
　　ⓑ サンプルサイズがかなり小さいときは，プロペンシティスコア法のほうがバイアスが小さい
　　ⓒ プロペンシティスコア法のほうが，妥当であるための条件が厳しい
　　ⓓ ⓐ，ⓑ，ⓒすべて誤り

3 曝露後に測定された因子（中間因子）を交絡因子として調整しなければならないときの考え方について，正しいものは次のうちどれでしょうか？

　　ⓐ 回帰モデルやプロペンシティスコア法以外の統計手法を用いるべき
　　ⓑ すべての交絡因子を調整すべきなので回帰モデルを用いるのが正しい
　　ⓒ 交絡因子を調整しないことよりも中間因子を調整することのほうが問題であるから，この解析結果は報告すべきではない
　　ⓓ ⓐ，ⓑ，ⓒすべて誤り

解答▶別冊
52ページ

オオサンショウウオ先生からのご挨拶

　30講にわたる長丁場にお付き合いいただき，ありがとうございました．
　この講義では，臨床試験，メタアナリシス，ケース・コントロール研究，コホート研究の基礎になっている方法論とその原理について，解説してきました．臨床研究は，「ランダム誤差」と「バイアス」との戦いです．この2つは，研究実施のあらゆるプロセスで生じうるため，それらに対抗するための手立ては，必然的に多種多様です（第30講 表1を復習すること！）．
　しかし，講義を通じて一貫した原理があったことに気付かれたでしょうか？ それは，ラテン語で"ceteris paribus"といいます．これは英語では"all other things being equal"，日本語では「すべての条件をそろえる」くらいの意味です．これまで取り上げたケーススタディは，いずれも原因（薬物療法，放射線被曝，喫煙）と結果（疾患発生や予後）との因果関係を，人間集団の比較を通じて調べようとしたものです．"ceteris paribus"をめざして工夫することこそが，比較の妥当性を高めるための原理なのです．
　もっと学びたいという方，臨床も研究もできる医師になりたいという方は，ぜひSchool of Public Health（SPH）への入学をご検討ください．SPHは，臨床研究や生物統計学などを学ぶ大学院です．東京大学（公共健康医学専攻），京都大学（社会健康医学系専攻）などいくつかの大学には，仕事を続けながら国内留学ができる制度が設けられています．京都大学SPHでは，臨床統計家育成コースという，臨床試験の統計専門家を育てるコースもあります（2018年4月開講）．SPHに行けば，オオサンショウウオ並みの絶滅危惧種である生物統計家に会えるかも？

+α! 教科書を教えて！

　さらに学びたい人のためには，世界的に定評のある教科書が翻訳されていますので，ぜひそちらにチャレンジしてください．

- この本を読んで，もう少し統計学を理論的に，ていねいに説明してほしいと思った方には，修士レベルの「医学研究における実用統計学」（Altman, DG/著　木船義久，佐久間 昭/訳），サイエンティスト社，1999 をお勧めします．
- 数学が得意で，本書の随所に出てきた回帰モデルを理解したい方は，修士レベルのコンパクトな教科書「一般化線形モデル入門 原著第2版」（Dobson, AJ/著　田中 豊，他/訳），共立出版，2008 がベストです．
- がん臨床試験に関心のある方には，「米国SWOGに学ぶがん臨床試験の実践 第2版（原書第3版）」（Green, S, 他/著　JCOGデータセンター/訳），医学書院，2013 が実践的です．
- もっとたくさんの研究事例を通じて疫学を学びたい方には，「疫学―医学的研究と実践のサイエンス」（Gordis, L/著　木原正博，他/訳），メディカルサイエンスインターナショナル，2010 をあげておきます．

+α! 統計ソフトウェアを教えて！

　定評のある統計ソフトウェアには，SAS, JMP, Stata, SPSS, R があります．この5つは第6講 表1の手法をほぼカバーしていますが，臨床試験，メタアナリシス，コホート研究，ケース・コントロール研究といった研究デザインや，がん，精神疾患，感染症など疾患領域によって統計手法が異なります．例えばSASはどちらかというと臨床試験の手法に強く，Stataはメタアナリシスでよく用いられます．

　あなたの研究領域でよく用いられており，マニュアルや参考書が充実している統計ソフトウェアを選ぶとよいでしょう．

索引

索引のうち，太字もしくは見出し語を下線で示す．

数　字

2値データ ………… <u>45</u>, 46, 47, 49, 84, 165, <u>166</u>, 170

25％点 ………………… 26, 29, 30

75％点 ………………… 26, 29, 30

95％信頼区間 ……………………
26, <u>27</u>, 28, 29, 30, 39, 43, 61, 83, 87, 88, 92, 113, 120, 122, 133, 134, 135, 137, <u>144</u>, 153, <u>169</u>, 175

ギリシャ文字

αエラー ……… 17, <u>55</u>, <u>56</u>, 57, 58, 61, 62, 63, 80

α消費関数 ………………… <u>72</u>

βエラー ……… <u>55</u>, 56, 58, 63, 71

χ^2検定 ……………… 46, 64, 87

Δ ………………………………… 86

欧　文

B・C

Bayes統計学 ………… 135, <u>137</u>

CochranのQ統計量 ………… 117

Cox回帰 …… 46, 49, 52, 60, <u>166</u>, 170, 183, <u>184</u>

Cox回帰モデル ………………… 51

CRC …………………………… 103

CRF (Case Report Form) … <u>103</u>

CTD (Common Technical Document) …………………… 99

D・E

data lock ……………………… 103

EDC (Electric Data Capture)
………………………………… <u>103</u>

EDCシステム ………………… 103

F

FAS (Full Analysis Set)
……………… <u>20</u>, <u>21</u>, 22, 24, <u>90</u>

Fisherの正確検定
……………… 45, 46, 47, 64, 75, 80

G

GCP (Good Clinical Practice)
…… 97, <u>98</u>, 100, 101, 102, 104

GCP実地調査 ………………… 104

I

I^2統計量 ……………… 117, 118

ITT (Intention-To-Treat) … <u>90</u>

ITT解析 ……… 21, <u>22</u>, 24, 60, 90

ITTの原則 ………… <u>20</u>, 21, 23, 24, 77, 80, 90, 93

K

Kaplan–Meier曲線
………………… <u>32</u>, 38, 172

Kaplan–Meier法 ……………………
33, <u>35</u>, 38, 39, 40, <u>43</u>, 49, 52, 183

M・O

McNemar検定 ………………… 46

O'Brien and Fleming型
………………………… <u>72</u>, 73

P

PECO ……………… 39, 149, 174

PICO ………… 14, <u>15</u>, 18, 39, <u>82</u>, <u>114</u>, 134, 149

Pocock型 ………………… <u>72</u>, 73

Poisson回帰
………………… 46, <u>166</u>, 167, 170

Poisson分布 …………………… 47

PPS (Per-protocol Set)
………………… <u>20</u>, <u>21</u>, 23, <u>90</u>

PPS 解析 ……… 20, 21, 22, 23, 60

p 値 … 16, 17, 19, 34, 45, 53, 54,
　　　55, 56, 57, 59, 60, 61, 62,
　　　63, 64, 73, 75, 78, 79, 80,
　　　83, 86, 137, 169, 180

T・V

t 検定 ………………………… 47, 60

VanderWeele-Shpitser ……… 179

VanderWeele-Shpitser の
　基準 ……………… 180, 181, 184

W

Wald 検定 … 30, 60, 61, 80, 169

Wilcoxon 順位和検定
　………………………… 45, 46, 47

Wilcoxon 符号付順位検定 … 46

和　文

あ行

アウトカム …… 15, 17, 45, 46, 84,
　　　115, 117, 125, 126, 127,
　　　177, 179, 180, 181, 182

アットリスク ………………………… 32

アットリスク数
　……………… 32, 33, 36, 37, 38

安全性の中止 ……………………… 73

安全性モニタリング ……………… 35

一貫性 … 136, 141, 142, 143, 145

一貫性の仮定 …………………… 144

一貫性の検定 …………………… 138

逸脱 ……………………………………… 21

イベント数 ……………………… 66

因果関係 …… 15, 148, 149, 150,
　　　　　151, 159, 162, 180

因果関係について合理的な
　可能性があるもの ……………… 15

因果関係を否定できないもの … 15

因果ダイアグラム ……………… 180

インフォームドコンセント 98, 104

打ち切り ……… 22, 23, 33, 36, 37,
　　　　38, 49, 51, 52, 170, 183

エラーバー …… 25, 26, 28, 30, 39

エンドポイント …… 15, 16, 17, 21,
　　　23, 59, 60, 78, 79, 81,
　　　84, 85, 87, 97, 105

エンリッチメントデザイン ……… 185

オーバーラップ
　………… 177, 178, 181, 183, 187

オッズ
　…… 84, 85, 154, 155, 166, 168

オッズ比 …… 84, 85, 110, 113,
　　　153, 154, 155, 157, 158,
　　　162, 163, 166, 168, 169,
　　　170, 172

思い出しバイアス ……… 156, 157,
　　　　　158, 182, 185, 186

重み付き平均 …………… 118, 132

か行

回帰係数 ………… 30, 80, 154, 165,
　　　　　166, 167, 168, 169,
　　　　　170, 172

回帰モデル ……… 30, 46, 48, 51, 60,
　　　80, 153, 154, 156, 165, 166,
　　　167, 168, 169, 170, 177, 178,
　　　179, 180, 181, 184, 187

回帰モデルの誤特定 ………… 156

解析対象集団
　……………… 19, 20, 24, 93, 105

確率分布 …………………………… 116

仮説検定 ……… 16, 45, 53, 54, 55,
　　　56, 60, 62, 66, 83, 87, 137

仮想的反復 ……………… 28, 29, 30,
　　　　　　61, 83, 137

片側 ……………………… 57, 61, 83

片側 (one-sided) 検定
　………………… 56, 57, 62, 63, 64

片側 p 値 ……………………… 53, 61

片側か両側か ……………………… 60

片側有意水準 …… 43, 56, 57, 61, 62, 67, 71, 72, 74, 92

監査 ……………………………… 100, 104

観察打ち切り ……………………… 33

観察研究 ……………………………… 122

観察人年 ……………………… 84, 85, 160

間接比較 …… 131, 132, 134, 135, 136, 137, 138, 139, 140, 141, 142, 143, 144, 146, 185

感度 ……………………………… 157, 158

感度解析 …………… 169, 170, 179, 183, 184

既知／未知 ………………………… 15

帰無仮説 ……… 54, 55, 60, 63, 67

局所管理 …………………………… 75

区間打ち切り ……………………… 184

区間打ち切りデータ ……………… 184

繰り返し …………………………… 75

クロスオーバー ………………… 22, 23

計数データ …… 45, 46, 47, 84, 166, 170

系統的レビュー登録データベース ……………………………… 109

ケース・コントロール研究 ………… 39, 47, 48, 80, 122, 149, 151, 152, 153, 154, 155, 156, 158, 159, 160, 162, 163, 164, 168, 172, 176, 178, 182, 183, 184, 185, 186

欠測データ ………………… 169, 170

研究実施計画書 ………………… 109

検出したい治療効果 …………… 68

検出したい治療効果が小さい …………………………………… 70

検出したい治療効果の大きさ ……………………………… 67, 70, 71

検出バイアス ……… 126, 127, 128, 182, 184

検出力 …… 43, 44, 47, 55, 67, 68, 70, 71, 122

原資料 ……………………… 99, 103, 104

検定 ……………………………… 69

効果安全性評価委員会 ……… 74

効果維持法 …………………… 89

交互作用 (interaction) ……… 120, 121, 122, 169, 185

交互作用p値 ………………… 121

交互作用の検定 ……… 120, 121, 122, 123, 169

公表バイアス …… 108, 109, 110, 111, 128, 136, 137, 146, 170, 182

交絡 …… 75, 150, 151, 159, 160, 161, 162, 163, 164, 165, 168, 174, 176, 177, 181, 182, 184, 185

交絡因子 …… 46, 159, 162, 168, 170, 171, 176, 177, 178, 179, 180, 181, 184, 187

交絡の調整 …… 45, 46, 47, 48, 80, 167, 176

合流点因子 ……………………… 180

国際共同臨床試験 ……………… 122

固定効果 ……………………… 116

固定効果モデル …… 112, 114, 116, 117, 118, 128, 135, 136, 146

誤特定 ……………………… 170

誤分類 …………………… 157, 158, 170

コホート …………………… 175

コホート研究 …… 39, 48, 80, 149, 151, 152, 155, 158, 160, 162, 164, 168, 174, 175, 176, 177, 182, 183, 184, 185

コホート研究やケース・コントロール研究 ……………… 48

コラプシビリティ ……………… 162

さ行

最小化法 ················ <u>76</u>, <u>77</u>, 78

最大の解析対象集団 (FAS)
················ <u>20</u>, 24, 90

最尤推定 ························ <u>30</u>

査察 ···························· 104

サブグループ
················ <u>120</u>, 121, <u>122</u>, 123

サブグループ解析 ········ 108, <u>120</u>,
122, 123, 146

サブグループ間 ·············· 120

サンプルサイズ ······ 27, <u>30</u>, 40, 43,
<u>55</u>, 56, 59, 60, 61, <u>66</u>,
<u>67</u>, 68, 69, <u>70</u>, 71, 83,
92, 93, 187

サンプルサイズの計算
················ 43, 44, 66, 69, 71

試験間分散 ··· <u>116</u>, 117, 118, <u>135</u>

試験実施計画書 ············ 21, 98

試験内分散 ········ <u>116</u>, 118, <u>135</u>

指数分布 ··········· 43, 48, 67, <u>68</u>

指数分布を仮定した回帰モデル
································ <u>184</u>

施設訪問モニタリング ······· 100

実験計画法 ····················· 75

質的交互作用 ················ <u>121</u>

市販後 ·························· 98

四分位範囲 ················ 26, 27

死亡率 ······················· 151

重症 ···························· <u>15</u>

重篤 ···························· <u>15</u>

重篤度 ······················ 15, 17

重篤な副作用 ················ 146

重篤な有害事象 ········ 15, 16,
45, 56, <u>57</u>, 58

主観確率 ···················· <u>137</u>

主効果 (main effect)
················ 121, 122, 169

主効果の検定 ········ <u>121</u>, 122

主要アウトカム ·············· 142

主要エンドポイント ······ <u>16</u>, <u>17</u>, 18,
34, 35, 43, 44, 49, 57,
82, 87, 89, 108

条件付きロジスティック回帰
··················· <u>153</u>, <u>168</u>

使用成績調査 ················ <u>97</u>

承認申請書類 ················ <u>104</u>

承認申請資料 ··········· 98, 104

症例数 ········ 27, 29, 43, 59, 66

症例報告書 ········ <u>103</u>, 104, 105

申請資料 ······················ 104

人年法 ······················ 50, 84

真の値 ····················· 27, 28

信頼区間 ········ <u>83</u>, <u>86</u>, 91, 117,
119, 136, 137, 146

信頼区間の係数 ··············· 83

信頼性 ························ <u>156</u>

推定値の分散 ··············· 116

スクリーニング効果 ········ <u>150</u>, 151

正規性 ························ 60

正規分布 ········ 26, <u>29</u>, 30, 40,
45, 47, 53, 60, <u>61</u>, 169

製造販売後臨床試験 ········ <u>97</u>

生存確率 ··········· 31, <u>34</u>, 35, 36,
<u>37</u>, 38, <u>49</u>, <u>50</u>, 51, 58, 68, 70

生存曲線 ········ 31, <u>32</u>, 33, 34, <u>35</u>,
37, 38, 43, 46, 49, <u>50</u>, 51, <u>54</u>,
55, 58, 61, 68, 74, 172,
183, <u>184</u>

生存時間解析
··········· 43, 49, 51, 52, 70, 125

生存時間データ ········ 23, 33, <u>45</u>,
46, 47, 48, 49, 68,
84, 85, 166, 170

生存割合 ····················· 50

製品製造 …………………… 98	脱落バイアス …… <u>33</u>, <u>51</u>, 52, 125, 126, 127, 128, 182, <u>183</u>	データ固定日 …………………… <u>103</u>
絶対リスク ………………… 84, 85	妥当性 ……………………… <u>156</u>, 162	データの型 …………… 45, 46, <u>47</u>, 48, 84, 170
線型モデル …………… 46, <u>165</u>, 166, 167, 170, 172	ダミー変数 ……………………… 167	データの品質管理 … 98, 101, 102
選択バイアス ……… <u>124</u>, 126, 127, 128, 182, <u>183</u>, <u>185</u>, <u>186</u>	置換ブロック法 …………………… 76	データモニタリング ………………… 35
相関 ……………………………… 46	治験 ……………………… <u>97</u>, 98, 101, 104	データモニタリング委員会 ……… <u>74</u>
相関関係 ………………… <u>150</u>, 151	治験審査委員会 …… 98, 101, 104	適合性書面調査 …………………… <u>104</u>
相対リスク ……… 83, 84, 85, 86, 110, 112, 113, 116, 117, 119, 120, <u>121</u>, 122, 125, 132, <u>135</u>, 154, 158, 160	治験薬 ………………………………… 104	同意説明文書 …………………… 100
	中央値 ……… 16, 27, 29, 30, 31, <u>32</u>, 34, 40, 59	統計学的に有意 …………………… 16
層別解析 ………………… <u>163</u>, 178	中間因子 ……… <u>179</u>, <u>180</u>, 181, <u>184</u>, 187	統計学的有意差 …………… 16, 92
層別ランダム化 …………………… 76	中間解析 …… 35, <u>43</u>, 44, 58, <u>72</u>, 73, 74	同等 ……………………………… 62
測定誤差 ………………………… 156	中心極限定理 …………………… <u>29</u>	同等性 ……………………………… 86
た行	直接比較 …… <u>131</u>, <u>132</u>, 134, 135, 136, <u>137</u>, 138, 139, 140, <u>141</u>, 142, 143, 146	同等性（equivalence）試験 ……………………… 59, <u>86</u>
第Ⅰ相試験 …………………… 97, 98	直接比較と間接比較の一貫性 …… 136, 137, 140, 141, 146, 170	特異度 …………………… 157, 158
第Ⅱ相試験 …………………… 97, 108	治療クロスオーバー ………… 59, 90	毒性 ……………………………… 98
第Ⅲ相試験 ……… 97, 98, 108, 109	治療ネットワーク ……… 131, 139, 140, 146, 185	閉じたコホート …………………… <u>155</u>
対応のあるt検定 …………………… 46	データ …………………………… 166	閉じたループ …………………… 144
対応のないt検定 ……… 45, 46, 64	データ固定 ……………… 93, <u>103</u>, 105	**な行**
対数ハザード比 …………………… 60		並び替え検定 …………………… 79, 80
対立仮説 …………………… 63, <u>67</u>		二項分布 …………………… 45, 47
		二重盲検 …………………… 125, 127

日米EU医薬品規制調和
　国際会議 98

ネットワークメタアナリシス ....
　130, 132, 134, 135, 136, 137,
　　　140, 142, 143, 145, 146

ノンパラメトリック 47, 48

は行

パーセンタイル 26, 30, 61

バイアス 34, 38, 51, 75, 76,
　77, 79, 124, 125, 126, 128,
　136, 143, 150, 151, 156, 157,
　158, 160, 162, 167, 168, 170,
　　176, 177, 179, 182, 183,
　　　184, 185, 186, 187

バイアスコイン法 76

ハザード
　............ 49, 50, 51, 68, 70, 166

ハザード性 68

ハザード比 28, 29, 43, 49, 50,
　51, 59, 60, 61, 66, 68, 70, 71,
　　80, 83, 84, 85, 87, 88, 89, 90,
　　92, 113, 154, 158, 166, 169,
　　　　170, 175, 177, 183

外れ値 26, 29, 30

発生率 ... 45, 46, 50, 82, 84, 85,
　87, 88, 112, 150, 151, 155,
　　　156, 160, 161, 166, 172

発生率比 84, 85, 113, 154,
　　　158, 166, 167, 169, 170

発生割合（リスク） 84

パフォーマンス 126

パフォーマンスバイアス
　........................ 127, 128, 182

パラメトリック 48

反復測定 23, 45, 46, 47, 48

反復測定データ 46, 166, 170

比 50, 170

被験者保護 96, 98, 100

人を対象とする医学系研究に
　関する倫理指針
　.................... 97, 98, 99, 101

標準誤差 26, 27, 29, 30,
　　　39, 60, 61, 110, 116, 169

標準正規分布 53, 60, 61

標準偏差
　...... 26, 27, 28, 29, 30, 39, 63

開いたコホート 155

非臨床開発 98

非臨床試験 97

比例ハザード 40

比例ハザード性 43, 50, 51,
　　　　52, 67, 68, 170

比例ハザードモデル 51

非劣性 81, 83, 86, 87, 88,
　　　89, 90, 91, 92, 93

非劣性（non-inferiority）試験
　23, 57, 59, 81, 82, 83, 86,
　　88, 90, 91, 92, 93, 112

非劣性から優越性への仮説の
　切り替え 88, 89, 91

非劣性マージン 83, 86, 87,
　　　88, 89, 90, 91, 92, 93

品質 98

品質管理 103, 104, 105

品質管理・保証 99

品質保証 104

ファンネルプロット 110, 111

不均一性
　................ 117, 135, 136, 137, 146

不均一性のI^2統計量 117

不均一性の検定 117, 118

複合エンドポイント 18

副作用 15, 51, 73, 81, 170

副次エンドポイント 17, 57

ブラインディング 126

ブラインド 99

プラセボ ……… 15, 16, 19, 43, 54, 55, 56, 57, 69, 70, 81, 83, 91, 130, 131, 133, 134, 136, 138, 139, 141, 144, 145, 146, 185

プラセボ群 ……………… 76, 77, 78

プロトコール …… 21, 98, 99, 100, 101, 103, 104, 122, 123

プロトコール逸脱 …… 20, 21, 24, 90, 103, 105

プロトコール遵守集団（PPS）
……………………… 20, 24, 90

プロペンシティスコア … 175, 176, 177, 178, 179, 181, 183, 184, 187

プロペンシティスコア解析 …… 178

プロペンシティスコア法 ……… 187

文献データベース … 109, 128, 137

平均 ……… 25, 26, 27, 29, 39, 46, 49, 61, 63, 75, 78, 79, 110, 112, 113, 115, 166, 167, 176

平均値 …… 29, 92, 112, 114, 132

変量効果 ……………………… 46, 166

変量効果ネットワークメタアナリシス ……………… 135

変量効果モデル …… 23, 46, 112, 114, 115, 116, 117, 118, 128, 135, 136, 166, 170

報告バイアス … 126, 127, 128, 182

母集団 ……………………… 27

保証 ……………… 98, 101, 102

ま行

マッチング ………… 168, 178, 187

マルコフ連鎖モンテカルロ法
……………………… 132, 135

未知/既知 …………………… 15

密度サンプリング ……………… 155

無益性 ……………………… 35

無益性の中止 …………………… 73

メタアナリシス … 17, 46, 89, 108, 109, 110, 111, 112, 113, 114, 115, 116, 119, 121, 124, 127, 130, 132, 133, 135, 136, 137, 141, 143, 145, 146, 149, 169, 182, 184, 185

モデルの誤特定 …… 80, 169, 170

モデルベース ……………… 79

モデルベースのアプローチ
……………………… 80, 169

モニタリング ………… 100, 104

モニタリングレポート ………… 21

や行

薬理 ……………………… 98

有意 ……………………… 144

有意差 … 16, 17, 22, 24, 35, 56, 58, 59, 62, 63, 64, 67, 69, 73, 81, 82, 88, 110, 120, 123, 134, 145

有意水準 ……… 44, 56, 57, 59, 60, 61, 62, 68, 71, 72, 73, 74, 80, 83, 137

優越性 ……………………… 86, 88

優越性から非劣性への仮説の
切り替え ……………… 89

優越性検定 …………… 88, 93

優越性試験 ……… 83, 86, 87, 88, 89, 91, 92, 93

有害事象 ……… 15, 45, 47, 56, 97, 98, 101, 104, 133, 134, 150

有効性の中止 …………………… 73

有病率 ……………… 161, 172

ら行

ランキング ………… 144, 145

ランキングの解釈 … 136, 137, 144

ランダム …………………… 176

ランダム化 …… 20, 22, 23, 35, 47, 48, 75, 76, 77, 78, 79, 80, 84, 90, 97, 124, 130, 136, 143, 159, 162, 164, 169, 176, 182

ランダム化調整因子 …… 76, 77, 78

ランダム化ベース ………………… 79

ランダム化ベースのアプローチ
　………………………………… 80, 169

ランダム化臨床試験 ……………… 182

ランダム誤差 …… 16, 26, 29, 34, 46, 54, 56, 58, 64, 125, 126, 145

ランダム誤差項 ……………………… 46

リスク ………… 50, 58, 84, 85, 131, 149, 153, 154, 155, 160, 161, 162, 163, 168, 174, 175

リスクオブバイアス評価ツール
　…………………………… 125, 126, 127

リスク差 ……………………………… 85

リスク比 ………… 84, 85, 113, 131, 132, 133, 134, 135, 137, 138, 141, 142, 144, 146, 154, 155, 158

率 …………………………… 50, 171, 172

両側 ………………………… 57, 68, 72, 83

両側（two-sided）検定
　……… 56, 57, 60, 62, 63, 64, 68

両側 p 値 ……………………………… 61, 79

両側か片側か ……………………… 60

両側片側 ……………………………… 57

両側有意水準 ……………… 57, 62, 71

量的交互作用 ……………………… 121

臨床開発 ……………………………… 98

臨床試験登録データベース
　…………………………………… 109, 111

倫理指針 ………………………… 97, 99

ループ …… 139, 140, 142, 143, 146

連続データ …… 29, 45, 46, 47, 49, 165, 166, 170

ログランク検定 ……… 34, 43, 45, 46, 47, 49, 52, 59, 60, 64, 68, 74

ロジスティック回帰 ………… 46, 47, 166, 169, 170, 172, 176, 177, 178, 179

わ行

割合 …………… 50, 154, 171, 172

割り付け …………………… 125, 127

短期集中！オオサンショウウオ先生の
医療統計セミナー　論文読解レベルアップ30

2016年11月10日　第1版　第1刷発行	著　者	田中司朗, 田中佐智子
2023年 7月10日　第1版　第4刷発行	発行人	一戸裕子
	発行所	株式会社　羊　土　社
		〒101-0052
		東京都千代田区神田小川町 2-5-1
		TEL　　03（5282）1211
		FAX　　03（5282）1212
		E-mail　eigyo@yodosha.co.jp
		URL　　www.yodosha.co.jp/
ⓒ YODOSHA CO., LTD. 2016	装　幀	トサカデザイン（戸倉 巌, 小酒保子）
Printed in Japan	カバー写真	アマナイメージズ
ISBN978-4-7581-1797-5	印刷所	株式会社 加藤文明社

本書に掲載する著作物の複製権, 上映権, 譲渡権, 公衆送信権（送信可能化権を含む）は（株）羊土社が保有します.
本書を無断で複製する行為（コピー, スキャン, デジタルデータ化など）は, 著作権法上での限られた例外（「私的使用のための複製」など）を除き禁じられています. 研究活動, 診療を含み業務上使用する目的で上記の行為を行うことは大学, 病院, 企業などにおける内部的な利用であっても, 私的使用には該当せず, 違法です. また私的使用のためであっても, 代行業者等の第三者に依頼して上記の行為を行うことは違法となります.

JCOPY ＜（社）出版者著作権管理機構 委託出版物＞
本書の無断複写は著作権法上での例外を除き禁じられています. 複写される場合は, そのつど事前に,（社）出版者著作権管理機構（TEL 03-3513-6969, FAX 03-3513-6979, e-mail：info@jcopy.or.jp）の許諾を得てください.

乱丁, 落丁, 印刷の不具合はお取り替えいたします. 小社までご連絡ください.

羊土社のオススメ書籍

実例から学ぶ！
臨床研究は「できない」が「できる！」に変わる本

片岡裕貴，青木拓也／編

診療現場で生まれたクリニカル・クエスチョンを研究につなげるための入門書!「何から始めればよいのかわからない」「やってみたけど上手くいかない」初学者の悩みを解決します！

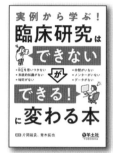

- 定価3,960円（本体3,600円＋税10%）　■ A5判
- 239頁　■ ISBN 978-4-7581-2383-9

あなたの臨床研究応援します
医療統計につながる正しい研究デザイン，観察研究の効果的なデータ解析

新谷 歩／著

臨床研究法が求めている「科学性」とはなにか，観察研究と介入研究のどちらをすればよいか…臨床医が陥りやすい事例を用い，臨床研究法下の注意，可能性，そして，どのような臨床研究を目指せばよいかをわかりやすく．

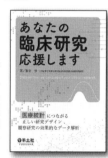

- 定価3,080円（本体2,800円＋税10%）　■ A5判
- 175頁　■ ISBN 978-4-7581-1851-4

基礎から学ぶ
統計学

中原 治／著

理解に近道はない．だからこそ，初学者目線を忘れないペース配分と励ましで伴走する入門書．可能な限り図に語らせ，道具としての統計手法を，しっかり数学として（一部は割り切って）学ぶ．独習・学び直しに最適．

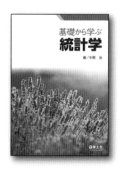

- 定価3,520円（本体3,200円＋税10%）　■ B5判
- 335頁　■ ISBN 978-4-7581-2121-7

スッキリわかる！
臨床統計はじめの一歩 改訂版
統計のイロハからエビデンスの読み解き方・活かし方まで

能登 洋／著

エビデンスを診療やケアに活かすための超入門書！「論文を読む際はどこを見る？」「臨床研究は何から始めるべき？」などの初歩的な疑問が数式なしでスッと理解できます．EBMを実践したい医師・看護師にオススメ！

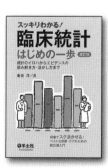

- 定価3,080円（本体2,800円＋税10%）　■ A5判
- 229頁　■ ISBN 978-4-7581-1833-0

発行　羊土社 YODOSHA

〒101-0052　東京都千代田区神田小川町2-5-1　TEL 03(5282)1211　FAX 03(5282)1212
E-mail：eigyo@yodosha.co.jp
URL：www.yodosha.co.jp/

ご注文は最寄りの書店，または小社営業部まで

プライマリケアと救急を中心とした総合誌
レジデントノート

☐ 年間定期購読料（国内送料サービス）
- 通常号（月刊）：
  定価 30,360円（本体 27,600円＋税10%）
- 通常号（月刊）＋増刊：
  定価 61,380円（本体 55,800円＋税10%）

医療現場での実践に役立つ研修医のための必読誌！

レジデントノート は，研修医・指導医にもっとも読まれている研修医のための雑誌です

月刊　毎月1日発行　B5判
定価 2,530円（本体 2,300円＋税10%）

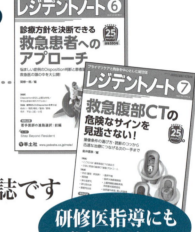

研修医指導にもご活用ください

特徴
① 医師となって最初に必要となる"基本"や"困ること"をとりあげ，ていねいに解説！
② 画像診断，手技，薬の使い方など，すぐに使える内容！日常の疑問を解決できます
③ 先輩の経験や進路選択に役立つ情報も読める！

増刊 レジデントノート

増刊　年6冊発行　B5判

月刊レジデントノートのわかりやすさで，1つのテーマをより広く，より深く解説！

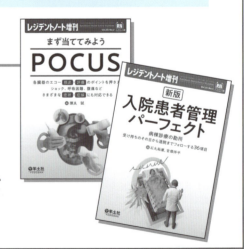

発行　羊土社 YODOSHA
〒101-0052 東京都千代田区神田小川町2-5-1　TEL 03(5282)1211　FAX 03(5282)1212
E-mail : eigyo@yodosha.co.jp
URL : www.yodosha.co.jp/

ご注文は最寄りの書店，または小社営業部まで

別冊

課題論文 &
演習問題の解答と解説

※この別冊は本体から取り外して使用できます

短期集中！
オオサンショウウオ先生の
医療統計セミナー
論文読解レベルアップ30

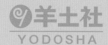

別冊目次

◆課題論文

課題論文1	Iijima K, et al：Lancet, 2014［腎疾患］	2
課題論文2	Ruff CT, et al：Lancet, 2014［循環器疾患］	12
課題論文3	Miura T, et al：Lancet Psychiatry, 2014［精神疾患］	22
課題論文4	Cardis E, et al：J Natl Cancer Inst, 2005［がん］	32
課題論文5	Tanaka S, et al：BMJ, 2015［歯科疾患］	42

◆演習問題の解答と解説　　51

課題論文1　Iijima K, et al：Lancet, 2014 ［腎疾患］

小児難治性頻回再発型またはステロイド依存性ネフローゼ症候群に対するリツキシマブ：多施設共同二重盲検ランダム化プラセボ対照試験

重要単語（Summaryより）

❶	frequently relapsing nephrotic syndrome	頻回再発型ネフローゼ症候群
❷	steroid-dependent nephrotic syndrome	ステロイド依存性ネフローゼ症候群
❸	multicenter, double-blind, randomized, placebo-controlled trial	多施設二重盲検ランダム化プラセボ対照試験
❹	eligible	適格
❺	computer-generated sequence	コンピューターで発生させた乱数列
❻	randomly assign patients (1:1)	患者を1:1の比でランダムに割り付ける
❼	adjustment factor	ランダム化調整因子
❽	primary endpoint	主要エンドポイント
❾	safety endpoint	安全性エンドポイント
❿	adverse event	有害事象
⓫	the University Hospital Medical Information Network clinical trials registry	UMIN臨床試験登録
⓬	95% CI (confidence interval)	95%信頼区間
⓭	hazard ratio	ハザード比

講義内容

確率分布

単変量分布
- 正規分布
- 二項分布
- Poisson分布
- 指数分布

交絡調整方法
- プロペンシティスコア
- VanderWeele-Shpitserの基準

多変量分布（回帰）
- 線型モデル
- ロジスティック回帰
- 条件付きロジスティック
- Poisson回帰
- Cox回帰※，指数回帰

誤差が階層構造の確率分布
- 変量効果モデル，Bayesモデル

誤差の表示
- 標準偏差
- パーセンタイル
- 標準誤差
- 95%信頼区間

データの型に応じた指標
- 平均
- 平均の差，回帰係数
- 発生リスク
- リスク比，オッズ比
- 発生率
- 発生率比
- 生存曲線，ハザード
- ハザード比

メタアナリシス
- 公表バイアス
- ファンネルプロット
- 不均一性
- リスクオブバイアス評価ツール

ネットワークメタアナリシス
- 直接比較，間接比較
- 間接比較への依存度
- 直接比較と間接比較の一貫性
- ランキングの解釈

仮説検定とp値
- 帰無仮説，対立仮説
- 優越性，非劣性
- 非劣性マージン
- 交互作用の検定
- 片側検定，両側検定
- αエラー，βエラー
- 有意水準
- サンプルサイズ

疫学
- コホート研究
- ケース・コントロール研究
- 比，率，割合
- 交絡
- 誤分類
- バイアスと感度解析

臨床試験
- 主要エンドポイント
- ランダム化
- ITTの原則
- プロトコル逸脱
- 有害事象，副作用
- 中間解析
- サブグループ解析
- GCP，倫理指針
- データの品質管理・保証

※正確にはセミパラメトリックモデルで，確率分布ではない

Articles

Rituximab for childhood-onset, complicated, frequently relapsing nephrotic syndrome or steroid-dependent nephrotic syndrome: a multicentre, double-blind, randomised, placebo-controlled trial

Kazumoto Iijima, Mayumi Sako, Kandai Nozu, Rintaro Mori, Nao Tuchida, Koichi Kamei, Kenichiro Miura, Kunihiko Aya, Koichi Nakanishi, Yoshiyuki Ohtomo, Shori Takahashi, Ryojiro Tanaka, Hiroshi Kaito, Hidefumi Nakamura, Kenji Ishikura, Shuichi Ito, Yasuo Ohashi, on behalf of the Rituximab for Childhood-onset Refractory Nephrotic Syndrome (RCRNS) Study Group

Summary

Background Rituximab could be an effective treatment for childhood-onset, complicated, frequently relapsing nephrotic syndrome (FRNS) and steroid-dependent nephrotic syndrome (SDNS). We investigated the efficacy and safety of rituximab in patients with high disease activity.

Methods We did a multicentre, double-blind, randomised, placebo-controlled trial at nine centres in Japan. We screened patients aged 2 years or older experiencing a relapse of FRNS or SDNS, which had originally been diagnosed as nephrotic syndrome when aged 1–18 years. Patients with complicated FRNS or SDNS who met all other criteria were eligible for inclusion after remission of the relapse at screening. We used a computer-generated sequence to randomly assign patients (1:1) to receive rituximab (375 mg/m²) or placebo once weekly for 4 weeks, with age, institution, treatment history, and the intervals between the previous three relapses as adjustment factors. Patients, guardians, caregivers, physicians, and individuals assessing outcomes were masked to assignments. All patients received standard steroid treatment for the relapse at screening and stopped taking immunosuppressive agents by 169 days after randomisation. Patients were followed up for 1 year. The primary endpoint was the relapse-free period. Safety endpoints were frequency and severity of adverse events. Patients who received their assigned intervention were included in analyses. This trial is registered with the University Hospital Medical Information Network clinical trials registry, number UMIN000001405.

Findings Patients were centrally registered between Nov 13, 2008, and May 19, 2010. Of 52 patients who underwent randomisation, 48 received the assigned intervention (24 were given rituximab and 24 placebo). The median relapse-free period was significantly longer in the rituximab group (267 days, 95% CI 223–374) than in the placebo group (101 days, 70–155; hazard ratio: 0·27, 0·14–0·53; p<0·0001). Ten patients (42%) in the rituximab group and six (25%) in the placebo group had at least one serious adverse event (p=0·36).

Interpretation Rituximab is an effective and safe treatment for childhood-onset, complicated FRNS and SDNS.

Funding Japanese Ministry of Health, Labour and Welfare.

Published Online
June 23, 2014
http://dx.doi.org/10.1016/
S0140-6736(14)60541-9

See Online/Comment
http://dx.doi.org/10.1016/
S0140-6736(14)60654-1

Department of Pediatrics, Kobe University Graduate School of Medicine, Chuo-ku, Kobe, Japan (Prof K Iijima MD, K Nozu MD, H Kaito MD); Division for Clinical Trials, Department of Development Strategy (M Sako MD, H Nakamura MD), and Department of Health Policy (R Mori MD), Center for Social and Clinical Research, National Research Institute for Child Health and Development, National Center for Child Health and Development, Setagaya-ku, Tokyo, Japan; Department of General Pediatrics and Interdisciplinary Medicine (N Tuchida MD) and Department of Nephrology and Rheumatology (K Kamei MD, S Ito MD), National Center for Child Health and Development, Setagaya-ku, Tokyo, Japan; Department of Pediatrics, Graduate School of Medicine, University of Tokyo, Bunkyo-ku, Tokyo, Japan (K Miura MD); Chuo University, Bunkyo-ku, Tokyo, Japan (Prof Y Ohashi PhD); Department of Pediatrics, Okayama University Graduate School of Medicine, Dentistry and Pharmaceutical Sciences, Shikata-cho, Okayama, Japan (K Aya MD); Department of Pediatrics, Wakayama Medical University, Wakayama, Japan (K Nakanishi MD); Department of Pediatrics, Juntendo University Nerima Hospital, Nerima-ku, Tokyo, Japan (Y Ohtomo MD);

Introduction

Childhood nephrotic syndrome is a disorder affecting the kidneys in which a large amount of protein passes through the glomerular filter, resulting in hypoproteinaemia and generalised oedema. Idiopathic nephrotic syndrome occurs in two or more of every 100 000 children[1] and is the most common chronic glomerular disease in paediatric nephrology practice. Minimal change nephrotic syndrome is the most common form of the disorder, for which steroid therapy is effective for most patients.[2] Those who respond well rarely progress to chronic renal failure, but up to half develop frequently relapsing nephrotic syndrome (FRNS) or steroid-dependent nephrotic syndrome (SDNS; table 1).[2] Moreover, 10–20% of patients with idiopathic nephrotic syndrome have steroid-resistant nephrotic syndrome (table 1).[2]

Standard treatments for FRNS, SDNS, and steroid-resistant nephrotic syndrome are immunosuppressive agents: cyclophosphamide, chlorambucil, ciclosporin, tacrolimus, and levamisole are used for paediatric FRNS and SDNS, and ciclosporin for paediatric steroid-resistant nephrotic syndrome.[3–5] Most children are effectively treated with these drugs; however, some have frequent relapses. In two studies,[6,7] 10–20% of children taking ciclosporin had frequent relapses, and in another study,[8] about 30% of the patients with steroid-resistant nephrotic syndrome after ciclosporin had steroid-sensitive, frequent relapses after complete remission. In addition to being ineffective in some patients, ciclosporin can cause side-effects—the most common of which is chronic nephrotoxicity[9,10]—suggesting that it should be discontinued within 24 months. However, discontinuation of ciclosporin almost always results in frequent relapses requiring long-term steroid treatment,[11]

Articles

Department of Pediatrics, Surugadai Nihon University Hospital, Chiyoda-ku, Tokyo, Japan (Prof S Takahashi MD); Department of Nephrology, Hyogo Prefectural Kobe Children's Hospital, Suma-Ku, Kobe, Japan (R Tanaka MD); and Department of Nephrology, Tokyo Metropolitan Children's Medical Center, Fuchu, Japan (K Ishikura MD)

Correspondence to:
Prof Kazumoto Iijima, Department of Pediatrics, Kobe University Graduate School of Medicine, 7-5-2 Kusunoki-cho, Chuo-ku, Kobe 650-0017, Japan
iijima@med.kobe-u.ac.jp

For the **trial protocol** see http://www.med.kobe-u.ac.jp/pediat/pdf/rcrn01.pdf

See Online for appendix

which also poses a long-term risk to children. Therefore, a new treatment that does not involve steroids or immunosuppressive agents is urgently needed.

In the past 10 years, rituximab has had some success in complicated FRNS and SDNS,[12,13] and several research groups have done single-arm or short-term studies of this drug.[14–16] The 2012 Kidney Disease: Improving Global Outcomes clinical practice guidelines[17] introduced rituximab as a treatment option for childhood-onset, complicated FRNS and SDNS. However, the efficacy and safety of rituximab for complicated FRNS and SDNS are yet to be established.[17] We aimed to assess the efficacy and safety of rituximab in patients with high disease activity.

Methods

Study design and participants

In a multicentre, double-blind, randomised, placebo-controlled trial, we enrolled patients at nine centres in Japan. Full eligibility criteria are listed in the appendix. Briefly, we screened patients aged 2 years or older experiencing a relapse of FRNS or SDNS, which had originally been diagnosed as nephrotic syndrome when aged 1–18 years (appendix). Patients with complicated FRNS or SDNS (table 1) who met all other criteria were eligible for inclusion after remission of the relapse they were experiencing at screening.

This study was approved by the institutional review boards at each centre and complied with the Declaration of Helsinki. Participants aged 20 years or older or parents of younger patients provided written informed consent.

Randomisation and masking

Once full eligibility was confirmed, patients were randomly assigned (1:1) to rituximab or placebo. We applied the minimisation method using a computer-generated sequence (SAS PROC PLAN), with age, institution, treatment history (whether a steroid or an immunosuppressive drug, or both, was given during the relapse immediately before randomisation), and the intervals between the previous three relapses as adjustment factors. Patients, patients' guardians, caregivers, treating physicians, and individuals assessing outcomes were masked to assignments. Investigators and patients (or their legal representatives) were masked to peripheral blood B-cell counts, which were centrally monitored. To maintain blinding, allocation codes were disclosed only after the entire clinical trial was completed and all data were locked. However, investigators could request the disclosure of a patient's allocation code urgently in the case of a serious adverse event that could lead to death or was life-threatening, a serious adverse event for which the information was essential to establish what treatment was necessary, or treatment failure.

Procedures

Patients received the first dose of their assigned drug within 2 weeks after randomisation. Patients assigned to rituximab received an intravenous dose of 375 mg/m² (maximum 500 mg) once weekly for 4 weeks. Because the optimum dose for paediatric FRNS and SDNS has not been established, we selected this dosing schedule on the basis of previous reports of rituximab's ability to prevent relapses in patients with immunosuppressant-resistant SDNS[12,13,18] and on the recommended dose for treating B-cell lymphoma, which has a known safety profile. Patients assigned to placebo received intravenous injections of a matched placebo at the same frequency. We used pretreatments to prevent infusion reaction (appendix). Patients could cease assigned treatment if they met discontinuation criteria (appendix).

Participants receiving prednisolone for the relapse at screening continued receiving the drug, taking 60 mg/m² orally three times a day (maximum of 80 mg per day) for 4 weeks. Participants not receiving prednisolone at screening received the same dose until 3 days after complete remission was achieved. After 4 weeks (in patients who received prednisolone at screening) or from 3 days after complete remission (in patients who did not receive prednisolone at screening), patients took 60 mg/m² prednisolone in the morning on alternate days (maximum

	Definition
FRNS	≥2 relapses of nephrotic syndrome within 6 months after initial remission, or ≥4 relapses within any 12-month period
SDNS	2 relapses of nephrotic syndrome during the reduction of steroid treatment or within 2 weeks of discontinuation of steroid treatment
SRNS	Persistent proteinuria after 60 mg/m² oral prednisolone per day for 4 weeks
Complicated FRNS or SDNS	Patients diagnosed with FRNS or SDNS when aged 2 years or older, who had ≥4 relapses in a 12-month period or steroid dependence at any point in the 2 years before relapse at screening, after completion of immunosuppressive drug treatment (eg, ciclosporin, cyclophosphamide, mizoribine, or mycophenolate mofetil); or patients diagnosed with FRNS or SDNS when aged 2 years or older, who had ≥4 relapses in a 12-month period or steroid dependence diagnosed at any point in the 2 years before relapse at screening, during immunosuppressive drug treatment (eg, ciclosporin, cyclophosphamide, mizoribine, or mycophenolate mofetil); or patients with a history of SRNS and diagnosed with FRNS or SDNS when aged 2 years or older, who had ≥4 relapses in a 12-month period or steroid dependence at any point in the 2 years before relapse at screening, during or after the completion of immunosuppressive drug treatment (eg, ciclosporin or a combination of ciclosporin and methylprednisolone)

FRNS=frequently relapsing nephrotic syndrome. SDNS=steroid-dependent nephrotic syndrome. SRNS=steroid-resistant nephrotic syndrome.

Table 1: Definitions

80 mg per day) for 2 weeks, then 30 mg/m² on alternate days (maximum 40 mg per day) for 2 weeks, and then 15 mg/m² on alternate days (maximum 20 mg per day) for 2 weeks. When patients had relapses during the study period (1 year of follow-up), they received 60 mg/m² oral prednisolone three times a day (maximum 80 mg per day) until 3 days after complete remission was obtained, when tapering began. If patients were receiving ciclosporin at screening, tapering of this drug began at day 85 (patients received their first dose of rituximab or placebo on day 1), with discontinuation by day 169 (figure 1). If patients were taking any other immunosuppressive drugs, these drugs were discontinued by day 85 (figure 1).

Patients were followed up for 1 year (figure 1). Study visits occurred at baseline; at weeks 1, 2, 3, and 4; and every 4 weeks from week 5. Patients were deemed to have treatment failure if a relapse had occurred by day 85, FRNS or SDNS was diagnosed between days 86 and 365, or steroid resistance was noted (figure 1, appendix). We designed the study protocol with consideration for the placebo group as much as possible. When patients had treatment failure, their allocation code was urgently disclosed. If a patient with treatment failure was in the placebo group, he or she could then choose to begin the treatment deemed the best by investigators—eg, new immunosuppressive drugs—and continue in our study, or to enter a separate rituximab pharmacokinetic study after discontinuation or completion of our trial.

Outcomes

The primary endpoint was the relapse-free period (time of randomisation to the time of first relapse after starting the study treatment). The prespecified secondary endpoints were time to treatment failure, relapse rate (number of relapses per person-year), time to four relapses of nephrotic syndrome in the study period, time to two relapses during reduction of steroid treatment or within 2 weeks of discontinuation of steroid treatment, time to transition to steroid resistance, steroid dose after randomisation, changes in steroid dose before and after randomisation, peripheral blood B-cell count, peripheral blood B-cell depletion period, human antichimeric antibody production rate, and rituximab blood concentration. Safety endpoints were frequency and severity of adverse events, and abnormal values in biochemical tests and haematology assessments. We did post-hoc analyses of the effects of age at time of treatment and age at disease onset on median relapse-free period, the effect of concomitant angiotensin-converting-enzyme inhibitors and angiotensin-receptor blockers on median relapse-free period, time to FRNS or SDNS, the proportion of patients who could discontinue steroid treatment after study drug infusion, the time between cessation of steroid treatment and first relapse, the frequency of infections that required treatment, the effect of B-cell depletion on infections that required treatment and relapses, and changes in characteristics between baseline and 1 year.

Statistical analysis

On the basis of previous reports,[12,13,18] we assumed that 40% of the patients in the rituximab group and 10% of the patients in the placebo group would maintain remission 6 months after registration. 30 patients in each group would be needed to establish the superiority of the test treatment for the primary endpoint with 90% power at a 2·5% one-sided significance level under the assumption of exponential distribution of relapse-free survival time and proportionality of hazards.

We used the log-rank test to analyse the primary endpoint and other time-to-event endpoints. We did an interim analysis (appendix) after 30 patients had relapsed, with a significance level set at 0·25% (one-sided). We summarised time-to-event data with the Kaplan-Meier method and estimated therapeutic effect hazard ratios (HRs) and their 95% CIs with Cox regression.

We made no multiplicity adjustment in the analysis of secondary endpoints. We set the significance level at 5% (two-sided) and report two-sided p values. We calculated the relapse rate and the frequency of infection with the number of events per person-years. We compared groups with the computer-based permutation test, and calculated

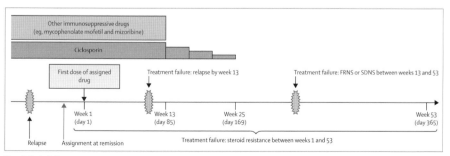

Figure 1: Study design
FRNS=frequently relapsing nephrotic syndrome. SDNS=steroid-dependent nephrotic syndrome.

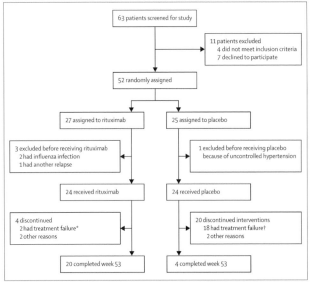

Figure 2: Trial profile
*One patient relapsed by week 13, and one was diagnosed with steroid resistance. †Ten relapsed by week 13, and eight were diagnosed with frequently relapsing nephrotic syndrome or steroid-dependent nephrotic syndrome after week 13.

the 95% CI of rate ratios fitting the negative binomial distribution and taking account of overdispersion. With the Wilcoxon rank-sum test, we compared daily steroid doses after randomisation and steroid doses before and after randomisation in both groups. We used the Kaplan-Meier method to assess the proportion of patients with human antichimeric antibody. Analyses were by modified intention to treat, including patients who received their assigned intervention. All analyses were done in SAS (version 9.1).

This trial is registered with the University Hospital Medical Information Network clinical trial registry, number UMIN000001405.

Role of the funding source

The funder of the study had no role in study design, data analysis, data interpretation, or writing of the report. The corresponding author had full access to all the data in the study and had final responsibility for the decision to submit for publication.

Results

Between Nov 13, 2008, and May 19, 2010, 52 patients were randomly assigned to rituximab or placebo. Follow-up ended on Nov 10, 2011. The preplanned interim analysis showed that rituximab was superior to placebo, after which the independent data and safety monitoring committee advised us to discontinue randomisation as specified in the protocol. Therefore, randomisation ended earlier than planned, on May 21, 2010.

52 patients underwent randomisation (figure 2). 48 patients received the assigned intervention (figure 2) and were included in analyses. 20 patients given rituximab and 23 given placebo received all four doses. No patient dropped out before the first relapse. All 20 patients with treatment failure in the placebo group were enrolled into a separate rituximab pharmacokinetic study after discontinuation (n=18) or completion (n=2) of this trial.

Baseline characteristics in the two groups were similar (table 2). The predominant histological type in both groups was minimal change nephrotic syndrome (table 2). All patients were given steroids or immunosuppressants, or both, at relapse immediately before assignment (table 2). More than 70% of patients in both groups reported side-effects of steroid treatment (table 2).

By the end of 1 year of follow-up, 17 patients in the rituximab group and 23 in the placebo group had relapsed. The median relapse-free period was significantly longer in the rituximab group (267 days, 95% CI 223–374) than in the placebo group (101 days, 70–155; HR 0·27, 95% CI 0·14–0·53; p<0·0001; figure 3A). Post-hoc analyses showed that age at disease onset and age at time of treatment did not affect the median relapse-free period in the rituximab group (appendix). Concomitant angiotensin-converting-enzyme inhibitors or angiotensin-receptor blockers, or both, decreased the median relapse-free period in the rituximab group, although the difference was marginally significant (appendix).

Treatment failure was reported in ten patients in the rituximab group and 20 in the placebo group. The time to treatment failure was significantly longer in the rituximab group than in the placebo group (HR 0·27, 95% CI 0·12–0·59; p=0·0005; figure 3B). The relapse rate was significantly lower in the rituximab group (1·54 relapses per person-year [29 relapses in 18·81 person-years]) than in the placebo group (4·17 relapses per person-year [46 relapses in 11·03 person-years]; HR 0·37, 95% CI 0·23–0·59; p<0·0001). Only two patients in each group had frequent relapses in the study period. Time to two relapses during reduction of steroid treatment or within 2 weeks of discontinuation of steroid treatment was significantly longer in the rituximab group than in the placebo group (HR 0·19, 95% CI 0·07–0·54; p=0·0005). A post-hoc analysis showed that significantly more patients in the rituximab group did not experience frequent relapses or steroid dependence than in the placebo group (0·17, 0·06–0·46; p=0·0001; figure 3C). Two patients in the rituximab group had steroid-resistant relapses, compared with no patients in the placebo group.

Mean daily steroid dose after randomisation was significantly lower in the rituximab group than in the placebo group (9·12 mg/m^2 per day [SD 5·88] vs 20·85 mg/m^2 per day [9·28]; p<0·0001). Mean daily steroid (prednisolone) dose in the rituximab group decreased significantly after randomisation, but did not change significantly in the placebo group (table 3). Exploratory analyses showed that the proportion of patients who could discontinue steroid treatment after the study drug infusion was similar in the rituximab group (21 of 24, 88%) and the placebo group (19 of 24, 79%; p=0·70). However, median time between cessation of steroid treatment and first relapse was significantly longer in the rituximab group (211 days, 95% CI 166–317) than in the placebo group (42 days, 14–98; HR 0·27, 95% CI 0·14–0·54; p<0·0001). The height-for-age Z score improved slightly 1 year after rituximab treatment compared with baseline, although the difference was not significant (appendix). Height Z score also seemed to improve in children with residual growth potential in the rituximab group, but again the difference was not significant (appendix).

Most adverse events were mild, and no patients died during the trial. Although more patients had serious adverse events in the rituximab group than in the placebo group (table 4), the difference was not significant (p=0·36). The most common grade 3–4 adverse events in the rituximab group were hypoproteinemia, lymphocytopenia, and neutropenia (table 5). Post-hoc analyses of adverse events showed that the incidence of infections that required treatment were similar in both groups (4·55 infections per person-year [105 infections in 23·08 person-years] vs 3·45 infections per person-year [42 infections in 12·18 person-years]; HR 1·27, 95% CI 0·77–2·07, p=0·21). More patients had mild infusion reactions in the rituximab group than in the placebo group (table 4), but the difference was not significant (p=0·12). No grade 3 or 4 infusion reactions were reported in either group (table 4).

The peripheral blood B-cell count decreased substantially immediately after the first dose of rituximab (figure 4), with a median period of B-cell depletion (<5 cells per μL) of 148 days (95% CI 131–170). B-cell counts returned to within the normal range in all patients given rituximab by day 253 (median 118 cells per μL, 95% CI 113–250). By contrast, peripheral blood B-cell count did not change in the placebo group (data not shown).

We did a post-hoc analysis of the effects of B-cell depletion on relapses and infections. No relapses were reported in the rituximab group during the period of B-cell depletion. However, the rate of infections requiring treatment was higher during the B-cell depletion period (8·43 infections per person-year [49 infections in 5·81 person-years]) than outside of this period (3·24 infections per person-year [56 infections in 17·27 person-years]; HR 0·39, 95% CI 0·27–0·58; p<0·0001); although most were grade 1 respiratory-tract infections. The cumulative proportion of patients with human antichimeric antibody at day 365 was 14% (95% CI 5–38). Blood concentrations of rituximab are shown in table 6.

Discussion

We have shown that the relapse-free period increases with rituximab in patients with childhood-onset, complicated FRNS and SDNS. Adverse events were generally mild and the frequency of serious adverse

	Rituximab (n=24)	Placebo (n=24)
Age (years)	11·5 (5·0)	13·6 (6·9)
Duration of disease (years)	7·9 (4·7)	8·0 (5·4)
Sex		
Male	18 (75%)	16 (67%)
Female	6 (25%)	8 (33%)
Height (cm)	137·7 (21·4)	143·4 (20·4)
Height-for-age Z score	−0·96 (1·37)	−0·88 (1·26)
Weight (kg)	44·0 (18·6)	47·5 (15·6)
Body-mass index	22·3 (4·9)	22·6 (4·3)
Systolic blood pressure (mm Hg)	112·3 (11·0)	111·0 (9·6)
Diastolic blood pressure (mm Hg)	65·6 (9·9)	66·8 (8·2)
Serum creatinine (μmol/L)	39·78 (13·26)	44·20 (15·91)
Estimated glomerular filtration rate (mL/m per 1·73 m²)	128·9 (20·6)	126·4 (26·0)
Serum total protein (g/L)	58 (6)	59 (6)
Serum albumin (g/L)	34 (6)	34 (5)
Urinary protein to creatinine ratio (mg/mg)	0·13 (0·11)	0·11 (0·10)
Steroid and immunosuppressant use at relapse immediately before assignment		
Ciclosporin, mycophenolate mofetil, and daily steroids	1 (4%)	0
Ciclosporin, mizoribine, and daily steroids	3 (13%)	3 (13%)
Ciclosporin and daily steroids	0	1 (4%)
Mycophenolate mofetil and daily steroids	0	1 (4%)
Mizoribine and daily steroids	1 (4%)	1 (4%)
Daily steroids with no immunosuppressant	1 (4%)	0
Ciclosporin, mycophenolate mofetil, and steroids on alternate days	2 (8%)	0
Ciclosporin, mizoribine, and steroids on alternate days	6 (25%)	4 (17%)
Ciclosporin and steroids on alternate days	2 (8%)	5 (21%)
Mycophenolate mofetil and steroids on alternate days	0	0
Mizoribine and steroids on alternate days	3 (13%)	3 (13%)
Steroids on alternate days with no immunosuppressant	1 (4%)	2 (8%)
Ciclosporin and mycophenolate mofetil, with no steroids	0	0
Ciclosporin and mizoribine, with no steroids	1 (4%)	1 (4%)
Ciclosporin, with no steroids	1 (4%)	2 (8%)
Mycophenolate mofetil, with no steroids	0	0
Mizoribine, with no steroids	2 (8%)	1 (4%)
No steroids or immunosuppressant	0	0
Renal histology		
Minimal change	21 (88%)	23 (96%)
Focal segmental glomerulosclerosis	2 (8%)	1 (4%)
Unknown	1 (4%)	0
Steroid toxicity*	17 (71%)	19 (79%)
Time between relapse immediately before screening and previous relapse		
<180 days	15 (63%)	18 (75%)
≥180 days	9 (38%)	6 (25%)
Time from assignment to start of assigned intervention (days)	6·3 (2·7)	6·3 (3·4)

Data are mean (SD) or n (%). *Complications induced by steroid treatments, such as hypertension, short stature, diabetes, glaucoma, cataract, central obesity, and osteoporosis.

Table 2: Baseline characteristics

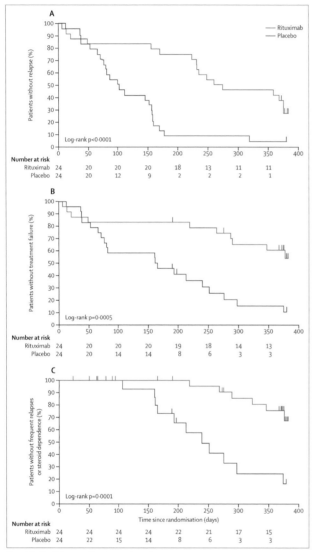

	Number of patients*	Daily prednisolone dose in the 365 days before randomisation (mg/m² per day)	Daily prednisolone dose after randomisation (mg/m² per day)	p value
Rituximab	19	19·13 (9·94)	8·37 (5·62)	<0·0001
Placebo	21	18·02 (10·15)	21·02 (9·81)	0·21

Data are mean (SD), unless otherwise stated. *Number of patients in each group for whom prednisolone doses were available for 365 days before randomisation.

Table 3: Change in daily prednisolone dose before and after randomisation, by group

	Rituximab (n=24)	Placebo (n=24)
Number of adverse events	357	251
Patients with ≥1 adverse event	24 (100%)	23 (96%)
Number of serious adverse events	16	7
Patients with ≥1 serious adverse event	10 (42%)	6 (25%)
Deaths	0	0
Number of grade 3 adverse events	24	15
Patients with ≥1 grade 3 adverse event	8 (33%)	3 (13%)
Number of grade 4 adverse events	3	0
Patients with ≥1 grade 4 adverse event	1 (4%)	0
Cases of infections that required treatment	105	42
Grade 1	1	0
Grade 2	101	42
Grade 3	3	0
Grade 4	0	0
Patients with ≥1 infection	23 (96%)	18 (75%)
Total number of infusion reactions	41	26
Grade 1	36	25
Grade 2	5	1
Grade 3	0	0
Grade 4	0	0
Patients with ≥1 infusion reaction	19 (79%)	13 (54%)

Data are n or n (%). Adverse events were categorised according to the National Cancer Institute's Common Terminology Criteria for Adverse Events (version 3.0).

Table 4: Adverse events

Figure 3: Kaplan-Meier curves for primary and secondary outcomes
(A) Patients without relapse. (B) Patients without treatment failure. (C) Patients without frequent relapses or steroid dependence. Vertical lines indicate censoring.

events did not differ significantly between groups. As far as we are aware, we are the first to show that rituximab is safe and effective for at least 1 year of treatment in a multicentre, double-blind, randomised, placebo-controlled trial (panel).

Patients with complicated FRNS or SDNS usually have a long history of the disease, and many of those included in our trial were receiving fairly high daily doses of steroids with or without immunosuppressive agents to prevent frequent relapses. Therefore, some patients did not meet the usual criteria for frequent relapses or steroid dependence before randomisation. However, more than 80% of patients in our study were treated with prednisolone at the relapse immediately before randomisation, and the mean daily prednisolone dose for 1 year before randomisation was about 20 mg/m². These facts indicate that overall disease activity was high. To allow enrolment of these patients into our trial, we modified the definitions of frequent relapses and steroid dependence immediately before the trial.

A fairly large study[16] of rituximab treatment for patients with steroid-dependent and calcineurin inhibitor-dependent idiopathic nephrotic syndrome, similar to those enrolled in our trial showed that the 6-month probability of remission after the first infusion was 48%. The relapse-free period was similar to that in our study, further emphasising the efficacy of the drug. Our finding that the age at disease onset and age at time of treatment did not greatly affect the outcome is fairly consistent with data from an uncontrolled study that also included adult patients.[19] The fact that patients in the rituximab group who were concomitantly treated with angiotensin-converting-enzyme inhibitors or angiotensin-receptor blockers, or both, had earlier relapses suggests that these drugs did not prevent relapses and patients treated with those drugs had more active disease.

More than half the patients in the rituximab group could discontinue steroids for more than 200 days without relapses after receiving rituximab. A long steroid-free period would allow patients to recover from side-effects, such as impaired growth. Indeed, the height Z score seemed to improve 1 year after treatment in the rituximab group, although the difference was not significant. Long-term follow-up studies are needed to clarify the effects of rituximab treatment for recovery from impaired growth.

Rituximab does not increase the frequency of infection when used to treat rheumatoid arthritis.[20,21] However, the rate of infections requiring treatment was higher during the period of B-cell depletion in the rituximab group in our study than when B cells were not depleted. Therefore, attention should be paid to infections during this phase, although most infections in our study were mild and treatable. In studies of patients with complicated nephrotic syndrome who had been taking rituximab, one child died because of pulmonary fibrosis[22] and another patient with fulminant myocarditis due to enterovirus underwent heart transplantation.[23] However, we recorded no deaths or cases of pulmonary fibrosis or myocarditis.

Although we recorded no relapses during B-cell depletion, a low B-cell count could offer clues about whether relapse is likely. Because our protocol did not specify that peripheral B-cell count should be established at time of relapse, a clear correlation between B-cell count and relapse could not be identified. We believe that continued monitoring of the B-cell count throughout the study period, especially at the time of relapse, will be necessary in future investigations. Another limitation of our study was the fairly short observation period. Therefore, the long-term prognosis of patients given rituximab is unclear. Specifically, we are aware of the possibility that not all rare and serious adverse effects were detected in our study—eg, progressive multifocal leukoencephalopathy is known to be a serious side-effect of rituximab.

All patients in our trial had relapsed by 19 months after randomisation. To extend the relapse-free period, further modification of the rituximab treatment and possibly adjunct immunosuppressive therapies might be necessary.

	Rituximab (n=24)		Placebo (n=24)	
	Grade 3	Grade 4	Grade 3	Grade 4
Gastritis	1 (4%)	0	0	0
Gastroenteritis	1 (4%)	0	0	0
Gum infection	1 (4%)	0	0	0
Cellulitis	1 (4%)	0	0	0
Hypertension	1 (4%)	0	0	0
Respiratory disturbance	1 (4%)	0	0	0
Acute kidney failure	1 (4%)	0	0	0
Haemorrhagic cystitis	1 (4%)	0	0	0
Hyperuricaemia	0	1 (4%)	0	0
Hypoproteinaemia*	6 (25%)	0	6 (25%)	0
Adrenal insufficiency	1 (4%)	0	0	0
Nettle rash	1 (4%)	0	0	0
Lymphocytopenia	4 (17%)	0	4	0
Neutropenia	2 (8%)	2 (8%)	0	0
Increased aspartate aminotransferase	0	0	1 (4%)	0
Increased alanine aminotransferase	1 (4%)	0	2 (8%)	0
Increased γ-glutamyl transpeptidase	0	0	1 (4%)	0
Increased creatine phosphokinase	1 (4%)	0	0	0
Hypophosphataemia	0	0	1 (4%)	0

Data are n (%). *Not known to be a side-effect of rituximab and was probably caused by the original disease rather than by rituximab or placebo, because occurred at time of relapse in both groups; other adverse events were known to be caused by the study drug.

Table 5: Grade 3–4 adverse events

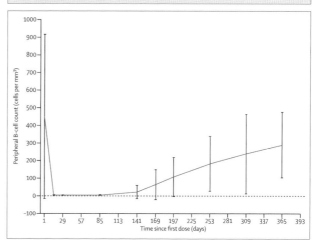

Figure 4: Mean peripheral B-cell counts in the rituximab group
Error bars show SD.

Additionally, a comparison of the efficacy, safety, and cost-effectiveness of various rituximab dosing regimens and B-cell-driven regimens still needs to be done.[24] An uncontrolled study[19] showed the importance of long-term follow-up after a core trial assessing the risk and benefit of rituximab treatment. We are preparing a retrospective

Articles

	Number of patients for whom data available	Mean rituximab blood concentration (ng/mL)
Day 1 (before the first infusion of rituximab)	24	0
Day 22 (before the fourth infusion of rituximab)	23	156 000 (53 700)
Day 85	24	28 800 (17 500)
Day 169	24	2320 (2680)
Day 365*	23	0

Data in parentheses are SD. *Three samples included here were not assessed on day 365; assessments occurred on days 189, 268, and 271, because these patients discontinued assigned treatment because of treatment failure. However, the values were less than the detectable range and so were included as data for day 365.

Table 6: Blood concentrations of rituximab

Panel: Research in context

Systematic review
On completion of our trial, we did a systematic review to identify any randomised controlled trial in which the effectiveness or safety of rituximab, or both, was assessed in children with complicated frequently relapsing nephrotic syndrome (FRNS) or steroid-dependent nephrotic syndrome (SDNS). We searched Medline, Embase, and the Cochrane Library for reports published in any language before Oct 5, 2013, with terms such as "nephrotic syndrome", "rituximab", and "child" (appendix). We identified two open-label, randomised controlled trial (appendix). Meta-analyses of remission frequency at 3 and 6 months confirmed the effectiveness of rituximab in these children, and showed an increase in the remission rate of about 50% at 3 months and of more than 300% at 6 months (appendix).

Interpretation
As far as we are aware, ours is the first randomised, placebo-controlled clinical trial in which the efficacy and safety of rituximab for childhood-onset, complicated FRNS and SDNS have been assessed. Rituximab should be considered as an effective treatment for children with these disorders.

---

long-term follow-up study of patients enrolled in our trial, with a focus on clinical courses, treatments after the clinical trial, growth, and late adverse effects.

The exact pathogenesis of nephrotic syndrome is unclear, but T-cell-mediated immunological abnormalities are thought to have a role.[25] Several studies[26–29] have shown that B cells can promote T-cell activation, mediate antibody-independent autoimmune damage, and provide costimulatory molecules and cytokines, which sustain T-cell activation in autoimmune diseases. Rituximab inhibits B-cell proliferation and induces B-cell apoptosis.[30] This action leads to B-cell depletion and hence suppression of interactions between B cells and T cells, which could prevent recurrences of nephrotic syndrome. Impaired function of regulatory T cells in patients with minimal change nephrotic syndrome and induction of remission in nephrotic syndrome by regulatory T cells have been reported previously.[31–33] Rituximab could induce an increase in the number and function of regulatory T cells.[34] Rituximab-maintained remission in nephrotic syndrome could be due to the restoration of function of regulatory T cells. Fornoni and colleagues reported[35] that rituximab binds directly to an acid sphingomyelinase-like phosphodiesterase 3b on the cell surface of podocytes, stabilising podocyte structure and function, which could lead to the prevention of recurrent focal segmental glomerulosclerosis. Whether a similar mechanism works in complicated FRNS and SDNS remains to be established.

Contributors
KIi and MS were responsible for the study concept. KIi, MS, and NT designed and managed the study. KNo, KK, KM, KA, KNa, YOht, ST, RT, HK, KIs, and SI collected and interpreted data. YOha did statistical analysis. RM did the systematic review. All authors were members of the writing group and agreed on the content of the report, reviewed drafts, and approved the final version.

Rituximab for Childhood-onset Refractory Nephrotic Syndrome Study Group investigators
Kandai Nozu, Hiroshi Kaito, Yuya Hashimura, Takeshi Ninchoji (Kobe University Graduate School of Medicine, Japan); Shori Takahashi, Hiroshi Saito (Surugadai Nihon University Hospital, Japan); Koichi Nakanishi, Yuko Shima (Wakayama Medical University, Japan); Ryojiro Tanaka, Kyoko Morinaga (Hyogo Prefectural Kobe Children's Hospital, Japan); Kenichiro Miura, Takashi Sekine (Graduate School of Medicine, University of Tokyo); Yoshiyuki Ohtomo, Daisuke Umino (Juntendo University Nerima Hospital, Japan); Kunihiko Aya, Takayuki Miyai (Okayama University Hospital, Japan); Kenji Ishikura, Hiroshi Hataya, Yuko Hamasaki (Tokyo Metropolitan Children's Medical Center, Japan); Shuichi Ito, Koichi Kamei, Masao Ogura, Tomohiro Udagawa, Akiko Tsutsumi (National Center for Child Health and Development, Japan).

Clinical trial steering committee
Kazumoto Iijima (Kobe University Graduate School of Medicine, Japan), Mayumi Sako (National Center for Child Health and Development, Japan), Nao Tsuchida (National Center for Child Health and Development, Japan).

Independent data and safety monitoring committee
Takashi Igarashi (Graduate School of Medicine, University of Tokyo, Japan), Masataka Honda (Tokyo Metropolitan Children's Medical Center, Japan), Satoshi Morita (Graduate School of Medicine, Yokohama City University, Japan).

Declaration of interests
KIi has received grants from the Japanese Ministry of Health, Labour and Welfare for the Large Scale Clinical Trial Network Project (Japan Medical Association Center for Clinical Trials: CCT-B-2001), research on rare and intractable diseases (H24-nanchitou (nan)-ippan-041), and clinical research (H25-iryogijutu-ippan-008); has received research grants from the Japanese Ministry of Education, Culture, Sports, Science and Technology (Grant-in-Aid for Scientific Research 23591192); has received research grants from Pfizer Japan, Kyowa Hakko Kirion, Abbot Japan, Takeda Pharmaceutical, Asahi Kasei Pharma, Astellas Pharma, Terumo, Chugai Pharmaceutical, Benesis, Dainippon Sumitomo Pharma, Genzyme Japan, Novartis Pharmaceuticals, Mizutori Clinic, AbbVie, and Janssen Pharmaceutical; has received lecture fees from Novartis Pharmaceuticals, Asahi Kasei Pharma, Baxter, Sanofi, Pfizer Japan, Meiji Seika Pharma, Taisho Toyama Pharmaceutical, Kyorin Pharmaceutical, Kyowa Hakko Kirion, Dainippon Sumitomo Pharma, Astellas Pharma, and Chugai Pharmaceutical; and is a paid adviser for Zenyaku Kogyo. MS has received grants from the Japanese Ministry of Health, Labour and Welfare, and is a paid adviser for Zenyaku Kogyo. RM has received research grants from WHO; the Japanese Ministry of Health, Labour and Welfare; the Japanese Ministry of Education, Culture, Sports, Science and Technology; the Gates Foundation; the Japanese Ministry of Foreign Affairs; and Save the Children. NT has received grants from Kaketsuken, GlaxoSmithKline, and Daiichi Sankyo. KA has received grants from JCR Pharmaceuticals and Teijin Pharma, and lecture fees from Boehringer Ingelheim Japan, JMS, Asahi Kasei Pharma, Ono Pharmaceutical, and Kyorin Pharmaceutical. KNa has received lecture fees from Asahi Kasei Pharma, Novartis Pharmaceuticals, Astellas Pharma, and Takeda Pharmaceutical. YOht has received grants from Asahi Kasei Pharma, Taiho Pharmaceutical, and Pfizer Japan; and lecture fees from Kyowa Hakko Kirin, Ferring Pharmaceuticals, Asahi Kasei Pharma, and Daiichi Sankyo. ST has received grants from Sanofi and Novartis Pharmaceuticals. RT has received lecture fees from Pfizer Japan and Novartis Pharmaceuticals. HK has received grants from the Danone

Institute of Japan Foundation, the Hyogo Prefecture Health Promotion Association, and Baxter; and lecture fees from Novartis Pharmaceuticals and Daiichi Sankyo. KIs has received lecture fees and travel expenses from Novartis Pharmaceuticals and Asahi Kasei Pharma. SI has received lecture fees from Asahi Kasei Pharma, Novartis Pharmaceuticals, and Chugai Pharmaceutical. YOha has received grants from the Japanese Ministry of Health, Labour and Welfare; received unlimited educational grants from Kowa Pharmaceutical, Astellas Pharma, Kyowa Hakko Kirin, and Takeda Pharmaceutical during the study period; received lecture fees and honorarium of more than US$5000 for consultations with Chugai Pharmaceutical, Shionogi, Sanofi, and DNP Media Create in the fiscal year of 2012; and has served as the chairman of the board of directors for Statcom, owning stock. The other authors declare no competing interests.

Acknowledgments
This study was funded by the Health and Labour Sciences Research Grants for the Large Scale Clinical Trial Network Project (Japan Medical Association Center for Clinical Trials: CCT-B-2001) from the Japanese Ministry of Health, Labour and Welfare. Zenyaku Kogyo provided rituximab and placebo (which they received from Genentech) free of charge. Zenyaku Kogy was responsible for measurement of human antichimeric antibodies and rituximab blood concentrations, which they delegated to Convence. The costs for these measurements was covered by a fund from the Japanese Ministry of Health, Labour and Welfare. This study was presented at Kidney Week 2012 (San Diego, CA, USA) on Nov 3, 2012, and was reported in abstract form. We thank all our patients and their families, the physicians who participated in this study, and Emma Barber for editing assistance.

References
1. Eddy AA, Symons JM. Nephrotic syndrome in childhood. *Lancet* 2003; **362:** 629–39.
2. Schulman SL, Kaiser BA, Polinsky MS, Srinivasan R, Baluarte HJ. Predicting the response to cytotoxic therapy for childhood nephrotic syndrome: superiority of response to corticosteroid therapy over histopathologic patterns. *J Pediatr* 1988; **113:** 996–1001.
3. The Scientific Committee of the Japanese Society for Pediatric Nephrology. The 2005 Japanese Society for Pediatric Nephrology treatment guideline for idiopathic nephrotic syndrome in children. http://www.jspn.jp/pdf/0505guideline.pdf (accessed Nov 20, 2013; in Japanese).
4. Hodson EM, Willis NS, Craig JC. Non-corticosteroid treatment for nephrotic syndrome in children. *Cochrane Database Syst Rev* 2013; **10:** CD002290.
5. Hodson EM, Willis NS, Craig JC. Interventions for idiopathic steroid-resistant nephrotic syndrome in children. *Cochrane Database Syst Rev* 2010; **11:** CD003594.
6. Ishikura K, Ikeda M, Hattori S, et al. Effective and safe treatment with cyclosporine in nephrotic children: a prospective, randomized multicenter trial. *Kidney Int* 2008; **73:** 1167–73.
7. Ishikura K, Yoshikawa N, Hattori S, et al, and Japanese Study Group of Renal Disease in Children. Treatment with microemulsified cyclosporine in children with frequently relapsing nephrotic syndrome. *Nephrol Dial Transplant* 2010; **25:** 3956–62.
8. Hamasaki Y, Yoshikawa N, Hattori S, et al, and the Japanese Study Group of Renal Disease. Cyclosporine and steroid therapy in children with steroid-resistant nephrotic syndrome. *Pediatr Nephrol* 2009; **24:** 2177–85.
9. Inoue Y, Iijima K, Nakamura H, Yoshikawa N. Two-year cyclosporin treatment in children with steroid-dependent nephrotic syndrome. *Pediatr Nephrol* 1999; **13:** 33–38.
10. Iijima K, Hamahira K, Tanaka R, et al. Risk factors for cyclosporine-induced tubulointerstitial lesions in children with minimal change nephrotic syndrome. *Kidney Int* 2002; **61:** 1801–05.
11. Ishikura K, Yoshikawa N, Nakazato H, et al. Two-year follow-up of a prospective clinical trial of ciclosporin for frequently relapsing nephrotic syndrome in children. *Clin J Am Soc Nephrol* 2012; **10:** 1576–83.
12. Benz K, Dötsch J, Rascher W, Stachel D. Change of the course of steroid-dependent nephrotic syndrome after rituximab therapy. *Pediatr Nephrol* 2004; **19:** 794–97.
13. Gilbert RD, Hulse E, Rigden S. Rituximab therapy for steroid-dependent minimal change nephrotic syndrome. *Pediatr Nephrol* 2006; **21:** 1698–700.
14. Guigonis V, Dallocchio A, Baudouin V, et al. Rituximab treatment for severe steroid- or cyclosporine-dependent nephrotic syndrome: a multicentric series of 22 cases. *Pediatr Nephrol* 2008; **23:** 1269–79.
15. Ravani P, Magnasco A, Edefonti A, et al. Short-term effects of rituximab in children with steroid- and calcineurin-dependent nephrotic syndrome: a randomized controlled trial. *Clin J Am Soc Nephrol* 2011; **6:** 1308–15.
16. Ravani P, Ponticelli A, Siciliano C, et al. Rituximab is a safe and effective long-term treatment for children with steroid and calcineurin inhibitor-dependent idiopathic nephrotic syndrome. *Kidney Int* 2013; **84:** 1025–33.
17. Kidney Disease: Improving Global Outcomes. KDIGO clinical practice guideline for glomerulonephritis. June, 2012. http://kdigo.org/home/glomerulonephritis-gn/ (accessed Nov 20, 2013).
18. Kemper MJ, Gellermann J, Habbig S, et al. Long-term follow-up after rituximab for steroid-dependent idiopathic nephrotic syndrome. *Nephrol Dial Transplant* 2012; **27:** 1910–15.
19. Ruggenenti P, Ruggiero B, Cravedi P, et al, for the Rituximab in Nephrotic Syndrome of Steroid-Dependent or Frequently Relapsing Minimal Change Disease Or Focal Segmental Glomerulosclerosis (NEMO) Study Group. Rituximab in steroid-dependent or frequently relapsing idiopathic nephrotic syndrome. *J Am Soc Nephrol* 2014; **25:** 850–63.
20. Kelesidis T, Daikos G, Boumpas D, Tsiodras S. Does rituximab increase the incidence of infectious complications? A narrative review. *Int J Infect Dis* 2011; **15:** e2–16.
21. Buch MH, Smolen JS, Betteridge N, et al, and the Rituximab Consensus Expert Committee. Updated consensus statement on the use of rituximab in patients with rheumatoid arthritis. *Ann Rheum Dis* 2011; **70:** 909–20.
22. Chaumais MC, Garnier A, Chalard F, et al. Fatal pulmonary fibrosis after rituximab administration. *Pediatr Nephrol* 2009; **24:** 1753–55.
23. Sellier-Leclerc AL, Belli E, Guérin V, Dorfmüller P, Deschênes G. Fulminant viral myocarditis after rituximab therapy in pediatric nephrotic syndrome. *Pediatr Nephrol* 2013; **28:** 1875–79.
24. Cravedi P, Ruggenenti P, Sghirlanzoni MC, Remuzzi G. Titrating rituximab to circulating B cells to optimize lymphocytolytic therapy in idiopathic membranous nephropathy. *Clin J Am Soc Nephrol* 2007; **2:** 932–37.
25. Shalhoub RJ. Pathogenesis of lipoid nephrosis: a disorder of T-cell function. *Lancet* 1974; **2:** 556–60.
26. Liu K, Mohan C. Altered B-cell signaling in lupus. *Autoimmun Rev* 2009; **8:** 214–18.
27. Chan OT, Hannum LG, Haberman AM, Madaio MP, Shlomchik MJ. A novel mouse with B cells but lacking serum antibody reveals an antibody-independent role for B cells in murine lupus. *J Exp Med* 1999; **189:** 1639–48.
28. Sfikakis PP, Boletis JN, Lionaki S, et al. Remission of proliferative lupus nephritis following B cell depletion therapy is preceded by down-regulation of the T cell costimulatory molecule CD40 ligand: an open-label trial. *Arthritis Rheum* 2005; **52:** 501–13.
29. Bugatti S, Codullo V, Caporali R, Montecucco C. B cells in rheumatoid arthritis. *Autoimmun Rev* 2007; **7:** 137–42.
30. Maloney DG. Mechanism of action of rituximab. *Anticancer Drugs* 2001; **12** (suppl 2)**:** S1–4.
31. Araya C, Diaz L, Wasserfall C, et al. T regulatory cell function in idiopathic minimal lesion nephrotic syndrome. *Pediatr Nephrol* 2009; **24:** 1691–98.
32. Hashimura Y, Nozu K, Kanegane H, et al. Minimal change nephrotic syndrome associated with immune dysregulation, polyendocrinopathy, enteropathy, X-linked syndrome. *Pediatr Nephrol* 2009; **24:** 1181–86.
33. Le Berre L, Bruneau S, Naulet J, et al. Induction of T regulatory cells attenuates idiopathic nephrotic syndrome. *J Am Soc Nephrol* 2009; **20:** 57–67.
34. Stasi R, Cooper N, Del Poeta G, et al. Analysis of regulatory T-cell changes in patients with idiopathic thrombocytopenic purpura receiving B cell-depleting therapy with rituximab. *Blood* 2008; **112:** 1147–50.
35. Fornoni A, Sageshima J, Wei C, et al. Rituximab targets podocytes in recurrent focal segmental glomerulosclerosis. *Sci Transl Med* 2011; **3:** 85ra46.

課題論文2　Ruff CT, et al：Lancet, 2014 ［循環器疾患］

心房細動患者における新規経口抗凝固薬のワルファリンに対する有効性と安全性の比較：ランダム化試験のメタアナリシス

重要単語（Summaryより）

❶	secondary outcome	副次アウトカム
❷	Medline	（文献データベースの名称）
❸	phase 3, randomised trial	第Ⅲ相ランダム化試験
❹	prespecified meta-analysis	事前に計画を規定したメタアナリシス
❺	main outcome	主要アウトカム
❻	relative risk	相対リスク
❼	95％ CI (confidence interval)	95％信頼区間
❽	subgroup analysis	サブグループ解析
❾	random-effects model	変量効果モデル
❿	test for heterogeneity	不均一性の検定
⓫	p for interaction	交互作用のp値

講義内容

確率分布
- 単変量分布
  - 正規分布
  - 二項分布
  - Poisson分布
  - 指数分布

交絡調整方法
- プロペンシティスコア
- VanderWeele-Shpitserの基準

多変量分布（回帰）
- 線型モデル
- ロジスティック回帰
- 条件付きロジスティック
- Poisson回帰
- Cox回帰*，指数回帰

誤差が階層構造の確率分布
- 変量効果モデル，Bayesモデル

誤差の表示
- 標準偏差
- パーセンタイル
- 標準誤差
- 95％信頼区間

データの型に応じた指標
- 平均
- 平均の差，回帰係数
- 発生リスク
- リスク比，オッズ比
- 発生率
- 発生率比
- 生存曲線，ハザード
- ハザード比

メタアナリシス
- 公表バイアス
- ファンネルプロット
- 不均一性
- リスクオブバイアス評価ツール

ネットワークメタアナリシス
- 直接比較，間接比較
- 間接比較への依存度
- 直接比較と間接比較の一貫性
- ランキングの解釈

仮説検定とp値
- 帰無仮説，対立仮説
- 優越性，非劣性
- 非劣性マージン
- 交互作用の検定
- 片側検定，両側検定
- αエラー，βエラー
- 有意水準
- サンプルサイズ

疫学
- コホート研究
- ケース・コントロール研究
- 比，率，割合
- 交絡
- 誤分類
- バイアスと感度解析

臨床試験
- 主要エンドポイント
- ランダム化
- ITTの原則
- プロトコール逸脱
- 有害事象，副作用
- 中間解析
- サブグループ解析
- GCP，倫理指針
- データの品質管理・保証

＊正確にはセミパラメトリックモデルで，確率分布ではない

Articles

Comparison of the efficacy and safety of new oral anticoagulants with warfarin in patients with atrial fibrillation: a meta-analysis of randomised trials

Christian T Ruff, Robert P Giugliano, Eugene Braunwald, Elaine B Hoffman, Naveen Deenadayalu, Michael D Ezekowitz, A John Camm, Jeffrey I Weitz, Basil S Lewis, Alexander Parkhomenko, Takeshi Yamashita, Elliott M Antman

Summary

Background Four new oral anticoagulants compare favourably with warfarin for stroke prevention in patients with atrial fibrillation; however, the balance between efficacy and safety in subgroups needs better definition. We aimed to assess the relative benefit of new oral anticoagulants in key subgroups, and the effects on important secondary outcomes.

Methods We searched Medline from Jan 1, 2009, to Nov 19, 2013, limiting searches to phase 3, randomised trials of patients with atrial fibrillation who were randomised to receive new oral anticoagulants or warfarin, and trials in which both efficacy and safety outcomes were reported. We did a prespecified meta-analysis of all 71 683 participants included in the RE-LY, ROCKET AF, ARISTOTLE, and ENGAGE AF–TIMI 48 trials. The main outcomes were stroke and systemic embolic events, ischaemic stroke, haemorrhagic stroke, all-cause mortality, myocardial infarction, major bleeding, intracranial haemorrhage, and gastrointestinal bleeding. We calculated relative risks (RRs) and 95% CIs for each outcome. We did subgroup analyses to assess whether differences in patient and trial characteristics affected outcomes. We used a random-effects model to compare pooled outcomes and tested for heterogeneity.

Findings 42 411 participants received a new oral anticoagulant and 29 272 participants received warfarin. New oral anticoagulants significantly reduced stroke or systemic embolic events by 19% compared with warfarin (RR 0·81, 95% CI 0·73–0·91; p<0·0001), mainly driven by a reduction in haemorrhagic stroke (0·49, 0·38–0·64; p<0·0001). New oral anticoagulants also significantly reduced all-cause mortality (0·90, 0·85–0·95; p=0·0003) and intracranial haemorrhage (0·48, 0·39–0·59; p<0·0001), but increased gastrointestinal bleeding (1·25, 1·01–1·55; p=0·04). We noted no heterogeneity for stroke or systemic embolic events in important subgroups, but there was a greater relative reduction in major bleeding with new oral anticoagulants when the centre-based time in therapeutic range was less than 66% than when it was 66% or more (0·69, 0·59–0·81 vs 0·93, 0·76–1·13; p for interaction 0·022). Low-dose new oral anticoagulant regimens showed similar overall reductions in stroke or systemic embolic events to warfarin (1·03, 0·84–1·27; p=0·74), and a more favourable bleeding profile (0·65, 0·43–1·00; p=0·05), but significantly more ischaemic strokes (1·28, 1·02–1·60; p=0·045).

Interpretation This meta-analysis is the first to include data for all four new oral anticoagulants studied in the pivotal phase 3 clinical trials for stroke prevention or systemic embolic events in patients with atrial fibrillation. New oral anticoagulants had a favourable risk–benefit profile, with significant reductions in stroke, intracranial haemorrhage, and mortality, and with similar major bleeding as for warfarin, but increased gastrointestinal bleeding. The relative efficacy and safety of new oral anticoagulants was consistent across a wide range of patients. Our findings offer clinicians a more comprehensive picture of the new oral anticoagulants as a therapeutic option to reduce the risk of stroke in this patient population.

Funding None.

Introduction

Atrial fibrillation, the most common sustained cardiac arrhythmia, predisposes patients to an increased risk of embolic stroke and has a higher mortality than sinus rhythm.[1,2] Until 2009, warfarin and other vitamin K antagonists were the only class of oral anticoagulants available. Although these drugs are highly effective in prevention of thromboembolism, their use is limited by a narrow therapeutic index that necessitates frequent monitoring and dose adjustments resulting in substantial risk and inconvenience. This limitation has translated into poor patient adherence and probably contributes to the systematic underuse of vitamin K antagonists for stroke prevention.[3,4]

Several new oral anticoagulants have been developed that dose-dependently inhibit thrombin or activated factor X (factor Xa) and offer potential advantages over vitamin K antagonists, such as rapid onset and offset of action, absence of an effect of dietary vitamin K intake on their activity, and fewer drug interactions. The

Lancet 2014; 383: 955–62

Published Online
December 4, 2013
http://dx.doi.org/10.1016/
S0140-6736(13)62343-0

See **Comment** page 931

Brigham and Women's Hospital and Harvard Medical School, Boston, MA, USA (C T Ruff MD, R P Giugliano MD, Prof E Braunwald MD, E B Hoffman PhD, N Deenadayalu MPH, Prof E M Antman MD); **Jefferson Medical College, Philadelphia, PA, and Cardiovascular Research Foundation, New York, NY, USA** (Prof M D Ezekowitz MBChB); **St George's University, London, UK** (Prof A J Camm MD); **McMaster University and the Thrombosis and Atherosclerosis Research Institute, Hamilton, ON, Canada** (Prof J I Wetiz MD); **Lady Davis Carmel Medical Center, Haifa, Israel** (Prof B S Lewis MD); **Institute of Cardiology, Kiev, Ukraine** (Prof A Parkhomenko MD); **and The Cardiovascular Institute, Tokyo, Japan** (Prof T Yamashita MD)

Correspondence to:
Dr Christian T Ruff, Thrombolysis in Myocardial Infarction (TIMI) Study Group, 350 Longwood Avenue, 1st Floor Offices, Boston, MA 02115, USA
cruff@partners.org

predictable anticoagulant effects of the new anticoagulants enable the administration of fixed doses without the need for routine coagulation monitoring, thereby simplifying treatment. Individually, new oral anticoagulants are at least as safe and effective as warfarin for prevention of stroke and systemic embolism in patients with atrial fibrillation.[5–8] Dabigatran, rivaroxaban, and apixaban have been approved by regulatory authorities, whereas edoxaban has completed late-stage clinical assessment.

Although previously published meta-analyses have been done of trials comparing new oral anticoagulants with warfarin in patients with atrial fibrillation,[9–13] this analysis is the first to include data from the Effective Anticoagulation with Factor Xa Next Generation in Atrial Fibrillation–Thrombolysis In Myocardial Infarction study 48 (ENGAGE AF-TIMI 48)[8,14] with edoxaban, the largest of the four trials. All four trials were powered to address their primary endpoints; however, the balance between efficacy and safety in important clinical subgroups needs better definition. We aimed to enhance precision in assessment of the relative benefit of new oral anticoagulants in key subgroups, and the effects of these drugs on important secondary outcomes, to offer clinicians a more comprehensive picture of the new oral anticoagulants as a therapeutic option to reduce the risk of stroke in patients with atrial fibrillation.

Methods
Study selection

We undertook a prespecified analysis of the four phase 3, randomised trials comparing the efficacy and safety of new oral anticoagulants with warfarin for stroke prevention in patients with atrial fibrillation: Randomized Evaluation of Long Term Anticoagulation Therapy (RE-LY; dabigatran),[5] Rivaroxaban Once Daily Oral Direct Factor Xa Inhibition Compared with Vitamin K Antagonism for Prevention of Stroke and Embolism Trial in Atrial Fibrillation (ROCKET AF),[6] Apixaban for Reduction in Stroke and Other Thromboembolic Events in Atrial Fibrillation (ARISTOTLE),[7] and the ENGAGE AF–TIMI 48 study (edoxaban).[8]

	RE-LY[5]			ROCKET-AF[6]		ARISTOTLE[7]		ENGAGE AF-TIMI 48[8]			Combined	
	Dabigatran 150 mg (n=6076)	Dabigatran 110 mg (n=6015)	Warfarin (n=6022)	Rivaroxaban (n=7131)	Warfarin (n=7133)	Apixaban (n=9120)	Warfarin (n=9081)	Edoxaban 60 mg (n=7035)	Edoxaban 30 mg (n=7034)	Warfarin (n=7036)	NOAC (n=42 411)	Warfarin (n=29 272)
Age (years)	71·5 (8·8)	71·4 (8·6)	71·6 (8·6)	73 (65–78)	73 (65–78)	70 (63–76)	70 (63–76)	72 (64–68)	72 (64–78)	72 (64–78)	71·6	71·5
≥75 years	40%	38%	39%	43%	43%	31%	31%	41%	40%	40%	38%	38%
Women	37%	36%	37%	40%	40%	36%	35%	39%	39%	38%	38%	37%
Atrial fibrillation type												
Persistent or permanent	67%	68%	66%	81%	81%	85%	84%	75%	74%	75%	76%	77%
Paroxysmal	33%	32%	34%	18%	18%	15%	16%	25%	26%	25%	24%	22%
CHADS2*	2·2 (1·2)	2·1 (1·1)	2·1 (1·1)	3·5 (0·94)	3·5 (0·95)	2·1 (1·1)	2·1 (1·1)	2·8 (0·97)	2·8 (0·97)	2·8 (0·98)	2·6 (1·0)	2·6 (1·0)
0–1	32%	33%	31%	0	0	34%	34%	<1%	<1%	<1%	17%	17%
2	35%	35%	37%	13%	13%	36%	36%	46%	47%	47%	35%	33%
3–6	33%	33%	32%	87%	87%	30%	30%	54%	53%	53%	48%	50%
Previous stroke or TIA*	20%	20%	20%	55%	55%	19%	18%	28%	29%	28%	29%	30%
Heart failure†	32%	32%	32%	63%	62%	36%	35%	58%	57%	58%	46%	47%
Diabetes	23%	23%	23%	40%	40%	25%	25%	36%	36%	36%	31%	31%
Hypertension	79%	79%	79%	90%	91%	87%	88%	94%	94%	94%	88%	88%
Prior myocardial infarction	17%	17%	16%	17%	18%	15%	14%	11%	12%	12%	15%	15%
Creatinine clearance‡												
<50 mL/min	19%	19%	19%	21%	21%	17%	17%	20%	19%	19%	19%	19%
50–80 mL/min	48%	49%	49%	47%	48%	42%	42%	43%	44%	44%	45%	45%
>80 mL/min	32%	32%	32%	32%	31%	41%	41%	38%	38%	37%	36%	36%
Previous VKA use§	50%	50%	49%	62%	63%	57%	57%	59%	59%	59%	57%	57%
Aspirin at baseline	39%	40%	41%	36%	37%	31%	31%	29%	29%	30%	34%	34%
Median follow-up (years)¶	2·0	2·0	2·0	1·9	1·9	1·8	1·8	2·8	2·8	2·8	2·2	2·2
Individual median TTR	NA	NA	67 (54–78)	NA	58 (43–71)	NA	66 (52–77)	NA	NA	68 (57–77)	NA	65 (51–76)

Data are mean (SD), median (IQR), or percent, unless otherwise indicated. NOAC=new oral anticoagulant. CHADS₂=stroke risk factor scoring system in which one point is given for history of congestive heart failure, hypertension, age ≥75 years, and diabetes, and two points are given for history of stroke or transient ischaemic attack. TIA=transient ischaemic attack. VKA=vitamin K antagonist. TTR=time in therapeutic range. NA=not available. *ROCKET-AF and ARISTOTLE included patients with systemic embolism. †ROCKET-AF included patients with left ventricular ejection fraction <35%; ARISTOTLE included those with left ventricular ejection fraction<40%. ‡RE-LY <50 mL/min, 50–79 mL/min, ≥80 mL/min; ARISTOTLE ≤50 mL/min, >50–80 mL/min, >80 mL/min. §RE-LY, ARISTOTLE, and ENGAGE AF-TIMI 48 patients who used VKAs for ≥61 days; ROCKET AF patients who used VKAs for ≥6 weeks at time of screening. ¶IQRs not available.

Table: Baseline characteristics of the intention-to-treat populations of the included trials

Statistical analysis

We obtained information about the following outcomes from the main trial publications, supplemental appendices, and relevant subsequent analyses:[5–8,15–23] stroke and systemic embolic events, ischaemic stroke, haemorrhagic stroke, all-cause mortality, myocardial infarction, major bleeding, intracranial haemorrhage (including haemorrhagic stroke, epidural, subdural, and subarachnoid haemorrhage), and gastrointestinal bleeding. When possible, we did analyses with the intention-to-treat population for efficacy outcomes and with the safety population for bleeding outcomes. In RE-LY[5] and ENGAGE AF–TIMI 48,[8] two doses of dabigatran and edoxaban, respectively, were compared with warfarin. Rather than combining data with both doses into one meta-analysis, which would merge the benefit and risk of different doses, potentially compromising interpretability, we undertook a meta-analysis with both higher doses (dabigatran 150 mg twice daily for RE-LY and edoxaban 60 mg once daily for ENGAGE AF–TIMI 48) combined with the single doses studied in ROCKET AF[6] (rivaroxaban 20 mg once daily) and ARISTOTLE[7] (5 mg twice daily). In a separate analysis we undertook a meta-analysis of the two lower doses (dabigatran 110 mg twice daily for RE-LY and edoxaban 30 mg once daily for ENGAGE AF–TIMI 48). We did two sensitivity analyses including a meta-analysis of only the factor Xa inhibitors, with removal of the thrombin inhibitor dabigatran, and an analysis combining all doses of all drugs (both high and low doses of dabigatran and edoxaban with rivaroxaban and apixaban). We did not use any data from phase 2 dose-ranging studies because of their small sample size and short follow-up, which precluded comparable ascertainment for all the outcomes analysed.

We calculated relative risks (RRs) and corresponding 95% CIs for each outcome and trial separately and checked findings against published data for accuracy. When necessary, we calculated numbers of outcome events on the basis of event rates, sample size, and duration of follow-up. Outcomes were then pooled and compared with a random-effects model.[24] We assessed the appropriateness of pooling of data across studies with use of the Cochran Q statistic and I^2 test for heterogeneity.[25]

We assessed comparative efficacy and safety for stroke or systemic embolic events and for major bleeding (the primary efficacy and safety outcomes) in important clinical subgroups: age (<75 vs ≥75 years), sex, history of previous stroke or transient ischaemic attack, history of diabetes, renal function (creatinine clearance <50 mL/min, 50–80 mL/min, >80 mL/min), $CHADS_2$ risk score (0–1, 2, 3–6), vitamin K antagonist status at study entry (naive or experienced), and centre-based time in therapeutic range (threshold of <66% vs ≥66%). The centre-based time in therapeutic range is the mean time in therapeutic range at each enrolling centre achieved in its patients randomised to warfarin. The range is used as a surrogate of the quality of control of international normalised ratio for all the patients receiving warfarin at that site. All four of the trials reported the centre-based time in therapeutic range achieved in their respective warfarin groups by quartiles. We selected our threshold of centre-based time in therapeutic range because RE-LY, ROCKET AF, and ARISTOTLE all had a quartile boundary near 66% and because the threshold differentiates the efficacy and safety of oral anticoagulants from dual antiplatelet therapy.[6,16,22] Because we had access to the clinical database in ENGAGE AF–TIMI 48, we could run this analysis at a threshold of 66%. We did all analyses with Comprehensive Meta-Analysis software (version 2).

Role of the funding source

There was no funding source for this study. All authors had full access to all the data in the study and had final responsibility for the decision to submit for publication.

Results

42 411 participants received a new oral anticoagulant and 29 272 participants received warfarin. The table shows baseline characteristics for each study. The average age of patients was similar between trials as was the proportion of women recruited (table). However, the underlying risk for stroke differed significantly across the trials as shown by the proportion of patients with $CHADS_2$ scores of 3–6 (table). Median follow-up ranged from 1·8 years to 2·8 years and the median time in

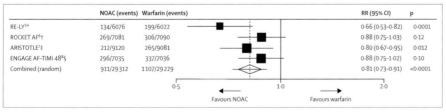

	NOAC (events)	Warfarin (events)		RR (95% CI)	p
RE-LY[5]*	134/6076	199/6022		0·66 (0·53–0·82)	0·0001
ROCKET AF[6]†	269/7081	306/7090		0·88 (0·75–1·03)	0·12
ARISTOTLE[7]‡	212/9120	265/9081		0·80 (0·67–0·95)	0·012
ENGAGE AF-TIMI 48[8]§	296/7035	337/7036		0·88 (0·75–1·02)	0·10
Combined (random)	911/29 312	1107/29 229		0·81 (0·73–0·91)	<0·0001

Figure 1: Stroke or systemic embolic events
Data are n/N, unless otherwise indicated. Heterogeneity: I^2=47%; p=0·13. NOAC=new oral anticoagulant. RR=risk ratio. *Dabigatran 150 mg twice daily. †Rivaroxaban 20 mg once daily. ‡Apixaban 5 mg twice daily. §Edoxaban 60 mg once daily.

therapeutic range in patients in the warfarin groups ranged from 58% to 68% (table).

Figure 1 shows the comparative efficacy of high-dose of new oral anticoagulants and warfarin. Allocation to a new oral anticoagulant significantly reduced the composite of stroke or systemic embolic events by 19% compared with warfarin (figure 1). The benefit was mainly driven by a large reduction in haemorrhagic stroke (figure 2). New oral anticoagulants were also associated with a significant reduction in all-cause mortality (figure 2). The drugs were similar to warfarin in the prevention of ischaemic stroke and myocardial infarction (figure 2).

Randomisation to a high-dose new oral anticoagulant was associated with a 14% non-significant reduction in major bleeding (figure 3). In line with the reduction in haemorrhagic stroke, a substantial reduction in intracranial haemorrhage was observed, which included haemorrhagic stroke, and subdural, epidural, and subarachnoid bleeding (figure 2). New oral anticoagulants were, however, associated with increased gastrointestinal bleeding (figure 2).

The benefit of new oral anticoagulants compared with warfarin in reducing stroke or systemic embolic events was consistent across all subgroups examined (figure 4). The safety of new oral anticoagulants compared with warfarin was generally consistent for the reduction of major bleeding across subgroups, with the exception of a significant interaction for centre-based time in therapeutic range (figure 4). We noted a greater relative reduction in bleeding with new oral anticoagulants at centres that achieved a centre-based time in therapeutic range of less than 66% than at those achieving a time in therapeutic range of 66% or more (figure 4).

The low-dose new oral anticoagulant regimens had similar efficacy to warfarin for the composite of stroke or systemic embolic events (appendix). When differentiated by stroke type, the low-dose regimens were associated with an increase in ischaemic stroke compared with warfarin, which was balanced by a large decrease in haemorrhagic stroke (appendix). Similar to the higher-dose regimens, the low doses showed a significant reduction in all-cause mortality (appendix). Significantly more myocardial infarctions were reported with the low-dose regimens than with warfarin (appendix). The low-dose regimens were associated with a non-significant reduction in major bleeding, but with a significant reduction in intracranial haemorrhage. Gastrointestinal bleeding was similar between low-dose new oral anticoagulants and warfarin (appendix).

A meta-analysis of only the factor Xa inhibitors, with removal of dabigatran, showed similar results to the

See **Online** for appendix

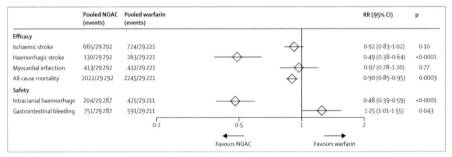

Figure 2: Secondary efficacy and safety outcomes
Data are n/N, unless otherwise indicated. Heterogeneity: ischaemic stroke I^2=32%, p=0·22; haemorrhagic stroke I^2=34%, p=0·21; myocardial infarction I^2=48%, p=0·13; all-cause mortality I^2=0%, p=0·81; intracranial haemorrhage I^2=32%, p=0·22; gastrointestinal bleeding I^2=74%, p=0·009. NOAC=new oral anticoagulant. RR=risk ratio.

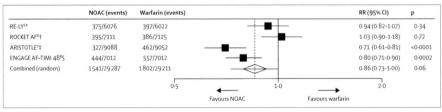

Figure 3: Major bleeding
Data are n/N, unless otherwise indicated. Heterogeneity: I^2=83%; p=0·001. NOAC=new oral anticoagulant. RR=risk ratio. *Dabigatran 150 mg twice daily. †Rivaroxaban 20 mg once daily. ‡Apixaban 5 mg twice daily. §Edoxaban 60 mg once daily.

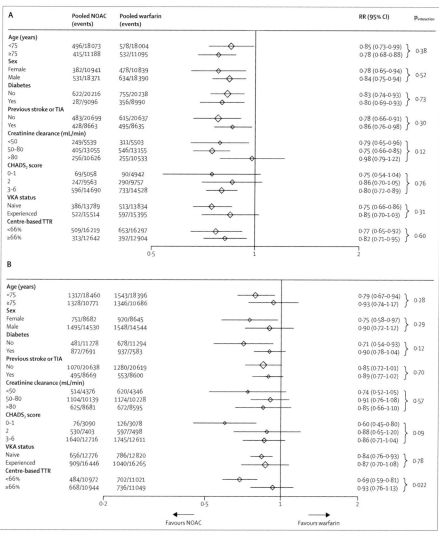

Figure 4: Stroke or systemic embolic events subgroups (A) and major bleeding subgroups (B)
Data are n/N, unless otherwise indicated. No data available from RE-LY for the following major bleeding subgroups: sex, creatinine clearance, diabetes, and CHADS$_2$ score. For ROCKET AF no major bleeding data available in the TTR and diabetes subgroup and major and non-major clinically relevant bleeding was used for subgroups of age, sex, CHADS$_2$ score, and creatinine clearance. NOAC=new oral anticoagulant. RR=risk ratio. TIA=transient ischaemic attack. VKA=vitamin K antagonist. TTR=time in therapeutic range

main meta-analysis for both stroke or systemic embolic events and major bleeding (appendix). An additional analysis was done combining all doses of all drugs in one meta-analysis (including both high and low doses of dabigatran and edoxaban with rivaroxaban and apixaban; appendix). Inclusion of low doses of dabigatran and edoxaban decreased the magnitude of the reduction in risk of stroke or systemic embolic events with new oral anticoagulants and resulted in less bleeding than warfarin (appendix).

Discussion

Our results show that stroke and systemic embolic events were significantly reduced in patients receiving new oral anticoagulants. This benefit was mainly driven by substantial protection against haemorrhagic stroke, which was reduced by half. Conceptually, haemorrhagic stroke is a complication of anticoagulant treatment even though it is part of the overall efficacy assessment of these drugs. Importantly, overall intracranial haemorrhage (which includes haemorrhagic stroke) was reduced by roughly half, which represents a substantial benefit of treatment with new oral anticoagulants. Intracranial haemorrhage is a feared and often fatal complication of anticoagulant treatment and about one in six first hospital admissions for this disorder are related to such treatment.[26] For the prevention of ischaemic stroke, the new oral anticoagulants had similar efficacy to warfarin, which itself is very effective in this regard and reduces ischaemic stroke by two-thirds compared with placebo.[27] In general, the new oral anticoagulants had a favourable safety profile compared with warfarin; however, they were associated with an increase in gastrointestinal bleeding. They were also associated with a significant reduction in all cause-mortality compared with warfarin.

A separate analysis of the two low-dose new oral anticoagulant regimens showed that although they have a similar efficacy to warfarin for protection against all stroke or systemic embolic events, they are not as effective for protection against ischaemic stroke in particular. However, they do have a safer profile than warfarin and preserve the mortality benefit noted with the high-dose regimens. Consequently, low-dose regimens might be an appealing option for frail patients or for those who have a high risk for bleeding with full-dose anticoagulation.

A criticism of meta-analyses in this specialty is that the large phase 3 trials for stroke prevention in patients with atrial fibrillation were well powered to evaluate the main treatment effect of their individual drug to reduce the risk of stroke or systemic embolic events compared with warfarin. However, most trials are underpowered to detect differences in secondary outcomes and subgroups. An example is the analysis of all-cause mortality; only apixaban and low-dose edoxaban were associated with significant reductions in all cause-mortality, yet the point estimates for the hazard ratios for all drugs (and doses) are very similar. The results of the meta-analysis support the premise that compared with warfarin, the new oral anticoagulants, as a class, reduce all-cause mortality by about 10% in the populations enrolled in the clinical trials.

Perhaps, more important than the provision of robust estimates of secondary outcomes is the ability of meta-analyses to enhance precision in assessment of the relative benefits of new oral anticoagulants in important, clinically relevant subgroups. Both risk of stroke and bleeding vary significantly across the range of patients with atrial fibrillation. For example, vulnerable populations, such as elderly people (aged ≥75 years),[28] patients with a previous history of stroke,[29,30] and those with renal dysfunction,[31,32] have an increased risk of both ischaemic and bleeding events. Inclusion of these individuals in trials is variable and they are often underrepresented. Consequently, each trial alone can only offer partial reassurance that the overall balance of efficacy and safety is preserved in these high-risk groups. For example, variations in the proportion of participants with a $CHADS_2$ score of 3–6 were mainly attributable to differential enrolment of patients with previous stroke or transient ischaemic attack.[33] This robust meta-analysis is the first to show that the relative efficacy and safety of new oral anticoagulants is consistent across a broad range of vulnerable patients (panel).

We investigated whether the benefit of new oral anticoagulants was dependent on whether patients had experience with use of vitamin K antagonists before enrolment in the trial. Previous findings suggested that patients with little to no prior exposure to vitamin K antagonists (ie, naive) had a higher risk of both ischaemic and bleeding events than experienced patients.[34] A concern has remained that new oral anticoagulants might have reduced benefit in experienced patients who have shown an ability to tolerate treatment with vitamin K antagonists. The results of our meta-analysis show that the benefit of new oral anticoagulants is consistent irrespective of a patient's history with vitamin K antagonists.

We also investigated whether the benefit of new oral anticoagulants was dependent on how well warfarin was managed during the trial, as assessed by the centre-based time in therapeutic range.[35,36] In the ACTIVE W trial,[37] anticoagulant treatment had no significant benefit compared with clopidogrel plus aspirin in centres with a centre-based time in therapeutic range that was less than

---

Panel: Research in context

Systematic review
We searched Medline from Jan 1, 2009 to Nov 19, 2013. Keywords were "atrial fibrillation", "dabigatran", "rivaroxaban", "apixaban", "edoxaban", "oral factor Xa inhibitor", "oral thrombin inhibitor", and "warfarin". We also did a search of ClinicalTrials.gov to identify relevant ongoing clinical studies. We restricted our analysis to phase 3, randomised trials that included patients with atrial fibrillation who were randomly assigned to receive new oral anticoagulants or warfarin, and trials in which both efficacy and safety outcomes were reported. We assessed the quality of identified studies to ensure minimisation of bias. No formal scoring system was used to assess the quality of the evidence.

Interpretation
This meta-analysis is the first to include results from all four new oral anticoagulants studied in the pivotal phase 3 clinical trials for stroke prevention in patients with atrial fibrillation. New oral anticoagulants showed a favourable risk-benefit profile with significant reductions in stroke, intracranial haemorrhage, and mortality with similar major bleeding as warfarin, but increased gastrointestinal bleeding. The relative efficacy and safety of the anticoagulants was consistent across a wide range of patients with atrial fibrillation. Our findings offer clinicians a more comprehensive picture of the new oral anticoagulants as a therapeutic option to reduce the risk of stroke in this patient population.

the median of 65%, whereas a reduction of more than two times was reported for vascular events in centres with a time in therapeutic range of more than 65%. The trials included in this meta-analysis had varying success in management of warfarin (median time in therapeutic range 58–68%), and although they reported no heterogeneity in the results across their trial-specific quartiles,[6,16,22] each trial was underpowered to detect a difference. In this meta-analysis, we examined a threshold of 66% for centre-based time in therapeutic range, which is similar to that used in the ACTIVE W analysis. We showed that the reduction in stroke or systemic embolism compared with warfarin is not dependent on how well warfarin is managed, within the limitations of analyses based on centre-based time in therapeutic range. However, an even more pronounced relative reduction in bleeding with new oral anticoagulants seems to take place in patients who have difficulty maintaining a therapeutic international normalised ratio.

Because we did not have individual participant data for all the trials, our statistical approach was done at a study level. We pooled the data for the factor Xa inhibitors (rivaroxaban, apixaban, edoxaban) and the thrombin inhibitor (dabigatran). Although these drugs inhibit different coagulation factors, we believe that pooling of the results is justified for several reasons: the drugs are all specific inhibitors of important factors in the coagulation cascade, the phase 3 warfarin-controlled trials of all four drugs are qualitatively similar in design, published guidelines refer to these drugs together as new oral anticoagulants, and previous meta-analyses have taken a similar approach. Additionally, sensitivity analyses removing dabigatran and including only factor Xa inhibitors showed similar results. Important differences also exist in drugs, patient demographics, and trial characteristics that might affect outcomes not accounted for in this analysis. We noted statistical heterogeneity across the trials with respect to major bleeding and gastrointestinal bleeding, which could show true differences across trials or between drugs. However, some heterogeneity is expected to be reported in large meta-analyses, and complete uniformity can show consistency in bias rather than consistency in real effects.[38] Use of a random-effects model and the robustness of the data across important clinical subgroups can help mitigate the potential effect of heterogeneity on the validity of the results. We included data from only clinical trials, which could affect the generalisability of the results because patients in clinical trials are often thought to be at lower risk for adverse events than are those in routine clinical practice.[39] However, post-approval experience with the new oral anticoagulants has approximated what was noted in the clinical trial population. For example, in a nationwide cohort study in Denmark with dabigatran, the first approved new oral anticoagulant, no excess of events in a clinical practice was reported compared with what was shown in the RE-LY trial.[40]

In summary, the new oral anticogulants show a favourable balance between efficacy and safety compared with warfarin, which is consistent across a wide range of patients with atrial fibrillation known to be at high risk for both ischaemic and bleeding events.

Contributors
CTR wrote the first draft of the manuscript; all authors contributed to subsequent drafts. CTR, ND, and EBH undertook the statistical analyses.

Conflicts of interest
CTR has served as a consultant and has received honoraria from Daiichi Sankyo, Boehringer Ingelheim, and Bristol-Myers Squibb. RPG has served as a consultant and has received honoraria from Bristol-Myers Squibb, Janssen, Daiichi Sankyo, Merck, Sanofi, and is a member of the TIMI Study Group, which has received research grant support from Daiichi Sankyo, Johnson & Johnson, and Merck. EB has riecived grants and personal fees for lectures from Daiichi Sankyo; grants from Duke University, AstraZeneca, Johnson & Johnson, Merck & Co, Sanofi-Aventis, GlaxoSmith Kline, Bristol-Myers Squibb, Beckman Coulter, Roche Diagnostics, and Pfizer; uncompensated personal fees for consultancy from Merck & Co; personal fees for consultancies from Genzyme, Amorcyte, Medicines Co, CardioRentis, and Sanofi-Aventis; uncompensated personal fees for lectures from Merck and CVRx; and personal fees for lectures from Eli Lilly, Menarini International, Medscape, and Bayer outside the submitted work. MDE has served as a consultant and has received honoraria from Boehringer Ingelheim, Bayer, Johnson & Johnson, Janssen, Bristol-Myers Squibb, Pfizer, Daiichi Sankyo, Sanofi, Portola, Medtronics, Aegerion, Merck, Gilead, and Pozen. AJC has served as a consultant and has received honoraria from Boehringer Ingelheim, Bayer, Bristol-Myers Squibb, Pfizer, and Daiichi Sankyo. JIW has served as a consultant and has received honoraria from Boehringer Ingelheim, Bayer, Janssen, Bristol-Myers Squibb, Pfizer, and Daiichi Sankyo. BSL has served as a consultant to Bayer, Bristol-Myers Squibb, and Pfizer and received research grants in these trials from Boehringer Ingelheim, Bayer, Bristol-Myers Squibb, Pfizer, and Daiichi Sankyo. AP has received a research grant from Daiichi Sankyo, Boehringer Ingelheim, Bayer, Bristol-Myers Squibb. TY has received honoraria from Boehringer Ingelheim, Bayer, Bristol-Myers Squibb, Pfizer, and Daiichi Sankyo. EMA has received a research grant from Daiichi Sankyo. All other authors declare that they have no conflicts of interest.

References
1. Camm AJ, Kirchhof P, Lip GY, et al, and the European Heart Rhythm Association, and the European Association for Cardio-Thoracic Surgery. Guidelines for the management of atrial fibrillation: the Task Force for the Management of Atrial Fibrillation of the European Society of Cardiology (ESC). *Eur Heart J* 2010; **31:** 2369–429.
2. Hylek EM, Go AS, Chang Y, et al. Effect of intensity of oral anticoagulation on stroke severity and mortality in atrial fibrillation. *N Engl J Med* 2003; **349:** 1019–26.
3. Birman-Deych E, Radford MJ, Nilasena DS, Gage BF. Use and effectiveness of warfarin in Medicare beneficiaries with atrial fibrillation. *Stroke* 2006; **37:** 1070–74.
4. Hylek EM, Evans-Molina C, Shea C, Henault LE, Regan S. Major hemorrhage and tolerability of warfarin in the first year of therapy among elderly patients with atrial fibrillation. *Circulation* 2007; **115:** 2689–96.
5. Connolly SJ, Ezekowitz MD, Yusuf S, et al, and the RE-LY Steering Committee and Investigators. Dabigatran versus warfarin in patients with atrial fibrillation. *N Engl J Med* 2009; **361:** 1139–51.
6. Patel MR, Mahaffey KW, Garg J, et al, and the ROCKET AF Investigators. Rivaroxaban versus warfarin in nonvalvular atrial fibrillation. *N Engl J Med* 2011; **365:** 883–91.
7. Granger CB, Alexander JH, McMurray JJ, et al, and the ARISTOTLE Committees and Investigators. Apixaban versus warfarin in patients with atrial fibrillation. *N Engl J Med* 2011; **365:** 981–92.
8. Giugliano RP, Ruff CT, Braunwald E, et al. Once-daily edoxaban versus warfarin in patients with atrial fibrillation. *N Engl J Med* 2013; **369:** 2093–104.

9 Dentali F, Riva N, Crowther M, Turpie AG, Lip GY, Ageno W. Efficacy and safety of the novel oral anticoagulants in atrial fibrillation: a systematic review and meta-analysis of the literature. *Circulation* 2012; **126:** 2381–91.
10 Baker WL, Phung OJ. Systematic review and adjusted indirect comparison meta-analysis of oral anticoagulants in atrial fibrillation. *Circ Cardiovasc Qual Outcomes* 2012; **5:** 711–19.
11 Lip GY, Larsen TB, Skjøth F, Rasmussen LH. Indirect comparisons of new oral anticoagulant drugs for efficacy and safety when used for stroke prevention in atrial fibrillation. *J Am Coll Cardiol* 2012; **60:** 738–46.
12 Dogliotti A, Paolasso E, Giugliano RP. Novel oral anticoagulants in atrial fibrillation: a meta-analysis of large, randomized, controlled trials vs warfarin. *Clin Cardiol* 2013; **36:** 61–67.
13 Miller CS, Grandi SM, Shimony A, Filion KB, Eisenberg MJ. Meta-analysis of efficacy and safety of new oral anticoagulants (dabigatran, rivaroxaban, apixaban) versus warfarin in patients with atrial fibrillation. *Am J Cardiol* 2012; **110:** 453–60.
14 Ruff CT, Giugliano RP, Antman EM, et al. Evaluation of the novel factor Xa inhibitor edoxaban compared with warfarin in patients with atrial fibrillation: design and rationale for the Effective aNticoaGulation with factor xA next GEneration in Atrial Fibrillation-Thrombolysis In Myocardial Infarction study 48 (ENGAGE AF-TIMI 48). *Am Heart J* 2010; **160:** 635–41.
15 Connolly SJ, Ezekowitz MD, Yusuf S, Reilly PA, Wallentin L, and the Randomized Evaluation of Long-Term Anticoagulation Therapy Investigators. Newly identified events in the RE-LY trial. *N Engl J Med* 2010; **363:** 1875–76.
16 Wallentin L, Yusuf S, Ezekowitz MD, et al, and the RE-LY investigators. Efficacy and safety of dabigatran compared with warfarin at different levels of international normalised ratio control for stroke prevention in atrial fibrillation: an analysis of the RE-LY trial. *Lancet* 2010; **376:** 975–83.
17 Ezekowitz MD, Wallentin L, Connolly SJ, et al, and the RE-LY Steering Committee and Investigators. Dabigatran and warfarin in vitamin K antagonist-naive and -experienced cohorts with atrial fibrillation. *Circulation* 2010; **122:** 2246–53.
18 Eikelboom JW, Wallentin L, Connolly SJ, et al. Risk of bleeding with 2 doses of dabigatran compared with warfarin in older and younger patients with atrial fibrillation: an analysis of the randomized evaluation of long-term anticoagulant therapy (RE-LY) trial. *Circulation* 2011; **123:** 2363–72.
19 Diener HC, Connolly SJ, Ezekowitz MD, et al, and the RE-LY study group. Dabigatran compared with warfarin in patients with atrial fibrillation and previous transient ischaemic attack or stroke: a subgroup analysis of the RE-LY trial. *Lancet Neurol* 2010; **9:** 1157–63.
20 Mahaffey KW, Wojdyla D, Hankey GJ, et al. Clinical outcomes with rivaroxaban in patients transitioned from vitamin K antagonist therapy: a subgroup analysis of a randomized trial. *Ann Intern Med* 2013; **158:** 861–68.
21 Hankey GJ, Patel MR, Stevens SR, et al, and the ROCKET AF Steering Committee Investigators. Rivaroxaban compared with warfarin in patients with atrial fibrillation and previous stroke or transient ischaemic attack: a subgroup analysis of ROCKET AF. *Lancet Neurol* 2012; **11:** 315–22.
22 Wallentin L, Lopes RD, Hanna M, et al, and the Apixaban for Reduction in Stroke and Other Thromboembolic Events in Atrial Fibrillation (ARISTOTLE) Investigators. Efficacy and safety of apixaban compared with warfarin at different levels of predicted international normalized ratio control for stroke prevention in atrial fibrillation. *Circulation* 2013; **127:** 2166–76.
23 Hohnloser SH, Hijazi Z, Thomas L, et al. Efficacy of apixaban when compared with warfarin in relation to renal function in patients with atrial fibrillation: insights from the ARISTOTLE trial. *Eur Heart J* 2012; **33:** 2821–30.
24 DerSimonian R, Laird N. Meta-analysis in clinical trials. *Control Clin Trials* 1986; **7:** 177–88.

25 Higgins JP, Thompson SG, Deeks JJ, Altman DG. Measuring inconsistency in meta-analyses. *BMJ* 2003; **327:** 557–60.
26 Flaherty ML, Kissela B, Woo D, et al. The increasing incidence of anticoagulant-associated intracerebral hemorrhage. *Neurology* 2007; **68:** 116–21.
27 Hart RG, Pearce LA, Aguilar MI. Meta-analysis: antithrombotic therapy to prevent stroke in patients who have nonvalvular atrial fibrillation. *Ann Intern Med* 2007; **146:** 857–67.
28 Hughes M, Lip GY, and the Guideline Development Group, National Clinical Guideline for Management of Atrial Fibrillation in Primary and Secondary Care, National Institute for Health and Clinical Excellence. Stroke and thromboembolism in atrial fibrillation: a systematic review of stroke risk factors, risk stratification schema and cost effectiveness data. *Thromb Haemost* 2008; **99:** 295–304.
29 Stroke Risk in Atrial Fibrillation Working Group. Independent predictors of stroke in patients with atrial fibrillation: a systematic review. *Neurology* 2007; **69:** 546–54.
30 Pisters R, Lane DA, Nieuwlaat R, de Vos CB, Crijns HJ, Lip GY. A novel user-friendly score (HAS-BLED) to assess 1-year risk of major bleeding in patients with atrial fibrillation: the Euro Heart Survey. *Chest* 2010; **138:** 1093–100.
31 Go AS, Fang MC, Udaltsova N, et al, and the ATRIA Study Investigators. Impact of proteinuria and glomerular filtration rate on risk of thromboembolism in atrial fibrillation: the anticoagulation and risk factors in atrial fibrillation (ATRIA) study. *Circulation* 2009; **119:** 1363–69.
32 Piccini JP, Stevens SR, Chang Y, et al, and the ROCKET AF Steering Committee and Investigators. Renal dysfunction as a predictor of stroke and systemic embolism in patients with nonvalvular atrial fibrillation: validation of the R(2)CHADS(2) index in the ROCKET AF (Rivaroxaban Once-daily, oral, direct factor Xa inhibition Compared with vitamin K antagonism for prevention of stroke and Embolism Trial in Atrial Fibrillation) and ATRIA (AnTicoagulation and Risk factors In Atrial fibrillation) study cohorts. *Circulation* 2013; **127:** 224–32.
33 Gage BF, Waterman AD, Shannon W, Boechler M, Rich MW, Radford MJ. Validation of clinical classification schemes for predicting stroke: results from the National Registry of Atrial Fibrillation. *JAMA* 2001; **285:** 2864–70.
34 Garcia DA, Lopes RD, Hylek EM. New-onset atrial fibrillation and warfarin initiation: high risk periods and implications for new antithrombotic drugs. *Thromb Haemost* 2010; **104:** 1099–105.
35 Morgan CL, McEwan P, Tukiendorf A, Robinson PA, Clemens A, Plumb JM. Warfarin treatment in patients with atrial fibrillation: observing outcomes associated with varying levels of INR control. *Thromb Res* 2009; **124:** 37–41.
36 Gallagher AM, Setakis E, Plumb JM, Clemens A, van Staa TP. Risks of stroke and mortality associated with suboptimal anticoagulation in atrial fibrillation patients. *Thromb Haemost* 2011; **106:** 968–77.
37 Connolly SJ, Pogue J, Eikelboom J, et al, and the ACTIVE W Investigators. Benefit of oral anticoagulant over antiplatelet therapy in atrial fibrillation depends on the quality of international normalized ratio control achieved by centers and countries as measured by time in therapeutic range. *Circulation* 2008; **118:** 2029–37.
38 Cleophas TJ, Zwinderman AH. Meta-analysis. *Circulation* 2007; **115:** 2870–75.
39 Cabral KP, Ansell J, Hylek EM. Future directions of stroke prevention in atrial fibrillation: the potential impact of novel anticoagulants and stroke risk stratification. *J Thromb Haemost* 2011; **9:** 441–49.
40 Larsen TB, Rasmussen LH, Skjøth F, et al. Efficacy and safety of dabigatran etexilate and warfarin in "real-world" patients with atrial fibrillation: a prospective nationwide cohort study. *J Am Coll Cardiol* 2013; **61:** 2264–73.

課題論文 3　Miura T, et al：Lancet Psychiatry, 2014 ［精神疾患］

双極性障害の維持療法における薬物療法の比較有効性と認容性：系統的レビューとネットワークメタアナリシス

重要単語（Summaryより）

❶	network meta-analysis	ネットワークメタアナリシス
❷	Embase, Medline, PreMedline, PsycINFO, the Cochrane Central Register of Controlled Trials	（いずれも文献データベースの名称）
❸	active treatment	実薬
❹	adverse event	有害事象
❺	a random-effects network meta-analysis within a Bayesian framework	Bayes（ベイズ）統計学の枠組みでの変量効果ネットワークメタアナリシス
❻	eligible	適格
❼	risk ratio	リスク比
❽	95% credible interval	95%信頼区間

講義内容

確率分布
- 単変量分布
  - 正規分布
  - 二項分布
  - Poisson 分布
  - 指数分布

交絡調整方法
- プロペンシティスコア
- VanderWeele-Shpitser の基準

多変量分布（回帰）
- 線型モデル
- ロジスティック回帰
- 条件付きロジスティック
- Poisson 回帰
- Cox 回帰*，指数回帰

誤差が階層構造の確率分布
- 変量効果モデル，Bayes モデル

誤差の表示
- 標準偏差
- パーセンタイル
- 標準誤差
- 95% 信頼区間

データの型に応じた指標
- 平均
- 平均の差，回帰係数
- 発生リスク
- リスク比，オッズ比
- 発生率
- 発生率比
- 生存曲線，ハザード
- ハザード比

メタアナリシス
- 公表バイアス
- ファンネルプロット
- 不均一性
- リスクオブバイアス評価ツール

ネットワークメタアナリシス
- 直接比較，間接比較
- 間接比較への依存度
- 直接比較と間接比較の一貫性
- ランキングの解釈

仮説検定とp値
- 帰無仮説，対立仮説
- 優越性，非劣性
- 非劣性マージン
- 交互作用の検定
- 片側検定，両側検定
- α エラー，β エラー
- 有意水準
- サンプルサイズ

疫学
- コホート研究
- ケース・コントロール研究
- 比，率，割合
- 交絡
- 誤分類
- バイアスと感度解析

臨床試験
- 主要エンドポイント
- ランダム化
- ITT の原則
- プロトコール逸脱
- 有害事象，副作用
- 中間解析
- サブグループ解析
- GCP，倫理指針
- データの品質管理・保証

*正確にはセミパラメトリックモデルで，確率分布ではない

Comparative efficacy and tolerability of pharmacological treatments in the maintenance treatment of bipolar disorder: a systematic review and network meta-analysis

Tomofumi Miura, Hisashi Noma, Toshi A Furukawa, Hiroshi Mitsuyasu, Shiro Tanaka, Sarah Stockton, Georgia Salanti, Keisuke Motomura, Satomi Shimano-Katsuki, Stefan Leucht, Andrea Cipriani, John R Geddes, Shigenobu Kanba

Summary

Background Lithium is the established standard in the long-term treatment of bipolar disorder, but several new drugs have been assessed for this indication. We did a network meta-analysis to investigate the comparative efficacy and tolerability of available pharmacological treatment strategies for bipolar disorder.

Methods We systematically searched Embase, Medline, PreMedline, PsycINFO, and the Cochrane Central Register of Controlled Trials for randomised controlled trials published before June 28, 2013, that compared active treatments for bipolar disorder (or placebo), either as monotherapy or as add-on treatment, for at least 12 weeks. The primary outcomes were the number of participants with recurrence of any mood episode, and the number of participants who discontinued the trial because of adverse events. We assessed efficacy and tolerability of bipolar treatments using a random-effects network meta-analysis within a Bayesian framework.

Findings We screened 114 potentially eligible studies and identified 33 randomised controlled trials, published between 1970 and 2012, that examined 17 treatments for bipolar disorder (or placebo) in 6846 participants. Participants assigned to all assessed treatments had a significantly lower risk of any mood relapse or recurrence compared with placebo, except for those assigned to aripiprazole (risk ratio [RR] 0·62, 95% credible interval [CrI] 0·38–1·03), carbamazepine (RR 0·68, 0·44–1·06), imipramine (RR 0·95, 0·66–1·36), and paliperidone (RR 0·84, 0·56–1·24). Lamotrigine and placebo were significantly better tolerated than carbamazepine (lamotrigine, RR 5·24, 1·07–26·32; placebo, RR 3·60, 1·04–12·94), lithium (RR 3·76, 1·13–12·66; RR 2·58, 1·33–5·39), or lithium plus valproate (RR 5·95, 1·02–33·33; RR 4·09, 1·01–16·96).

Interpretation Although most of the drugs analysed were more efficacious than placebo and generally well tolerated, differences in the quality of evidence and the side-effect profiles should be taken into consideration by clinicians and patients. In view of the efficacy in prevention of both manic episode and depressive episode relapse or recurrence and the better quality of the supporting evidence, lithium should remain the first-line treatment when prescribing a relapse-prevention drug in patients with bipolar disorder, notwithstanding its tolerability profile.

Funding None.

Introduction

Bipolar disorder is a complex disorder characterised by recurrent episodes of depression and mania (bipolar I disorder) or hypomania (bipolar II disorder).[1,2] The lifetime prevalence of bipolar I and II disorders has been estimated at about 0·5% and 1·5%, respectively.[3] Bipolar disorder is often chronic: results of long-term prospective follow-up studies show that the proportions of bipolar I patients who remain in remission are very low: 28% for 4 years and about 10% for 5 years.[4–6]

Long-term treatment is usually needed to minimise the risk of serious relapse or recurrence and to stabilise mood. Pharmacotherapy is the standard therapeutic approach. Lithium has been the standard long-term therapy for 40 years, but antiepileptics, antipsychotics, and antidepressants are also recommended and widely used in clinical practice. As the number and variety of available drugs increase, uncertainty about their comparative efficacy and tolerability increases, and questions remain about which agent should be used for which patient.[7–9]

When several treatment options are available for a specific indication, having a reliable estimate of comparative efficacy (prevention of any mood episode, of manic, hypomanic, or mixed episode, and of depressive episode), tolerability, and acceptability is clinically useful. In the absence of direct comparisons between all available treatments, a network meta-analysis can be used to synthesise the available direct and indirect evidence. This method has been successfully applied to guide clinical practices in medicine and psychiatry.[10–12] We did a systematic review and network meta-analysis of the efficacy and tolerability of pharmacological treatments for bipolar disorder to provide the most up-to-date, methodologically sound summary of the available evidence and to inform decisions about long-term treatment.

Lancet Psychiatry 2014
Published Online
September 16, 2014
http://dx.doi.org/10.1016/
S2215-0366(14)70314-1

See Online/Comment
http://dx.doi.org/10.1016/
S2215-0366(14)70350-5

Department of Neuropsychiatry Graduate School of Medical Sciences, Kyushu University, Fukuoka, Japan (T Miura MD, H Mitsuyasu MD, K Motomura MD, S Shimano-Katsuki MD, Prof S Kanba MD); Department of Data Science, The Institute of Statistical Mathematics, Tokyo, Japan (H Noma PhD); Department of Health Promotion and Human Behavior, Kyoto University Graduate School of Medicine and School of Public Health, Kyoto, Japan (Prof T A Furukawa MD); Department of Pharmacoepidemiology, Kyoto University School of Public Health, Kyoto, Japan (S Tanaka PhD); Department of Psychiatry, University of Oxford, Oxford, UK (S Stockton BA, A Cipriani PhD, Prof J R Geddes MD); Department of Hygiene and Epidemiology, University of Ioannina School of Medicine, Ioannina, Greece (G Salanti PhD); Department of Psychiatry and Psychotherapy, Technische Universität München, Munich, Germany (Prof S Leucht MD); and Department of Public Health and Community Medicine, Section of Psychiatry and Clinical Psychology, University of Verona, Verona, Italy (A Cipriani PhD)

Correspondence to:
Dr Tomofumi Miura, Department of Neuropsychiatry Graduate School of Medical Sciences, Kyushu University, 3-1-1 Maidashi, Higashi-ku, Fukuoka 812-8582, Japan
tmiura@npsych.med.
kyushu-u.ac.jp

Methods
Search strategy and selection criteria
Before beginning the review, we registered the study protocol with the PROSPERO database of systematic reviews (number CRD42012002739; appendix pp 2–11), and we did our systematic review in accordance with PRISMA (Preferred Reporting Items for Systematic Reviews and Meta-Analyses) guidelines. Subsequent changes to the protocol are shown in the appendix (p 12). The overall dataset is available online.

We searched Embase, Medline, PreMedline, PsycINFO, and the Cochrane Central Register of Controlled Trials (CENTRAL) to identify eligible studies published between the date of the databases' inception and July 26, 2012, and we updated the search on June 28, 2013. We also searched international trial registers via the WHO's International Clinical Trials Registry Platform (ICTRP) and the US Food and Drug Administration (FDA) website on July 4, 2013, and asked pharmaceutical companies to provide additional information about their studies. Full details of the search strategies are given in the appendix (pp 13–26).

We included all randomised controlled trials comparing any pharmacological agent with placebo or active comparator, with at least 12 weeks of follow-up, for the maintenance treatment of patients with a primary diagnosis of bipolar disorder, irrespective of whether the patients' subtypes were specified or not. We also included trials in which the investigators did not use operationalised criteria, but apparently discriminated between bipolar illness and unipolar depression and provided the data separately for bipolar patients. We excluded studies focusing on child or adolescent bipolar disorder. The eligible pharmacological agents included not only the so-called mood stabilisers, but also any antipsychotics, antidepressants, and antiepileptic drugs. We included combination or augmentation studies when the two drugs used were specified, but excluded studies whose treatment group allowed either lithium or valproate as the baseline treatment. We included open trials and those with any level of blinding. We included blinded drugs, open-label drugs, and also open-label drugs plus blinded placebo into the same drug node in the network meta-analysis, because these three treatment groups should not differ in their pharmacological activities. To investigate the effect of blinding, we did a sensitivity analysis restricted to trials using double blinding. We excluded studies in which participants were randomly assigned to a maintenance treatment regimen while in an acute mood episode (so-called continuation studies); however, we included prophylaxis design (euthymic participants were eligible) and relapse prevention design (only those who responded to the investigational drug during the acute-phase treatment were eligible to be randomly assigned to either remain on the drug or be switched to placebo or comparator).

Outcome measures and data extraction
The primary outcomes were the number of participants with any recurrent mood episode (depressive, manic, hypomanic, or mixed) as defined by the study investigators (treatment efficacy) and the number of participants who dropped out of treatment because of adverse events (treatment tolerability), both at the longest available follow-up. Secondary outcomes included the number of participants who had a depressive episode, those who had a manic, hypomanic, or mixed episode, and those who discontinued treatment for any reason including relapse (treatment acceptability). We also examined the number of participants who completed suicide and the social functioning of all patients.

At least two of three reviewers (TM, HM, and TAF) selected the studies, and TM and HM, independently, were responsible for data extraction. We contacted the corresponding author or sponsor of the original article for further information when necessary. Any disagreements were resolved through discussion within the review team. We assessed the risk of bias in the included studies using the Cochrane Collaboration method, with an additional item to assess whether definitions of the mood episode relapse or recurrence were explicit or operationalised, or not.[13]

Statistical analysis
Network meta-analysis combines direct and indirect evidence for all relative treatment effects and provides estimates with maximum power.[14–18] Although an odds ratio (OR) is a frequently used effect measure in network meta-analyses, it is not necessarily an approximation to a risk ratio (RR), which is generally easier to interpret for clinicians. We therefore used RRs in our network meta-analysis since event rates were not small in some trials.

First, we did pair-wise meta-analyses of direct evidence using the random-effects model, with R version 3.0.0 and the metafor package.[19,20] Second, we did a random-effects network meta-analysis within a Bayesian framework using Markov chain Monte Carlo in OpenBUGS 3.2.2.[21] Comparative RRs are reported with their 95% credible intervals (CrIs). The network meta-analysis model and the BUGS codes are shown in the appendix (pp 27–30).

The assumption of transitivity[17,22] in the network (a prime requisite of network meta-analysis) was first assessed by considering the distributions of major effect modifiers (publication year, subtypes of bipolar disorder, percentage of female participants, inclusion of rapid-cycling bipolar disorder, mood state at recruitment, and treatment before randomisation) for all the comparisons in the networks. Consistency between direct and indirect sources of evidence was then statistically assessed globally (by comparing the fit and parsimony of consistency and inconsistency models) and locally (by calculating the difference between direct and indirect estimates in all closed loops in the network).[23–25] We graphically presented the data and evaluated inconsistency using computational and graphical tools with STATA version 13.0.[23]

The treatment network will consist of closed loops and single-standing nodes. Because transitivity of single-standing nodes cannot be assessed, and its effect size estimates do not benefit from the network (ie, they cannot borrow strength from the entire network), but are often based on only one trial, analyses mainly focused on the treatment nodes constituting the closed-loop network.

We assessed the quality of evidence contributing to each network estimate with the GRADE framework, which characterises the quality of a body of evidence on the basis of the study limitations, imprecision, heterogeneity or inconsistency, indirectness, and publication bias.[26] The starting point for confidence in each network estimate was high, but was downgraded according to the assessments of these five aspects. We quantified the limitation of studies contributing to each network estimate by calculating the contributions from studies with an enrichment design and secondly by calculating those from studies at high risk of bias. The judgment of precision was based on whether the CrI around the point estimate overlapped with the clinically meaningful threshold.

We did sensitivity analyses using publication year, subtypes of bipolar disorder, rapid-cycling course of illness, enrichment design, sponsorship bias, duration of follow-up, and blinding of the treatment group.

Role of the funding source
This study received no external funding. The corresponding author had full access to all the data in the study and had final responsibility for the decision to submit for publication.

Results
We identified 10815 references through the electronic searches and retrieved 114 potentially eligible studies to analyse in detail (figure 1). We excluded 83 reports that did not meet the eligibility criteria, and identified two further studies when we updated our search. We also found one candidate trial from the WHO ICTRP search; however, insufficient information was available and we therefore regarded the study as awaiting assessment. We found another candidate trial[27] from inquiries to pharmaceutical companies and requested detailed information about it, but the clinical data of the study were not available from the company. We did not find any unpublished trials from the FDA website.

In our network meta-analysis, we included 33 trials published between 1970 and 2012, including 6846 participants. Table 1 lists the included studies (for details and references, see appendix pp 31–46) and table 2 reports their summary characteristics. The mean age of

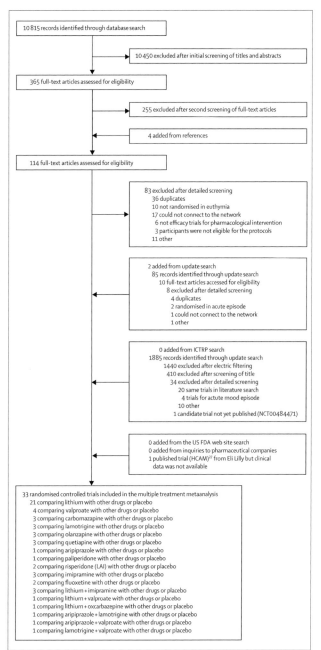

Figure 1: PRISMA flowchart
ICTRP=WHO International Clinical Trials Registry Platform. FDA=Food and Drug Administration. LAI=longacting injection. PRISMA=Preferred Reporting Items for Systematic Reviews and Meta-Analyses.

Articles

	Interventions (number of participants)	Included diagnosis	Mood status at recruitment	Blinding	Enrichment design
Melia, 1970	Lithium (5) vs placebo (6)	BP	Euthymia	Double-blind	No
Cundall, 1972	Lithium (8) vs placebo (5)	BP	Unknown	Double-blind	Yes
Prien, 1973a	Lithium (18) vs imipramine (13) vs placebo (13)	BP	Depressive episode	Double-blind	No
Prien, 1973b	Lithium (101) vs placebo (104)	BP	Manic episode/hypomanic episode	Double-blind	Yes
Dunner, 1976	Lithium (16) vs placebo (24)	BP-II, BP other	Euthymia	Double-blind	No
Fieve, 1976	Lithium (24) vs placebo (29)	BP-I, BP-II	Euthymia	Double-blind	No
Kane, 1981	Lithium + imipramine (37) vs lithium + placebo (38)	BP-I	Euthymia	Double-blind	No
Kane, 1982	Lithium + imipramine (6) vs lithium (4) vs imipramine (5) vs placebo (7)	BP-II	Euthymia	Double-blind	No
Prien, 1984	Lithium + imipramine (36) vs imipramine (36) vs lithium (42)	BP	Manic episode/hypomanic episode/mixed episode/depressive episode	Double-blind	Yes
Coxhead, 1992	Lithium (16) vs carbamazepine (15)	BP	Euthymia	Double-blind	No
Bowden, 2000	Valproate (187) vs lithium (91) vs placebo (94)	BP-I	Manic episode/mixed episode/euthymia	Double-blind	No
Calabrese, 2000	Lamotrigine (93) vs placebo (89)	BP-I, BP-II	Manic episode/hypomanic episode/mixed episode/depressive episode/euthymia	Double-blind	Yes
Kleindienst, 2000	Lithium (86) vs carbamazepine (85)	BP-I, BP-II, BP-NOS	Manic episode/hypomanic episode/mixed episode/depressive episode	Open	No
Bowden, 2003	Lamotrigine (59) vs lithium (46) vs placebo (70)	BP-I	Manic episode/hypomanic episode	Double-blind	Yes
Calabrese, 2003	Lamotrigine (171) vs lithium (121) vs placebo (121)	BP-I	Depressive episode	Double-blind	Yes
Hartong, 2003	Carbamazepine (30) vs lithium (23)	BP-I, BP-II	Euthymia	Double-blind	No
Amsterdam, 2005	Fluoxetine (8) vs placebo (4)	BP-II	Depressive episode	Double-blind	Yes
Calabrese, 2005	Lithium (32) vs valproate (28)	BP-I, BP-II	Manic episode/hypomanic episode/mixed episode/depressive episode/euthymia	Double-blind	No
Tohen, 2005	Olanzapine (217) vs lithium (214)	BP-I	Manic episode/mixed episode	Double-blind	No
Tohen, 2006	Olanzapine (225) vs placebo (136)	BP-I	Manic episode/mixed episode	Double-blind	Yes
Keck, 2007	Aripiprazole (78) vs placebo (83)	BP-I	Manic episode/mixed episode	Double-blind	Yes
Vieta, 2008	Lithium + oxcarbazepine (26) vs lithium (29)	BP-I, BP-II	Euthymia	Double-blind	No
Amsterdam, 2010	Fluoxetine (28) vs lithium (26) vs placebo (27)	BP-II	Depressive episode	Double-blind	Yes
Geddes, 2010	Lithium (110) vs valproate (110) vs lithium + valproate (110)	BP-I	Euthymia	Open	No
Quiroz, 2010	Risperidone LAI (140) vs placebo (135) for efficacy outcome; risperidone LAI (154) vs placebo (149) for safety outcome	BP-I	Manic episode/mixed episode/euthymia	Double-blind	Yes
Koyama, 2011	Lamotrigine (45) vs placebo (58)	BP-I	Manic episode/mixed episode/depressive episode/euthymia	Double-blind	Yes
Weisler, 2011	Quetiapine (404) vs lithium (364) vs placebo (404)	BP-I	Manic episode/mixed episode/depressive episode/euthymia	Double-blind	Yes
Woo, 2011	Valproate + aripiprazole (40) vs valproate (43)	BP-I	Manic episode/mixed episode	Double-blind	Yes
Carlson, 2012	Aripiprazole + lamotrigine (178) vs lamotrigine (173)	BP-I	Manic episode/mixed episode	Double-blind	Yes
Berwaerts, 2012	Paliperidone (152) vs placebo (148)	BP-I	Manic episode/mixed episode	Double-blind	Yes
Young, 2012	Quetiapine (291) vs placebo (294)	BP-I, BP-II	Depressive episode	Double-blind	Yes
Bowden, 2012	Lamotrigine (45) vs lamotrigine + valproate (41)	BP-I, BP-II	Depressive episode/euthymia	Double-blind	Yes
Vieta, 2012	Risperidone LAI (132) vs placebo (135) vs olanzapine (131)	BP-I	Manic episode/mixed episode/euthymia	Double-blind	Yes

See appendix (pp 31–46) for more details and references. BP=bipolar disorder. LAI=longacting injection.

Table 1: Summary of randomised controlled trials of treatments for bipolar disorder with at least 12 weeks' follow-up

participants was 40·2 years (SD 12·8) and 3633 (55%) of 6655 participants for whom data were reported were women. The eligible diagnoses in primary studies were bipolar I disorder (15 [45%] trials), bipolar II disorder (four [12%] trials), both bipolar I and II disorder (eight [24%] trials), and unspecified bipolar disorder (six [18%] trials). Rapid-cycling bipolar disorder was excluded in five (15%) studies and included in 12 (36%) studies; no mention of it was made in the remaining 16 (48%) trials.

Participants were assigned to placebo or to one of the following 17 treatment interventions: aripiprazole, carbamazepine, fluoxetine, imipramine, lithium, lithium plus imipramine, lithium plus oxcarbazepine, lithium plus valproate, lamotrigine, aripiprazole plus lamotrigine, valproate plus lamotrigine, olanzapine, paliperidone, quetiapine, risperidone longacting injection (LAI), valproate, and valproate plus aripiprazole. Two non-blinded randomised trials were included. The mean of the study durations of the included studies was 74·0 weeks (SD 37·6; range 17·3–171·4). We noted considerable differences across studies in mood states of the participants at study recruitment (table 2) and in treatments to stabilise

	Studies (N=33)
Recruitment area	
Cross-continental	11 (33%)
North America	14 (42%)
Europe	6 (18%)
Asia	2 (6%)
Number of treatment groups	
Two	23 (70%)
Three or more	10 (30%)
Blinding	
Open-label	2 (6%)
Single-blind	0
Double-blind	31 (94%)
Diagnostic criteria	
Not operationalised	4 (12%)
Feighner criteria	2 (6%)
Research Diagnostic Criteria	3 (9%)
DSM-III	1 (3%)
DSM-III-R	2 (6%)
DSM-IV	14 (42%)
DSM-IV-TR	7 (21%)
Included diagnosis	
Bipolar I disorder	15 (45%)
Bipolar II disorder	4 (12%)
Bipolar I and II disorder	8 (24%)
Bipolar disorder (subtype not specified)	6 (18%)
Inclusion of rapid cycling	
Included	12 (36%)
Excluded	5 (15%)
Unclear	16 (48%)
Mood statuses at recruitment	
Acute mood episode	16 (48%)
Depressive episode	5 (15%)
Manic/hypomanic/mixed episode	8 (24%)
Any acute mood episode	3 (9%)
Acute mood episode or euthymia	7 (21%)
Euthymia	6 (18%)
Unclear	4 (12%)
Mood statuses of most recent episode	
Reported*	23 (70%)
Not reported	10 (30%)
Enrichment design	
Yes	19 (58%)
No	14 (42%)
Sponsorship	
Unclear	3 (9%)
Yes	22 (67%)
No	8 (24%)

DSM=Diagnostic and Statistical Manual of Mental Disorders. *Depressive episode was reported for 1970 participants and a manic/hypomanic/mixed episode was reported for 3660 participants.

Table 2: Summary characteristics of the 33 included studies

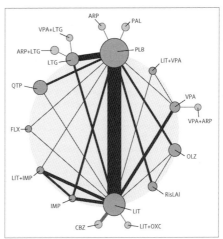

Figure 2: Network of all eligible comparisons for the network meta-analysis
Each node (circle) corresponds to a drug included in the analysis, with the size proportional to the number of participants randomly assigned to that drug. Each line represents direct comparisons between drugs, with the width of the lines proportional to the number of trials comparing each pair of treatments. The treatment nodes in the closed-loop network are purple, whereas single-standing nodes and their connections are light blue. All the monotherapies, except for ARP, PAL, and CBZ, were compared with at least two other treatment nodes (ie, were in the closed-loop network). 12 (50%) of 24 comparisons for the primary efficacy outcome and seven (29%) of 24 comparisons for tolerability were done in more than one trial. ARP=aripiprazole. CBZ=carbamazepine. FLX=fluoxetine. IMP=imipramine. LIT=lithium. LTG=lamotrigine. OLZ=olanzapine. OXC=oxcarbazepine. PAL=paliperidone. PLB=placebo. QTP=quetiapine. RisLAI=risperidone longacting injection. VPA=valproate.

mood episodes before randomisation (appendix pp 55–58). An enrichment design—ie, selection of patients who responded acutely to treatment—was used in 19 (58%) trials, whereas treatment before randomisation was not restricted in six (18%) trials.[28] In eight (24%) trials, neither one of the treatment groups had an advantage from the active run-in design (any one of the study drugs or both of them were used to stabilise mood episodes) or participants were recruited in a euthymic mood. 22 (67%) studies were done, at least in part, under industry sponsorship. Other risks of bias of the included studies are presented in the appendix (pp 47–50).

Figure 2 shows the network of eligible comparisons for the network meta-analysis. Of 153 possible pair-wise comparisons among 18 interventions, 24 direct comparisons were made for our primary outcomes (the networks for each outcome are provided in the appendix pp 51–54). Distributions of the major effect modifiers in each comparison are shown in the appendix (pp 55–58). The summaries of pair-wise meta-analyses (primary and secondary outcomes, test of heterogeneity, and funnel plots in comparison with lithium and placebo) are shown in the appendix (pp 59–67).

Figure 3 presents the results of the network meta-analyses for the primary outcomes. The heterogeneity variances of the random-effects network meta-analysis models for primary outcomes were 0·147 for any mood episode relapse or recurrence and 0·366 for tolerability.

Also, the assumption of global consistency was supported by a better trade-off between model fit and complexity when consistency was assumed than when it was not. Tests of local inconsistency revealed that the percentages for inconsistent loops were to be expected according to empirical data (one of ten comparison loops for the primary efficacy outcome and zero of seven for tolerability; for details of the assessments of consistency, see appendix pp 68–75).

For any mood episode relapse or recurrence, most of the drugs were better than placebo except for aripiprazole, carbamazepine, imipramine, and paliperidone (figure 3). Of the active drugs that were better than placebo, olanzapine and quetiapine were significantly better than lamotrigine (figure 3). For tolerability, lamotrigine and placebo were significantly better tolerated than carbamazepine, lithium, or lithium plus valproate (figure 3). The results of secondary outcomes are presented in the appendix (pp 76–80).

Figure 4 presents ranked forest plots of RRs for compounds that are included in the closed-loop network in comparison with placebo. The quality of evidence for any mood episode relapse or recurrence was rated as moderate for lithium and olanzapine, very low for lithium plus imipramine, and low for all the others (for details of the estimation of the quality of the evidence, see appendix pp 81–106). Lithium was better than placebo in the prevention of both manic and depressive relapse or recurrence, but less well tolerated than placebo. Quetiapine was also better than placebo in the prevention of both manic and depressive relapse or recurrence. Olanzapine was significantly better than placebo in the prevention of manic but not depressive relapse or recurrence. In the other interventions, either one or both of the secondary efficacy outcomes were statistically non-significant.

We also presented results in a two-dimensional plot of RR of each drug in comparison with placebo for any mood relapse or recurrence versus tolerability, and depressive relapse or recurrence versus manic, hypomanic, or mixed relapse or recurrence (appendix pp 107–09). The cumulative probability plots and SUCRAs (surface under the cumulative ranking curve) for all the included treatment groups are presented in the appendix (pp 110–20).

Because the number of completed suicides was zero or one in most of the trials, we did not calculate their RRs, and showed the raw numbers in the appendix (pp 121–24). Only five trials reported social functioning as measured by the Global Assessment of Functioning scale or the Global Assessment Scale.

Tolerability (discontinuation due to adverse event; 95% CrI) | Comparison | Efficacy (any mood episode relapse; 95% CrI)

ARP+VPA	0·04 (0·00–1·64)	0·07 (0·00–2·01)	0·13 (0·00–3·56)	0·04 (0·00–1·01)	0·15 (0·00–5·77)	0·02 (0·00–1·88)	0·06 (0·00–1·49)	0·04 (0·00–1·69)	0·12 (0·01–2·40)	0·09 (0·00–2·87)	0·04 (0·00–1·33)	0·23 (0·01–7·41)	0·14 (0·00–4·88)	0·06 (0·00–9·80)	0·16 (0·00–4·28)	0·11 (0·00–4·93)	1·15 (0·01–>100)
0·71 (0·22–2·27)	LIT+OXC	1·82 (0·24–12·20)	3·24 (0·44–23·26)	0·97 (0·11–8·77)	3·80 (0·33–44·39)	0·45 (0·01–19·81)	1·54 (0·26–9·16)	0·85 (0·05–13·79)	2·95 (0·34–25·00)	2·23 (0·24–19·23)	1·10 (0·14–8·78)	5·78 (0·65–50·00)	3·37 (0·29–40·00)	1·41 (0·02 to134·69)	3·98 (0·60–27·00)	2·65 (0·17–45·65)	28·57 (0·51–>100)
0·58 (0·22–1·55)	0·81 (0·40–1·63)	OLZ	1·78 (0·64–6·13)	0·53 (0·13–2·67)	2·08 (0·35–13·89)	0·25 (0·01–7·58)	0·84 (0·40–2·19)	0·47 (0·05–4·43)	1·62 (0·42–7·58)	1·22 (0·36–4·55)	0·61 (0·17–2·47)	3·17 (0·84–13·63)	1·85 (0·33–11·76)	0·77 (0·01–48·91)	2·18 (0·95–6·13)	1·45 (0·15–14·28)	15·52 (0·43–>100)
0·55 (0·20–1·49)	0·77 (0·38–1·57)	0·96 (0·66–1·34)	QTP	0·30 (0·07–1·38)	1·17 (0·18–7·13)	0·14 (0·00–4·24)	0·48 (0·19–1·14)	0·26 (0·03–2·25)	0·91 (0·21–4·02)	0·69 (0·16–2·79)	0·34 (0·09–1·34)	1·78 (0·44–6·99)	1·04 (0·19–5·71)	0·44 (0·01–27·06)	1·23 (0·57–2·73)	0·82 (0·09–7·77)	8·74 (0·23–>100)
0·55 (0·20–1·49)	0·77 (0·37–1·64)	0·96 (0·62–1·48)	1·00 (0·64–1·60)	LIT+VPA	3·91 (0·45–31·69)	0·46 (0·01–16·35)	1·58 (0·45–5·37)	0·88 (0·08–10·06)	3·03 (0·83–11·11)	2·29 (0·36–13·51)	1·14 (0·22–5·61)	**5·95 (1·02–33·33)**	3·46 (0·43–27·78)	1·45 (0·02–>100)	**4·09 (1·01–16·96)**	2·72 (0·24–33·22)	29·41 (0·65–>100)
0·55 (0·18–1·62)	0·76 (0·33–1·77)	0·95 (0·54–1·66)	0·99 (0·56–1·77)	0·99 (0·52–1·86)	ARP+LTG	0·12 (0·00–5·05)	0·41 (0·07–2·24)	0·22 (0·02–3·13)	0·78 (0·10–6·29)	0·59 (0·08–4·41)	0·29 (0·04–2·17)	1·52 (0·47–5·13)	0·89 (0·09–8·70)	0·37 (0·00–31·25)	1·05 (0·20–5·84)	0·70 (0·05–10·42)	7·46 (0·23–>100)
0·46 (0·16–1·32)	0·65 (0·30–1·41)	0·81 (0·49–1·30)	0·84 (0·51–1·39)	0·84 (0·48–1·44)	0·85 (0·43–1·65)	LIT+IMP	3·41 (0·12–89·12)	1·89 (0·04–94·44)	6·54 (0·20–>100)	4·95 (0·15–>100)	2·45 (0·07–73·77)	12·82 (0·37–>100)	7·46 (0·18–>100)	3·13 (0·10–84·61)	8·82 (0·31–>100)	5·87 (0·11–>100)	62·50 (0·43–>100)
0·47 (0·18–1·21)	0·65 (0·34–1·26)	0·81 (0·62–1·03)	0·84 (0·64–1·13)	0·84 (0·58–1·21)	0·85 (0·51–1·44)	1·00 (0·66–1·53)	LIT	0·55 (0·07–4·64)	1·92 (0·60–6·37)	1·45 (0·39–5·32)	0·72 (0·25–2·04)	**3·76 (1·13–12·66)**	2·19 (0·41–11·90)	0·92 (0·02–54·05)	**2·58 (1·33–5·39)**	1·72 (0·20–15·00)	18·52 (0·54–>100)
0·46 (0·16–1·36)	0·65 (0·28–1·49)	0·80 (0·46–1·38)	0·84 (0·48–1·46)	0·84 (0·44–1·56)	0·85 (0·41–1·70)	1·00 (0·52–1·93)	0·99 (0·59–1·66)	ARP	3·46 (0·30–38·46)	2·62 (0·23–29·41)	1·30 (0·12–13·89)	6·80 (0·65–66·67)	3·95 (0·33–47·62)	1·66 (0·02–>100)	4·67 (0·64–34·26)	3·11 (0·16–55·56)	33·33 (0·61–>100)
0·46 (0·18–1·16)	0·64 (0·32–1·29)	0·79 (0·56–1·13)	0·83 (0·58–1·23)	0·83 (0·58–1·19)	0·84 (0·47–1·50)	0·98 (0·61–1·62)	0·98 (0·77–1·28)	0·99 (0·56–1·78)	VPA	0·76 (0·12–4·29)	0·38 (0·08–1·79)	1·96 (0·36–10·76)	1·14 (0·14–8·79)	0·48 (0·01–34·54)	1·35 (0·35–5·32)	0·90 (0·08–10·83)	9·61 (0·23–>100)
0·45 (0·17–1·24)	0·63 (0·31–1·32)	0·79 (0·55–1·10)	0·82 (0·56–1·22)	0·82 (0·50–1·32)	0·83 (0·46–1·49)	0·98 (0·58–1·64)	0·97 (0·70–1·34)	0·98 (0·55–1·75)	0·99 (0·66–1·47)	RisLAI	0·50 (0·09–2·66)	2·59 (0·50–14·15)	1·51 (0·22–11·13)	0·63 (0·01–42·48)	1·78 (0·54–6·41)	1·19 (0·09–14·18)	12·70 (0·32–>100)
0·43 (0·15–1·22)	0·60 (0·27–1·30)	0·74 (0·45–1·19)	0·77 (0·46–1·27)	0·77 (0·44–1·32)	0·78 (0·40–1·51)	0·92 (0·51–1·65)	0·91 (0·60–1·38)	0·92 (0·47–1·78)	0·93 (0·56–1·51)	0·94 (0·55–1·57)	CBZ	**5·24 (1·07–26·32)**	3·05 (0·44–21·74)	1·28 (0·02–83·33)	**3·60 (1·04–12·94)**	2·40 (0·22–27·78)	25·64 (0·62–>100)
0·38 (0·14–1·01)	0·53 (0·27–1·06)	**0·66 (0·48–0·89)**	**0·69 (0·50–0·96)**	0·68 (0·44–1·04)	0·69 (0·43–1·10)	0·81 (0·51–1·31)	0·81 (0·64–1·02)	0·82 (0·47–1·41)	0·83 (0·59–1·15)	0·83 (0·59–1·19)	0·89 (0·56–1·44)	LTG	0·58 (0·08–4·20)	0·24 (0·00–17·78)	0·69 (0·21–2·35)	0·46 (0·04–5·18)	4·90 (0·19–>100)
0·34 (0·12–0·99)	0·48 (0·22–1·05)	**0·60 (0·37–0·94)**	0·63 (0·39–1·01)	0·62 (0·36–1·08)	0·63 (0·33–1·20)	0·74 (0·42–1·34)	0·74 (0·48–1·13)	0·75 (0·39–1·41)	0·76 (0·46–1·22)	0·76 (0·47–1·25)	0·81 (0·45–1·47)	0·91 (0·58–1·43)	PAL	0·42 (0·01–31·12)	1·18 (0·26–5·47)	0·79 (0·06–10·78)	8·41 (0·19–>100)
0·30 (0·11–0·84)	**0·43 (0·20–0·89)**	**0·53 (0·34–0·80)**	**0·55 (0·36–0·86)**	**0·55 (0·33–0·90)**	0·56 (0·30–1·03)	0·66 (0·43–1·00)	**0·65 (0·46–0·92)**	0·66 (0·36–1·21)	0·67 (0·43–1·01)	0·67 (0·42–1·06)	0·72 (0·42–1·23)	0·80 (0·54–1·20)	0·88 (0·51–1·50)	IMP	2·82 (0·05–>100)	1·88 (0·02–>100)	20·00 (0·09–>100)
0·29 (0·11–0·76)	**0·40 (0·21–0·79)**	**0·50 (0·39–0·63)**	**0·52 (0·40–0·68)**	**0·52 (0·35–0·77)**	**0·53 (0·32–0·88)**	**0·62 (0·40–0·96)**	**0·62 (0·53–0·72)**	0·62 (0·38–1·03)	**0·63 (0·47–0·83)**	**0·64 (0·48–0·85)**	0·68 (0·44–1·06)	**0·76 (0·62–0·94)**	0·84 (0·56–1·24)	0·95 (0·66–1·36)	PLB	0·67 (0·08–5·62)	7·14 (0·21–>100)
..	..	..	..	..	..	..	..	..	..	..	..	..	..	..	..	FLX	10·75 (0·19–>100)
..	..	..	..	..	..	..	..	..	..	..	..	..	..	..	..	..	VPA+LTG

***Figure 3*: Efficacy (any mood episode relapse or recurrence) and tolerability (discontinuation due to adverse event) according to the network meta-analysis**
Comparisons between treatments should be read from left to right and the estimates are in the cell in common between the column-defining treatment and the row-defining treatment. Drugs are reported in order of efficacy (any mood episode relapse or recurrence) ranking estimated by SUCRA (surface under the cumulative ranking curve). For tolerability, a risk ratio (RR) lower than 1·00 favours the row-defining treatment. For any mood episode relapse or recurrence, a RR lower than 1·00 favours the column-defining treatment. Significant results are in bold. The RR of drug B over drug A can be obtained by calculating the inverse of the RR of drug A over drug B. ARP=aripiprazole. CBZ=carbamazepine. CrI=credible interval. FLX=fluoxetine. IMP=imipramine. LIT=lithium. LTG=lamotrigine. OLZ=olanzapine. QTP=quetiapine. OXC=oxcarbazepine. PAL=paliperidone. PLB=placebo. RisLAI= risperidone longacting injection. VPA=valproate.

We did sensitivity analyses with respect to publication year, bipolar disorder subtype, rapid-cycling course of illness, enrichment design, sponsorship from pharmaceutical company, study duration, and blinding of the trial (appendix pp 125–31). When analyses were restricted to trials with bipolar I disorder, lithium plus imipramine seemed to increase manic relapse or recurrence. Exclusion of the studies without rapid-cycling bipolar disorder participants left 12 trials, and we noted no differences in the conclusions of primary and secondary outcomes when assessing these trials only. Giving less weight to studies with enrichment design, sponsorship from a pharmaceutical company had no or little effect on estimates of all the outcomes across the network. When the studies were restricted to those that had at least 52 weeks of follow-up or those with a double-blind design, the results showed little or no effect on estimates of any outcomes (appendix pp 125–31).

Discussion

Our comprehensive search for relevant trials identified 33 randomised controlled trials (6846 participants) of drug therapies in the maintenance treatment of bipolar disorder.

Within the main network consisting of closed loops (figure 2), all drugs or combinations, except for imipramine, were significantly more efficacious in the prevention of any mood episode relapse or recurrence than was placebo, by sizeable margins. With respect to the secondary outcomes of prophylactic efficacy, only quetiapine and lithium prevented relapse or recurrence of both polarities of the mood episode, compared with placebo (figure 4). However, we noted considerable differences in design features of the included trials (table 1). Lithium was the dominant node in the evidence network, and the evidence for lithium was well balanced in terms of mood states at recruitment, with small (or possibly null) contributions from enrichment design trials (despite its discovery about 60 years ago, most evidence about lithium has been produced in the past 15 years and lithium has often been the reference drug in registration studies about second-generation antipsychotics, ruling out the potential for sponsorship bias). In quetiapine and lamotrigine studies, the participants were more balanced in terms of mood states at study entry than were participants in olanzapine trials, but they were enriched; in olanzapine trials only participants with an acute or recent manic or mixed episode were recruited, but they were more balanced in terms of enrichment than were quetiapine and lamotrigine trials (table 1; appendix p 90). In risperidone longacting injection and fluoxetine studies, participants with specific polarity were recruited and only those responding to the investigational drug were eligible (table 1; appendix pp 55–58). Olanzapine, lithium plus valproate, and risperidone longacting injection seemed to be more prophylactic for manic episodes than for depressive episodes, whereas lamotrigine might be more prophylactic for depressive episodes (figure 4). These

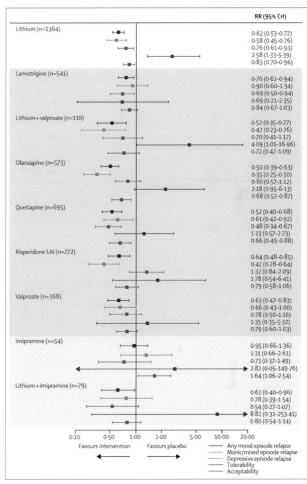

Figure 4: Efficacy according to type of mood episode recurrence or relapse, and tolerability and acceptability, compared with placebo

Results from the main closed-loop network are shown for any mood episode relapse or recurrence (dark blue line), manic, hypomanic, or mixed episode relapse or recurrence (green line), depressive episode relapse or recurrence (light blue line), tolerability (dark red line), and acceptability (red line). Fluoxetine is excluded from the plot because the result for manic, hypomanic, or mixed episode relapse or recurrence was not reported. The interventions are divided into three groups: the white background shows that all three efficacy outcomes are statistically significant and the confidence in estimate of RR to prevent any mood episode relapse is moderate; the light blue background shows that either one of three efficacy outcomes is statistically non-significant or the confidence in estimate is low; and the light green background shows that two or more of the efficacy outcomes are statistically non-significant or the confidence in estimates is low or very low. Treatments are presented in alphabetical order in each group. RR=risk ratio. CrI=credible interval. LAI=longacting injection.

drugs could be a second choice for a patient who has a specific dominant polarity.

We then examined the single-standing nodes, which do not form closed loops and are often connected to the main network by one trial only with a relatively small sample size (figure 2). In our evidence network, several combination treatments seem to have favourable point estimates of RRs for efficacy, tolerability, or acceptability. However, they were not statistically significant, with wide CrIs (figure 3; appendix pp 76–80). Therefore, further investigation is needed for these single-standing nodes to confirm or disconfirm their relative efficacy and safety.

Three systematic reviews of maintenance treatment for bipolar disorder, namely one network meta-analysis and two pairwise meta-analyses,[29–31] have been previously reported in the scientific literature. A substantial number of important trials have been published even since the most recent of these reviews, and the results therefore cannot be directly compared with ours, but the main differences can be summarised as follows. First, in the previous reviews, lithium was reported to be better than placebo in prevention of any mood episode, but not necessarily in prevention of manic or mixed episode or depressive episode relapse or recurrence. By contrast, results of our systematic review show the superiority of lithium in all three efficacy outcomes. Our analysis seems to have had higher statistical power than previous analyses, because several new trials have been published since the previous reviews were done and because we used the network meta-analytical method. Second, we were able to delineate the efficacy profiles of some newly examined compounds including quetiapine, olanzapine, risperidone longacting injection, or lamotrigine, for which the previous reviews did not have enough randomised evidence.

This study is not without limitations. First, the evidence network in our network meta-analyses was well connected overall, but had a relatively small number of trials and participants in comparison with the other network meta-analyses previously undertaken in psychiatry.[10–12] Second, we were unable to do separate analyses for bipolar II disorder or for rapid-cycling bipolar disorder, and different drugs might have different efficacy profiles for different subtypes. However, exclusion of the few studies that focused on these disorders or inclusion of them in the total evidence network did not materially change the results. Third, many of the studies of maintenance treatment for bipolar disorder were funded by pharmaceutical companies and used the enrichment design to select patients who responded to treatment in the acute phase (tables 1, 2), which might give clear advantage to the investigational drug and cause a sponsorship bias. The effect of these study limitations were taken into account when we assessed the quality of evidence behind major comparisons. However, sensitivity analyses taking into account the effect of potentially favouring the newest treatments across the network did not produce materially different results.

In conclusion, even though the generalisation of our study's findings to real-world clinical practice will be difficult, some important clinical implications can be drawn. Lithium seems to be the most reasonable candidate for a first-line treatment option for the long-term treatment of bipolar disorder (it is one of the most effective treatments in the prevention of both manic and depressive episodes, with the most robust and unbiased evidence, with a higher rate of adverse events than placebo, but not substantially more dropout due to any cause). Quetiapine might also be a suitable choice, but because the quetiapine studies were heavily biased by enrichment design, the evidence supporting quetiapine should be interpreted with caution. Additionally, when a patient's dominant polarity is known, evidence suggests that olanzapine is more antimanic than is quetiapine and lithium, and lamotrigine is more effective than placebo in the prevention of depressive relapse or recurrence. The other drugs in the closed-loop network—except for imipramine and lithium plus imipramine—should be considered as third-line treatments even though they are all more effective than placebo in the prevention of any mood episode. All these drugs have very different side-effect profiles and this important clinical issue has to be taken into account at the individual patient level.

Two research implications follow. First, our results suggest that some drugs could be divided into two classes according to their relative efficacy of prophylactic activity against depressive episodes or manic, hypomanic, or mixed episodes. The relation between patients' polarity and drugs' characteristics should be more clearly recognised and researched in future trials. Second, because none of the examined and available monotherapies is clearly effective for all required aspects of bipolar maintenance therapy, and because some of the trialled cotherapies provide hopeful leads (albeit with wide CrIs), future research in this domain should focus on the above-mentioned stronger candidates and their combinations.

Contributors
TM, HN, TAF, HM, ST, GS, KM, SS-K, AC, JRG, and SK were involved in the design of the meta-analysis. TM, TAF, HM, SS, KM, and SS-K identified and acquired reports of relevant trials. TM, TAF, and HM extracted the data. TM and TAF contacted trial investigators and pharmaceutical companies to request additional information. TM, HN, TAF, HM, and ST analysed the data. TM, TAF, HN, ST, GS, KM, AC, SL, JRG, and SK contributed to the interpretation of the data. TM, TAF, HN, and ST drafted the report and all other authors critically reviewed the report. All authors saw and approved the final submitted version.

Declaration of interests
TM has received honoraria for lectures from GlaxoSmithKline, Eli Lilly Japan, Meiji Seika Pharma, Otsuka, Pfizer, Dainippon Sumitomo, Chugai Pharmaceutical, and Mochida, royalties from the Japan Council for Quality Health Care. HN has received a lecture fee from Boehringer Ingelheim, and grants from the Japan Society of the Promotion of Science KAKENHI, the Japanese Ministry of the Environment, and the Japanese Ministry of Health, Labour and Welfare. TAF has received lecture fees from Eli Lilly, Meiji, Mochida, MSD, Pfizer, and Tanabe-Mitsubishi; consultancy fees from Sekisui and Takeda Science Foundation; and royalties from Igaku-Shoin, Seiwa-Shoten, and Nihon Bunka Kagaku-sha. HM has received honoraria from Mitsubishi Tanabe, Meiji Seika Pharma, GlaxoSmithKline, Pfizer, MSD, Astellas, Otsuka, and Dainippon Sumitomo. ST has received honoraria from AstraZeneca, Ono Pharmaceutical, and CanBas, and grant or research support from Asahi Kasei Pharma and the Japanese Ministry

of Health, Labour and Welfare. KM has received grant or research support from Ono and Eli Lilly, and honoraria from Eli Lilly, Meiji Seika Pharma, Otsuka, Pfizer, and Shionogi. SL has received honoraria for lectures from AbbVie, AstraZeneca, Bristol-Myers Squibb, ICON, Eli Lilly, Janssen, Johnson & Johnson, Roche, Sanofi-Aventis, Lundbeck, and Pfizer; honoraria for consulting or advisory boards from Roche, Eli Lilly, Medavante, Bristol-Myers Squibb, Alkermes, Janssen, Johnson & Johnson, and Lundbeck; and Eli Lilly has provided medication for a study with SL as primary investigator. JRG is an UK National Institute of Health Research senior investigator and chief investigator on the independent, UK Medical Research Council-funded CEQUEL trial, to which GlaxoSmithKline contributed the investigational drugs. SK has received honoraria from Pfizer, Janssen, GlaxoSmithKline, Eli Lilly Japan, Eisai, Meiji Seika Pharma, Taisho Toyama, Astellas, Ono, Mochida, Otsuka, Abott Japan, Shionogi, Dainippon Sumitomo, Nippon-Chemifa, Yoshitomiyakuhin, and MSD; and has received grant or research support from Pfizer, Ono, GlaxoSmithKline, Astellas, Janssen, Yoshitomiyakuhin, Eli Lilly Japan, Otsuka, Mochida, Daiichi-Sankyo, Dainippon Sumitomo, Meiji Seika Pharma, Shionogi, Eisai, and the Japanese Ministry of Health, Labour and Welfare. All other authors declare no competing interests.

Acknowledgments
We thank the following authors and pharmaceutical companies for providing additional information for the included studies: Eduard Vieta, Joseph Calabrese, AstraZeneca, Otsuka, and Eli Lilly. We also thank for Vladimir Saenko for helping us to translate Russian articles into English. TM acknowledges support from the Japan Society of the Promotion of Science Grants-in-Aid for Scientific Research C (KAKENHI, grant number 24591722). SK acknowledges support from the Health and Labour Science Research Grants programme (number H24-Seishin-Jitsuyouka (Seishin)-Ippan-001). GS acknowledges support from the European Research Council Starting Grant IDEAS (project IMMA 260559). AC acknowledges support from the UK National Institute for Health Research (NIHR) Oxford Cognitive Health Clinical Research Facility. JRG acknowledges support from the NIHR Collaboration for Leadership in Applied Health Research and Care Oxford at Oxford Health National Health Service (NHS) Foundation Trust. The views expressed are those of the authors and not necessarily those of the NHS, the NIHR, or the Department of Health.

References
1 American Psychiatric Association. Diagnostic and statistical manual of mental disorders, 5th edn. Arlington, VA: American Psychiatric Association, 2013.
2 Phillips ML, Kupfer DJ. Bipolar disorder diagnosis: challenges and future directions. *Lancet* 2013; **381**: 1663–71.
3 Merikangas KR, Jin R, He JP, et al. Prevalence and correlates of bipolar spectrum disorder in the world mental health survey initiative. *Arch Gen Psychiatry* 2011; **68**: 241–51.
4 Goodwin FK, Jamison KR. Manic-depressive illness, 2nd edn. Oxford, UK: Oxford University Press, 2007.
5 Keller MB, Lavori PW, Coryell W, Endicott J, Mueller TI. Bipolar I: a five-year prospective follow-up. *J Nerv Ment Dis* 1993; **181**: 238–45.
6 Tohen M, Waternaux CM, Tsuang MT. Outcome in mania. A 4-year prospective follow-up of 75 patients utilizing survival analysis. *Arch Gen Psychiatry* 1990; **47**: 1106–11.
7 National Institute for Health and Care Excellence. Bipolar disorder: the management of bipolar disorder in adults, children and adolescents, in primary and secondary care, July 2006. http://www.nice.org.uk/CG038 (accessed April 14, 2014).
8 Yatham LN, Kennedy SH, Parikh SV, et al. Canadian Network for Mood and Anxiety Treatments (CANMAT) and International Society for Bipolar Disorders (ISBD) collaborative update of CANMAT guidelines for the management of patients with bipolar disorder: update 2013. *Bipolar Disord* 2013; **15**: 1–44.
9 Geddes JR, Miklowitz DJ. Treatment of bipolar disorder. *Lancet* 2013; **381**: 1672–82.
10 Cipriani A, Barbui C, Salanti G, et al. Comparative efficacy and acceptability of antimanic drugs in acute mania: a multiple-treatments meta-analysis. *Lancet* 2011; **378**: 1306–15.
11 Cipriani A, Furukawa TA, Salanti G, et al. Comparative efficacy and acceptability of 12 new-generation antidepressants: a multiple-treatments meta-analysis. *Lancet* 2009; **373**: 746–58.
12 Leucht S, Cipriani A, Spineli L, et al. Comparative efficacy and tolerability of 15 antipsychotic drugs in schizophrenia: a multiple-treatments meta-analysis. *Lancet* 2013; **382**: 951–62.
13 Higgins JP, Green S, eds. Cochrane handbook for systematic reviews of interventions, version 5.1.0, updated March, 2011. www.cochrane-handbook.org (accessed Aug 5, 2013).
14 Caldwell DM, Ades AE, Higgins JP. Simultaneous comparison of multiple treatments: combining direct and indirect evidence. *BMJ* 2005; **331**: 897–900.
15 Higgins JP, Whitehead A. Borrowing strength from external trials in a meta-analysis. *Stat Med* 1996; **15**: 2733–49.
16 Lu G, Ades AE. Combination of direct and indirect evidence in mixed treatment comparisons. *Stat Med* 2004; **23**: 3105–24.
17 Salanti G. Indirect and mixed-treatment comparison, network, or multiple-treatments meta-analysis: many names, many benefits, many concerns for the next generation evidence synthesis tool. *Res Synth Methods* 2012; **3**: 80–97.
18 Salanti G, Higgins JP, Ades AE, Ioannidis JP. Evaluation of networks of randomized trials. *Stat Methods Med Res* 2008; **17**: 279–301.
19 DerSimonian R, Laird N. Meta-analysis in clinical trials. *Control Clin Trials* 1986; **7**: 177–88.
20 Viechtbauer W. Conducting meta-analyses in R with the metafor package. *J Stat Softw* 2010; **36**: 1–48.
21 Lunn D, Spiegelhalter D, Thomas A, Best N. The BUGS project: evolution, critique and future directions. *Stat Med* 2009; **28**: 3049–67.
22 Cipriani A, Higgins JP, Geddes JR, Salanti G. Conceptual and technical challenges in network meta-analysis. *Ann Intern Med* 2013; **159**: 130–7.
23 Chaimani A, Higgins JP, Mavridis D, Spyridonos P, Salanti G. Graphical tools for network meta-analysis in STATA. *PloS One* 2013; **8**: e76654.
24 Dias S, Welton NJ, Sutton AJ, Caldwell DM, Lu G, Ades AE. Evidence synthesis for decision making 4: inconsistency in networks of evidence based on randomized controlled trials. *Med Decis Making* 2013; **33**: 641–56.
25 Salanti G, Marinho V, Higgins JP. A case study of multiple-treatments meta-analysis demonstrates that covariates should be considered. *J Clin Epidemiol* 2009; **62**: 857–64.
26 Balshem H, Helfand M, Schunemann HJ, et al. GRADE guidelines: 3. Rating the quality of evidence. *J Clin Epidemiol* 2011; **64**: 401–06.
27 Amsterdam JD, Garcia-España F, Fawcett J, et al. Efficacy and safety of fluoxetine in treating bipolar II major depressive episode. *J Clin Psychopharmacol* 1998; **18**: 435–40.
28 Cipriani A, Barbui C, Rendell J, Geddes JR. Clinical and regulatory implications of active run-in phases in long-term studies for bipolar disorder. *Acta Psychiatr Scand* 2014; **129**: 328–42.
29 Soares-Weiser K, Bravo Vergel Y, Beynon S, et al. A systematic review and economic model of the clinical effectiveness and cost-effectiveness of interventions for preventing relapse in people with bipolar disorder. *Health Technol Assess* 2007; **11**: iii–iv, ix–206.
30 Smith LA, Cornelius V, Warnock A, Bell A, Young AH. Effectiveness of mood stabilizers and antipsychotics in the maintenance phase of bipolar disorder: a systematic review of randomized controlled trials. *Bipolar Diord* 2007; **9**: 394–412.
31 Vieta E, Günther O, Locklear J, et al. Effectiveness of psychotropic medications in the maintenance phase of bipolar disorse: a meta-analysis of randomized controlled trials. *Int J Neuropsychopharmacol* 2011; **14**: 1029–49.

課題論文4　Cardis E, et al：J Natl Cancer Inst, 2005［がん］

小児におけるヨウ素131曝露後の甲状腺がんリスク

重要単語（Abstractより）

❶	Chernobyl nuclear power plant accident	チェルノブイリ原発事故
❷	iodine isotope	放射性ヨウ素
❸	^{131}I	ヨウ素131
❹	population-based case-control study	一般住民ベースのケース・コントロール研究
❺	stable iodine status	安定ヨウ素の摂取状況
❻	conditional logistic regression	条件付きロジスティック回帰
❼	statistical test	仮説検定
❽	two-sided	両側
❾	radiation dose	放射線線量
❿	Gy	グレイ（放射線線量の単位）
⓫	odds ratio	オッズ比
⓬	95% confidence interval	95%信頼区間
⓭	iodine-deficient	ヨウ素欠乏
⓮	relative risk	相対リスク
⓯	potassium iodide	ヨウ化カリウム

講義内容

交絡調整方法
- プロペンシティスコア
- VanderWeele-Shpitser の基準

誤差の表示
- 標準偏差
- パーセンタイル
- 標準誤差
- 95%信頼区間

仮説検定とp値
- 帰無仮説，対立仮説
- 優越性，非劣性
- 非劣性マージン
- 交互作用の検定
- 片側検定，両側検定
- αエラー，βエラー
- 有意水準
- サンプルサイズ

確率分布

単変量分布	多変量分布（回帰）	データの型に応じた指標
・正規分布	・線型モデル	・平均 ・平均の差，回帰係数
・二項分布	・ロジスティック回帰 ・条件付きロジスティック	・発生リスク ・リスク比，オッズ比
・Poisson分布	・Poisson回帰	・発生率 ・発生率比
・指数分布	・Cox回帰*，指数回帰	・生存曲線，ハザード ・ハザード比

誤差が階層構造の確率分布
- 変量効果モデル，Bayesモデル

メタアナリシス
- 公表バイアス
- ファンネルプロット
- 不均一性
- リスクオブバイアス評価ツール

ネットワークメタアナリシス
- 直接比較，間接比較
- 間接比較への依存度
- 直接比較と間接比較の一貫性
- ランキングの解釈

疫学
- コホート研究
- ケース・コントロール研究
- 比，率，割合
- 交絡
- 誤分類
- バイアスと感度解析

臨床試験
- 主要エンドポイント
- ランダム化
- ITTの原則
- プロトコール逸脱
- 有害事象，副作用
- 中間解析
- サブグループ解析
- GCP, 倫理指針
- データの品質管理・保証

＊正確にはセミパラメトリックモデルで，確率分布ではない

ARTICLES

Risk of Thyroid Cancer After Exposure to ^{131}I in Childhood

Elisabeth Cardis, Ausrele Kesminiene, Victor Ivanov, Irina Malakhova, Yoshisada Shibata, Valeryi Khrouch, Vladimir Drozdovitch, Evaldas Maceika, Irina Zvonova, Oleg Vlassov, André Bouville, Guennadi Goulko, Masaharu Hoshi, Alexander Abrosimov, Jadvyga Anoshko, Larisa Astakhova, Sergey Chekin, Evgenyi Demidchik, Rosaria Galanti, Masahiro Ito, Elena Korobova, Evgenyi Lushnikov, Marat Maksioutov, Vladimir Masyakin, Alexander Nerovnia, Vladimir Parshin, Evgenyi Parshkov, Nikolay Piliptsevich, Aldo Pinchera, Semyon Polyakov, Nina Shabeka, Eero Suonio, Vanessa Tenet, Anatoli Tsyb, Shunichi Yamashita, Dillwyn Williams

Background: After the Chernobyl nuclear power plant accident in April 1986, a large increase in the incidence of childhood thyroid cancer was reported in contaminated areas. Most of the radiation exposure to the thyroid was from iodine isotopes, especially ^{131}I. We carried out a population-based case–control study of thyroid cancer in Belarus and the Russian Federation to evaluate the risk of thyroid cancer after exposure to radioactive iodine in childhood and to investigate environmental and host factors that may modify this risk. *Methods:* We studied 276 case patients with thyroid cancer through 1998 and 1300 matched control subjects, all aged younger than 15 years at the time of the accident. Individual doses were estimated for each subject based on their whereabouts and dietary habits at the time of the accident and in following days, weeks, and years; their likely stable iodine status at the time of the accident was also evaluated. Data were analyzed by conditional logistic regression using several different models. All statistical tests were two-sided. *Results:* A strong dose–response relationship was observed between radiation dose to the thyroid received in childhood and thyroid cancer risk ($P<.001$). For a dose of 1 Gy, the estimated odds ratio of thyroid cancer varied from 5.5 (95% confidence interval [CI] = 3.1 to 9.5) to 8.4 (95% CI = 4.1 to 17.3), depending on the risk model. A linear dose–response relationship was observed up to 1.5–2 Gy. The risk of radiation-related thyroid cancer was three times higher in iodine-deficient areas (relative risk [RR]= 3.2, 95% CI = 1.9 to 5.5) than elsewhere. Administration of potassium iodide as a dietary supplement reduced this risk of radiation-related thyroid cancer by a factor of 3 (RR = 0.34, 95% CI = 0.1 to 0.9, for consumption of potassium iodide versus no consumption). *Conclusion:* Exposure to ^{131}I in childhood is associated with an increased risk of thyroid cancer. Both iodine deficiency and iodine supplementation appear to modify this risk. These results have important public health implications: stable iodine supplementation in iodine-deficient populations may substantially reduce the risk of thyroid cancer related to radioactive iodines in case of exposure to radioactive iodines in childhood that may occur after radiation accidents or during medical diagnostic and therapeutic procedures. [J Natl Cancer Inst 2005;97:724–32]

Until the Chernobyl accident, the carcinogenic effect of exposure to ^{131}I was considered to be small compared with that of external photon exposure *(1,2)*. In fact, little information about the effects of exposure of the child's thyroid to radioactive iodine isotopes was then available, because most studies on the risk of cancer associated with exposure to ^{131}I had been conducted in adult populations with underlying thyroid disease. It was, however, well known that the child's thyroid was sensitive to external x-rays *(3,4)*.

Affiliations of authors: International Agency for Research on Cancer, Lyon, France (EC, AK, VD, VT); Medical Radiological Research Center RAMS, Obninsk, the Russian Federation (VI, OV, AA, SC, EL, MM, VP, EP, AT); Belarusian Center for Medical Technologies, Computer Systems, Administration and Management of Health, Minsk, Belarus (IM, SP, NS); Nagasaki University, Nagasaki, Japan (YS, SY); State Research Center—Institute of Biophysics, Moscow, the Russian Federation (VK); Institute of Physics, Vilnius, Lithuania (EM); Research Institute of Radiation Hygiene, St. Petersburg, the Russian Federation (IZ); National Cancer Institute, Bethesda, MD (AB); Clinic and Policlinic for Nuclear Medicine, Bayerische Julius-Maximilians University of Würzburg, Germany (GG); Research Institute for Radiation Biology and Medicine, Hiroshima University, Hiroshima, Japan (MH); Institute of Geological Sciences of the National Academy of Sciences of Belarus, Minsk, Belarus (JA); Center of Laser Medicine, Childhood Polyclinic No. 8, Minsk, Belarus (LA); Belarusian State Medical University, Minsk, Belarus (ED); Centre for Tobacco Prevention, Stockholm Centre of Public Health and Clinical Epidemiology Unit, Karolinska University Hospital, Sweden (RG); National Nagasaki Medical Center, Nagasaki, Japan (MI); Vernadsky Institute of Geochemistry and Analytical Chemistry, Russian Academy of Sciences, Moscow, the Russian Federation (EK); Republican Research Centre of Radiation Medicine and Human Ecology, Gomel, Belarus (VM); Belarusian State Medical University, Minsk, Belarus (AN, NP); Department of Endocrinology and Metabolism, University of Pisa, Italy (AP); Clinic of Oncology, Turku University Hospital, Turku, Finland (ES); Strangeways Research Laboratory, Cambridge, U.K. (DW).

Correspondence to: E. Cardis, PhD, International Agency for Research on Cancer, Lyon, France (e-mail: cardis@iarc.fr).

See "Notes" following "References."

DOI: 10.1093/jnci/dji129

Journal of the National Cancer Institute, Vol. 97, No. 10, © Oxford University Press 2005, all rights reserved.

The accident that occurred in reactor 4 of the Chernobyl nuclear power plant in the Ukraine in April 1986 resulted in widespread radioactive contamination, particularly of the territories of Belarus, the Russian Federation, and the Ukraine. For most persons living in these territories, the main contribution to the radiation dose to the thyroid was from radioactive isotopes of iodine, mainly ^{131}I. It is estimated that, in Belarus, the thyroids of several thousand children received ^{131}I doses of at least 2 Gy (5).

A very large increase in the incidence of thyroid cancer in young people was observed as early as 5 years after the accident in Belarus (6,7) and slightly later in the Ukraine and the Russian Federation (8–10). Before the accident, incidence rates in children were, as in most countries in the world, less than one case per million per year; this rate increased to more than 90 per million in Gomel, the most contaminated region of Belarus, in the period from 1991 through 1994 (10). By the end of 2003, a total of 740 cases of childhood thyroid cancer had been observed in Belarus alone among those who were exposed as children (i.e., aged 0–14 years); about half of these were residents of Gomel region at the time of the accident (E. Demidchik, personal communication). An increased incidence of thyroid cancer continues to be observed in this population as it ages into adolescence and young adulthood. The evidence that this increase is related to the fallout of radioactive iodine from the Chernobyl accident is compelling (11–16). Questions remain, however, concerning the magnitude of the risk of thyroid cancer associated with these exposures (5) and the role of iodine deficiency, which was present in most of the affected areas at the time of the accident (17) and which has been postulated as a possible modifier of radiation-related thyroid cancer risk (18,19).

The Chernobyl experience provides the most important source of information for the quantification of risks to young people from exposure to ^{131}I and shorter-lived radioactive isotopes and for the study of factors—both environmental and host factors—that may play a role in the risk of radiation-related thyroid cancer in these areas (18,20,21). We carried out a case–control study of thyroid cancer in young people to evaluate the risk of thyroid cancer related to exposure to ^{131}I in childhood and to study environmental and host factors that may modify this risk, in particular iodine deficiency and stable (nonradioactive) iodine intake.

SUBJECTS AND METHODS

Study Design and Collection of Information

The study was designed as a population-based case–control study of thyroid cancer in young people. It was carried out in the regions of Belarus and the Russian Federation that were most contaminated by fallout from the Chernobyl accident.

We present risk estimates of thyroid cancer associated with exposure to ^{131}I that are based on 276 case patients and 1300 control subjects who resided in the Gomel and Mogilev administrative regions (i.e., oblasts) of Belarus or the Tula, Orel, Kaluga, and Bryansk administrative regions of the Russian Federation and were aged younger than 15 years at the time of the Chernobyl accident. The case patients were diagnosed with histologically verified thyroid carcinoma between January 1, 1992 [to avoid overlap with a previous case-control study in Belarus (13)], and December 31, 1998, and underwent surgery in Belarus or the Russian Federation. We included patients ascertained retrospectively as having been diagnosed with incident thyroid cancer between January 1, 1992, and December 31, 1996, as well as patients with new incident thyroid cancers diagnosed from January 1, 1997, through December 31, 1998. In Bryansk region, the study was restricted to patients with new incident thyroid cancers diagnosed from January 1, 1998, through December 31, 1998, to avoid overlap with a separate study coordinated by the U.S. International Consortium for Research on the Health Effects of Radiation (16), because such overlap would have entailed too heavy a burden (reinterviewing and reexamining) on patients previously interviewed and examined in that study. In Gomel region, where the largest number of thyroid cancers has been diagnosed, it was not possible to include all cases diagnosed before 1997 for logistic and financial reasons. Therefore, a representative sample of these patients was included as follows: all patients who were younger than 2 years at the time of the Chernobyl accident and a 50% random sample, stratified by age at the time of the accident and by sex, of those who were 2 years old or older at the time of the accident. In Belarus, prospective case patients with thyroid cancer were identified directly from the Republican Scientific and Practical Center for Thyroid Tumors in Minsk, where most young people diagnosed with thyroid cancer in Belarus are referred to for surgery. The records of the oblast oncological dispensaries and of surgical departments of oblast hospitals were also consulted to ensure completeness of ascertainment of eligible cases. In the Russian Federation, prospective case patients with thyroid cancer were identified directly from the oblast oncologic dispensaries and surgical departments of the central hospitals of the regions under study. Collaboration was established with the hospitals in Belarus and the Russian Federation to ensure rapid identification of new cases of thyroid cancer in our study population. An international panel of pathologists from Belarus, the Russian Federation, Japan, and the United Kingdom reviewed histologic slides from the case patients included in the study and found that all but 11 of these tumors were papillary carcinomas.

To maximize statistical power, we interviewed at least four population-based control subjects for each case patient in the study. Control subjects were matched to case patients by age (within 1 year for those who were 18 months or older at the time of the accident, within 6 months for those aged 12–18 months, and within 1 month for those who were younger than 12 months at the time of the accident), sex, and administrative region of residence at the time of the accident. Control subjects were randomly drawn from records of the birth registry centralized at the region level in all regions except Kaluga and Orel, where access to the birth registry records was denied by local administrative authorities. In these regions, therefore, control subjects were selected from the records of the computerized medical insurance system, which covers virtually the entire population.

Information was collected on study subjects by use of a detailed questionnaire that was administered by a trained interviewer during an in-person interview. The interview included questions about selected lifestyle factors of the subject at the time of the accident and in the days and the first 2 months after the accident, as well as questions about the consumption of stable iodine immediately after the accident and during the following years. Questions were also included about other known or suspected risk factors for thyroid cancer. Subjects who were younger than 12 years at the time of the Chernobyl accident were mostly interviewed with their mothers. Because the scars from thyroidectomy are generally visible, it was not possible to blind the interviewers to the case–control status of the interviewees. The interview was complemented by a clinical and ultrasound examination and analyses of blood and urine samples of subjects who consented to donate such samples. Response rates were very high among case patients in both Belarus (98%) and the Russian Federation (99%); the rate was lower among control subjects in Belarus (84.5%) and the Russian Federation (58%).

Radiation Dose Estimation

For each study subject, individual radiation doses to the thyroid were reconstructed by taking into account knowledge of the whereabouts and dietary habits of the subjects, which was obtained by questionnaire, and information on environmental contamination and on dates when cattle were put out for pasture, which were available for each settlement where the subject resided during the period after the accident until interview. The following pathways of exposure were considered: 1) internal irradiation arising from the intake of ^{131}I via inhalation or ingestion of contaminated foodstuffs; 2) internal irradiation arising from the intake of short-lived radioactive iodine isotopes (^{132}I, ^{133}I, and ^{135}I) and radioactive tellurium isotopes (^{131m}Te and ^{132}Te) via inhalation and ingestion; 3) external irradiation from radionuclides deposited on the ground and other materials; and 4) internal irradiation resulting from the intake of radionuclides other than iodine and tellurium (essentially, ^{134}Cs and ^{137}Cs). The total radiation dose to the thyroid was estimated as the sum of the doses from these different radiation types.

The approach taken to estimate the individual thyroid ^{131}I dose combined individual information on period and length of residence in each settlement, on dietary patterns, and on stable iodine prophylaxis immediately after the accident with the average age-specific doses for each settlement. Because ^{131}I decayed before sufficient contamination surveys could be performed, a semiempirical model for the estimation of settlement level dose (22,23), modified to take into account specificities of deposition in different territories (24), was used. Details of the model and of its implementation will be presented elsewhere (V. T. Khrouch, V. V. Drozdovitch, E. Maceika, I. A. Zvonova, O. K. Vlasov, A. Bouville, et al., unpublished results). The semiempirical model used was based on the relation between environmental contamination and thyroid dose estimated from 130 000 direct thyroid exposure rate measurements carried out in territories with different contamination levels and in populations of all ages (infants, children, adolescents, and adults).

The radiation dose reconstruction was validated through a series of intercomparison exercises. Group radiation doses were evaluated by calculating the average radiation doses to the thyroid in populations of specific age groups for several settlements where direct thyroid measurements were available. The calculated group radiation doses were compared with average radiation doses to the thyroid derived from direct thyroid measurements in these settlements, assuming the same lifestyle and dietary habits as used in the calculation of doses from direct thyroid measurements; agreement was very good (correlation coefficient = .98). Validation of individual thyroid radiation dose estimation was then carried out by comparing predicted individual doses with doses calculated from direct thyroid measurements for subjects for whom information on lifestyle and diet was obtained from the study questionnaire; again, the agreement was good. A detailed description of the intercomparison study results will be presented elsewhere (V. T. Khrouch, V. V. Drozdovitch, E. Maceika, I. A. Zvonova, O. K. Vlasov, A. Bouville, et al., unpublished results).

Evaluation of Iodine-deficiency Status

For each subject in the study, the level of stable iodine in soil in the settlement of residence at the time of the Chernobyl accident was used as a surrogate of stable iodine status. This level was derived from the estimated average iodine content in the predominant soil types in the land used for agriculture in the area around the settlements and was based on a relation between soil type and iodine level established by Lozovsky (25). The majority of the subjects in the study resided in rural areas, and local vegetables, meat, and milk provided most of the daily iodine intake in the diet of such areas of the former Soviet Union (26,27). The determination of iodine status of a settlement also took into account whether the location was rural or urban. Because, at the time of the Chernobyl accident, the food supply in large cities was dependent mainly on foodstuffs imported from other regions of the former Soviet Union (notably non–iodine-deficient regions of the Ukraine and Kazakhstan, for example, for wheat), the populations of large cities were assumed to be iodine sufficient. For smaller towns, we assumed that half of the diet was composed of locally produced foodstuffs and half of imported foodstuffs.

Assurances

Written informed consent to participate in the study was obtained from each study subject or from his or her guardian, as appropriate. The study was approved by the IARC Ethical Review Committee, the Belarus Coordinating Council for Studies of the Medical Consequences of the Chernobyl Accident, and the Ethical Committee of the Medical Radiological Research Centre of the Russian Academy of Medical Sciences, Obninsk. The procedures followed were in accordance with the ethical standards of the responsible committee on human experimentation (institutional or regional) and with the Helsinki Declaration of 1975, as revised in 1983. Data analyses for this paper were carried out in Lyon, France, by E. Cardis, A. Kesminiene, and V. Tenet.

Statistical Analysis

Data were analyzed by conditional logistic regression. The primary risk model used was the excess relative risk model, a model commonly used in radiation risk estimation (5,28,29,30), where the estimate of the relative risk, the odds ratio (OR), at a dose d, is expressed as $OR(d) = 1 + \beta d + \gamma d^2 + ...$, where β and γ denote, respectively, the slope coefficients of the linear and quadratic dose terms in the model. Analyses were also carried out with a model more commonly used in environmental epidemiology, the log-linear risk model, in which the odds ratio at a dose d is expressed as $OR(d) = \exp(\beta d + \gamma d^2 + ...)$. As indicated below, both risk models yielded very similar risk estimates. However, convergence problems are sometimes encountered in fitting excess relative risk models, particularly when interaction terms are included in the model. Consequently, the log-linear risk model was used for the exploration of interactions.

The main analyses were carried out by assuming that β is constant and by using dose as a continuous variable. Departures from linearity of risk were explored by fitting polynomial equations in dose. Departures from a constant relative risk model were explored by carrying out analyses that address the possible modifying effects of other variables (including soil iodine content and iodine supplementation) by the introduction of interaction terms. The statistical significance of model parameters was tested with the likelihood ratio test. For descriptive purposes, analyses of risk in 11 distinct radiation dose categories (the lower bounds of the intervals were respectively 0, 0.016, 0.20, 0.40, 0.60, 0.80, 1.0, 1.25, 1.5, 2.0, and 3.0 Sv) were carried out; the lowest, reference category represents the lowest decile of the dose distribution. Estimated odds ratios and 95% confidence intervals (CIs) were calculated for the mean of each dose class. For analyses of the impact of soil iodine level, this variable was categorized into tertiles. All risk models were fit by use of the EPICURE software package *(31)*. All statistical tests were two-sided.

RESULTS

The majority of case patients were from the Gomel region in Belarus (Table 1). Case patients from the regions of Kaluga, Orel, and Tula, which had the lowest contamination levels in the study, tended to be older (mean age = 7.4 years; standard deviation [SD] = 4.2 years) at the time of the accident than case patients from other regions (mean = 4.4 years; SD = 3.9 years); consequently, a higher proportion of these cases may have been spontaneous thyroid cancers, because the baseline incidence of thyroid cancer is extremely low in very young children and increases with age *(32)*. As shown in Table 1, the number of boys and girls with thyroid cancer were similar in Bryansk and Kaluga regions; in all other regions, the number of girls was much greater than the number of boys.

The distribution of thyroid radiation doses was highly skewed for all subjects (Fig. 1). The median radiation dose from all radiation types was estimated to be 365 mGy (95% intercentile ranges = 7 to 3109 mGy) in Belarus and 40 mGy (95% intercentile ranges = 3 to 1691 mGy) in the Russian Federation. The highest doses were about 10.2 Gy in Belarus and 5.3 Gy in the Russian Federation. Most of the dose was from ^{131}I: The median dose from ^{131}I in Belarus was 356 mGy and in the Russian Federation was 39 mGy (maximum dose from ^{131}I was 9.5 and 5.3 Gy, respectively). The median estimated dose from short-lived iodine and tellurium isotopes was 1.2 mGy (1.6 in Belarus and 0.1 mGy in the Russian Federation) and the highest dose was 534 mGy (95% intercentile range in Belarus = 0.1 to 32 mGy, and 95% intercentile range in Russia = 0 to 9 mGy). Individual estimated thyroid doses from external exposure ranged from close to 0 to 98 mGy (median = 2.2 mGy, 95% intercentile range = 0.2 to 24 mGy) and from internal exposure from cesium ingestion up to 42 mGy (median = 1 mGy, 95% intercentile range = 0.1 to 7 mGy). The total dose to the thyroid decreased with increasing age at exposure: the median doses were 400, 365, 124, and 43 mGy, respectively, in the age groups of younger than 2, 2–4, 5–9, and 10–14 years.

Figure 2 shows the variation in odds ratios as a function of dose level. A strong dose–response relationship was observed ($P<.001$); the odds ratio appeared to increase linearly with dose up to 1.5–2 Gy and then to plateau at higher doses. Statistically significant increases in risk were associated with all radiation dose categories greater than 0.2 Gy.

The statistical models that best describe these data are the linear excess relative risk model up to 1 Gy, the linear excess relative risk model up to 2 Gy, and the linear-quadratic excess relative risk model over the entire dose range. As shown in Fig. 2, however, the latter model tended to underestimate risks up to 2 Gy. The estimated odds ratios of thyroid cancer at 1 Gy calculated with the best fitting log-linear and excess relative risk models in different dose ranges were similar, however (Table 2). Estimates derived from analyses restricted to doses of less than 1 Gy were slightly higher than, but statistically compatible with, those derived from analyses carried out on a wider dose range. Because of the absence of a consistent pattern in risk at greater doses, further analyses were restricted to subjects who received doses of less than 2 Gy.

The odds ratios at 1 Gy estimated for total thyroid dose, as well as dose from ^{131}I alone and in combination with short-lived isotopes of iodine and tellurium, are shown in Table 3. These odds ratios are very similar, indicating that the risk is related mainly to ^{131}I exposure. Adjusting for doses from longer-lived radionuclides and external radiation had little effect on the risk estimate.

We investigated the possible modifying effect of the stable iodine deficiency on the radiation-related thyroid cancer risk based on estimated average level of soil iodine in the areas in which study participants resided at the time of the accident. We found a statistically significant interaction between radiation dose to the thyroid and iodine level in soil on the risk of thyroid cancer (χ^2 for interaction = 25.0, 2 degrees of freedom; $P<.001$). There was no statistically significant difference in radiation risk estimates between settlements in the highest and middle tertiles of soil iodine. However, for subjects living in settlements in the lowest tertile of soil iodine, the odds of developing thyroid cancer after a 1-Gy exposure was 3.2 (95% CI = 1.9 to 5.5) times higher than that for subjects living in areas of greater soil iodine.

Table 1. Characteristics and distribution of study subjects

	Belarus		Russian Federation				
Characteristic	Gomel	Mogilev	Bryansk	Kaluga	Orel	Tula	Total
Case patients, No.	188	32	11	10	18	17	276
Region control subjects, No.	877	167	49	39	87	81	1300
Age at exposure*, No.							
<2 y	69	10	4	1	1	2	87
2–4 y	59	8	3	2	3	5	80
5–9 y	45	3	2	4	6	6	66
10–14 y	15	11	2	3	8	4	43
Sex*, No.							
Boys	74	7	6	4	6	5	102
Girls	114	25	5	6	12	12	174

*Distribution shown is for case patients only. Because control subjects were matched to case patients by age at exposure and sex, the proportion of control subjects and case patients in the different age and sex categories are identical.

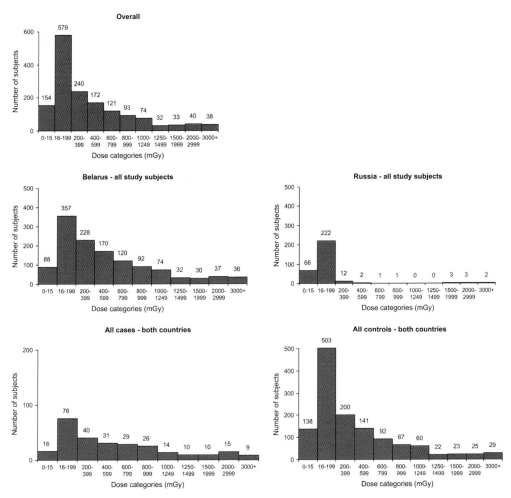

Fig. 1. Total thyroid dose among study subjects (overall, by country, and by case–control status). The lowest, reference category represents the lowest decile of the dose distribution; other dose cutpoints were chosen to be equally spaced in different dose ranges (every 200 mSv up to 1 Sv, every 250 mSv up to 1.5 Sv, and every 1000 mSv above). Intervals are larger in the higher dose categories because of the small number of subjects.

We also investigated the possible modifying effect of the stable iodine consumption on radiation-related thyroid cancer risk based on information collected on the consumption of potassium iodide as antistrumin, a preparation that was used in the former Soviet Union for goiter prophylaxis and that was distributed, mainly in Belarus, to children evacuated after the Chernobyl accident. The usual doses for goiter prophylaxis were as follows: 0.5 mg every 15 days for children aged 1–3 years, 0.5 mg weekly for children aged 3–7 years, and 1 mg weekly for children older than 7 years *(33)*. Consumption of potassium iodide appeared to be associated with a statistically significantly reduced risk of radiation related thyroid cancer (χ^2 for interaction = 5.16, 1 degree of freedom; P = .02). The odds of developing thyroid cancer after a 1-Gy exposure in subjects who consumed potassium iodide was about 3 times less (0.34, 95% CI = 0.1 to 0.9) than in those who did not.

The effects of these variables were similar when both were included in the model: Consumption of potassium iodide was again associated with a threefold reduction (OR = 0.31, 95% CI = 0.1 to 0.9) in risk of thyroid cancer at 1 Gy, compared with no consumption. Residence in the areas of lowest tertile of soil iodine content was associated with a threefold increase (OR = 3.1, 95% CI = 1.7 to 5.4) in thyroid cancer risk at 1 Gy, compared with residence in areas of higher soil iodine content (highest and middle tertiles). Both variables appeared to act independently (P for interaction = .99). Table 4 shows the resulting estimated odds ratios at 1 Gy, cross-classified by potassium iodide consumption status and soil iodine. As shown, consumption of potassium iodide reduced the odds ratio at 1 Gy from 3.5 to 1.1 in areas of higher iodine soil content and from 10.8 to 3.3 in areas of low iodine soil content.

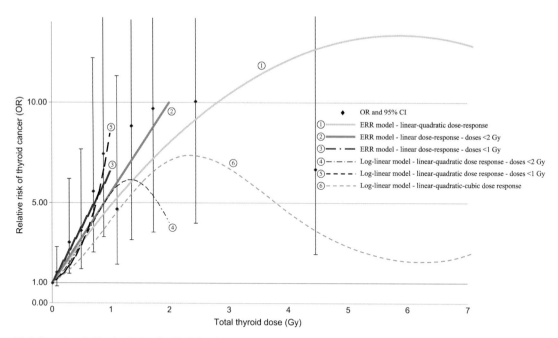

Fig. 2. Comparison of odds ratios (ORs) predicted by the best-fitting risk models with categorical odds ratios estimated in 11 dose categories. Results from the following models are presented: the excess relative risk (ERR) model—linear-quadratic (L-Q) dose–response model over the entire dose range (**curve 1**); the ERR model—linear dose-response model for doses of <2 Gy (**curve 2**); the ERR model—linear dose–response model for doses of <1 Gy (**curve 3**); the log-linear model—linear-quadratic dose-response model for doses of <2 Gy (**curve 4**); the log-linear model—linear-quadratic dose–response model for doses of <1 Gy (**curve 5**); the log-linear model—linear-quadratic-cubic dose–response model over the entire dose range (**curve 6**). **Error bars** = 95% confidence intervals.

Similar modifying effects of soil iodine level and potassium iodide consumption were seen (data not shown) when analyses included all subjects, regardless of their radiation dose level, and when analyses were restricted to subjects who received doses of less than 1 Gy. Among subjects who received less than 1 Gy, however, the interactions between radiation dose and potassium iodide and between radiation dose and soil iodine levels were no longer statistically significant. The modifying effects of soil iodine level and of potassium iodide consumption on the risk of radiation-related thyroid cancer were also similar when an excess relative risk model was used. The radiation-related risk of thyroid cancer was not statistically significantly different between males and females (OR at 1 Gy, compared with no exposure, in girls = 5.3, 95% CI = 2.8 to 10.1; OR at 1 Gy, compared with no exposure, in boys = 5.7, 95% CI = 2.8 to 11.8; $P = .86$), by country (OR at 1 Gy in Belarus = 5.1, 95% CI = 2.9 to 8.9; and OR at 1 Gy in the Russian Federation = 31.5, 95% CI = 1.3 to 761; $P = .11$), by region (P for heterogeneity = .20), or by time since the accident ($P = .75$).

DISCUSSION

A very strong dose–response relationship was observed in this study between radiation dose to the thyroid received in childhood and the risk of a subsequent thyroid cancer. This relation appears to be mainly related to exposure to ^{131}I. The estimated odds ratio of thyroid cancer in children who received a thyroid dose of 1 Gy compared with unexposed children varied from 5.5 to 8.4, depending on the model used (Table 2). This estimate is slightly lower than, but similar to, that (i.e., OR at 1 Gy = 8.7, 95% CI = 3.1 to 29.7) observed in studies of children exposed to external radiation *(3)*.

We provide evidence of nonlinearity in the relationship between radiation dose and the risk of thyroid cancer for doses greater than 1.5–2 Gy. Although flattening of the dose–response relationship has been observed in other populations (e.g., atomic bomb survivors and patients treated with radiotherapy) and attributed mainly to cell killing, doses in the range of 1–3 Gy are not thought to be sufficiently high to kill a substantial number of cells. Other explanations of the nonlinearity are therefore needed. Errors in the dose estimates or possible recall bias among case

Table 2. Risk of thyroid cancer at a 1-Gy radiation dose, from different models*

Model	OR at 1 Gy (95% CI)
Logistic regression—excess relative model	
L-Q* model over the entire dose range	4.9 (2.2 to 7.5)
Linear model up to 2 Gy	5.5 (2.2 to 8.8)
Linear model up to 1.5 Gy	5.8 (2.1 to 9.4)
Linear model up to 1 Gy	6.6 (2.0 to 11.1)
Logistic regression—log-linear risk model	
L-Q model up to 2 Gy	5.5 (3.1 to 9.5)
L-Q model up to 1.5 Gy	5.9 (3.3 to 10.5)
Linear model up to 1 Gy	8.4 (4.1 to 17.3)

*L-Q = linear–quadratic; OR = odds ratio at 1 Gy compared with no exposure; CI = confidence interval.

Table 3. Risk of thyroid cancer at a 1-Gy radiation dose by radiation type (analyses restricted to subjects with radiation doses to the thyroid of <2 Gy)

Radiation type	OR at 1 Gy (95% CI)*
Total dose	5.5 (2.2 to 8.8)
^{131}I	5.2 (2.2 to 8.2)
All iodine isotopes	5.2 (2.2 to 8.3)
All iodine isotopes, adjusting for external and long-lived nuclides	5.9 (1.6 to 10.2)

*OR = odds ratio at 1 Gy compared with no exposure; CI = confidence interval.

Table 4. Estimated risk of developing thyroid cancer after a radiation dose of 1 Gy, by level of soil iodine in the settlement of residence at the time of the accident and by potassium iodide (i.e., antistrumin) consumption status (analyses restricted to subjects with radiation doses to the thyroid of less than 2 Gy)*

Consumption of potassium iodide	OR at 1 Gy (95% CI)	
	Highest two tertiles of soil iodine	Lowest tertile of soil iodine
No	3.5 (1.8 to 7.0)	10.8 (5.6 to 20.8)
Yes	1.1 (0.3 to 3.6)	3.3 (1.0 to 10.6)

*Levels of iodine in soil in settlement of residence at time of accident were divided into tertiles. OR = odds ratio at 1 Gy compared with no exposure; CI = confidence interval.

patients who may have overestimated their milk consumption (and for whom dose would, therefore, be overestimated) could account for this result. The relatively small number of subjects in the highest dose categories may also affect the apparent dose–response relationship in this range (24 case patients received doses of >2 Gy, but only nine of them received doses of >3 Gy). The possibility of differential levels of iodine supplementation (through the use of iodized salt and/or distribution of iodine supplements) between territories with different contamination levels also may have contributed to this result.

Our results also indicate that iodine deficiency increases the risk of ^{131}I-related thyroid cancer. Because no reliable population indicators of iodine-deficiency status at the time of the Chernobyl accident were available for all of the areas under study, soil iodine concentration in settlements of residence at the time of the Chernobyl accident was used as a surrogate marker for iodine status of study subjects. It is noted that measurements of thyroid volume and urinary iodine levels also provide an indication of the stable iodine status of a population. Measurements of thyroid volume were in fact carried out in control subjects, and measurements of urinary iodine in all study subjects, at the time of interview in this study. However, although these measurements provide information on recent iodine status of the subjects, they do not necessarily reflect iodine status at the time of the accident because changes in dietary habits, in the availability of iodized food, and in commercial food distribution circuits that have occurred since the accident are likely to have modified the iodine status of study subjects. Population studies of iodine deficiency have been carried out in the years after the Chernobyl accident by several national and international organizations (19,34). Although they provide important information, they do not cover all of the territories included in this study. Data from these studies are being sought to validate the classification of iodine status based on soil iodine content used in this study. Nevertheless, any error in iodine status classification is likely to be random and, therefore, would tend to bias estimates toward the null. Thus, it is unlikely that the observed effect of iodine deficiency is artifactual. We note, moreover, that our findings support the results of a recent ecologic study carried out in Bryansk region of the Russian Federation (19), in which the excess relative risk per Gy from ^{131}I in areas of severe iodine deficiency was found to be approximately twice that in areas with normal iodine intake.

Our findings also indicate that use of a dietary iodine supplement containing potassium iodide can reduce the risk of ^{131}I-related thyroid cancer. Unlike Poland, where the rapid, countrywide distribution of potassium iodide was organized to reduce the dose from iodine isotopes to the thyroid (35), no widespread systematic prophylaxis occurred in the most contaminated areas of Belarus and the Russian Federation immediately after the accident (5). Several different measures were, however, taken months and years after the Chernobyl accident to provide stable iodine to children in exposed regions, including the distribution of potassium iodide as antistrumin, multivitamins containing iodine, and iodized salt. More detailed analyses are also under way to evaluate the effect of these measures, in particular those of the timing, dose, and length of administration of iodine-containing supplements on the risk of ^{131}I-related thyroid cancer. Potassium iodide (which was administered to evacuated children in the days after the accident and continued to be given to some school children in the following years) alone, however, appears to reduce the risk of ^{131}I-related thyroid cancer by a factor of approximately 3.

There are two mechanisms through which dietary iodine supplementation could be related to the incidence of thyroid cancer after exposure to radioiodines. First, stable iodine given shortly before, during, or immediately after exposure reduces the uptake of radioactive iodine by the thyroid and, therefore, reduces the radiation dose to the thyroid (35,36). However, as indicated above, no widespread systematic iodine administration occurred in the regions under study. Second, long-term dietary iodine supplementation reduces the size of the thyroid in iodine-deficient areas, and a reduction in thyroid growth, particularly in children, would be expected to be associated with reduced incidence of cancer.

We found that iodine deficiency and consumption of potassium iodide appeared to act independently as modifiers of radiation-related thyroid cancer risk. This result is somewhat surprising because we expected that iodine supplementation in iodine-sufficient areas would have little or no additional benefit. Most of the areas studied are mildly to moderately deficient in soil iodine, and so the comparison group (highest two tertiles of soil iodine) is not really iodine sufficient. Furthermore, the number of subjects who lived in the most iodine-deficient areas and consumed potassium iodide is small ($n = 12$ subjects). Consequently, this study did not have the statistical power to detect a difference associated with potassium iodide consumption among residents of areas with different iodine soil contents.

Uncertainties in thyroid dose estimates and possible biases resulting from selection, recall, confounding, or effect modifiers need to be considered carefully when interpreting the results of this study. The main sources of dosimetric uncertainty are as follows: 1) variability of model parameters related to the transfer of ^{131}I from deposition on the ground to the human thyroid; 2) uncertainties in information on individual lifestyle and dietary habits obtained by questionnaire; and 3) uncertainties in the original direct thyroid measurements made some days or weeks after the accident and in the dose estimates derived from these measurements. These uncertainties are currently being estimated, and their impact on the risk estimates will be reported elsewhere.

The low participation rate among control subjects, particularly in the Russian Federation, is of concern because it may have introduced a selection bias. Although it is not possible to estimate individual doses for nonrespondents because information on their dietary intake is not available, an estimation of the average age-specific "settlement doses" is possible, using age and place of residence at the time of the accident and standard assumptions about food consumption in different age groups. We compared the distribution of these settlement doses among participating control subjects and nonrespondent controls; the distribution was similar, with the median dose among nonrespondents slightly lower (198 mGy) than among participating control subjects (245 mGy). Thus, although a small selection bias is possible, its most likely effect would have been to artificially increase the dose among control subjects, and so bias the risk estimates downward.

Interviews were carried out with case patients and control subjects (or their mothers) years after the Chernobyl accident, and the possibility that recall bias may have played a role in the magnitude of the observed risk estimate cannot be excluded. Although a few study subjects have had direct thyroid measurements and were interviewed about their dietary habits shortly after the accident, it has not been logistically possible in this study to obtain the questionnaire data for intercomparison. A comparison was made, however, of the estimated doses for these subjects. For case patients, the dose derived from model estimates tended to be somewhat lower than the dose derived from direct thyroid measurements, and hence a recall bias related to case patients systematically overestimating their dietary habits appears unlikely.

This study, to our knowledge, is the largest population-based case–control study of thyroid cancer in young people. The very large increase in the risk of thyroid cancer after the Chernobyl accident has provided a unique opportunity to 1) estimate the magnitude of the thyroid cancer risk associated with exposure to ^{131}I in childhood and 2) evaluate the modifying effect of stable iodine on the risk of radiation-related thyroid cancer. The risk from ^{131}I appears to be similar to that observed after external radiation exposures and to that reported by Davis et al. *(16)* in a case–control study (including 26 case patients) in the Bryansk region of the Russian Federation.

Both iodine deficiency and iodine supplementation appear to be important and independent modifiers of the risk of thyroid cancer after exposure to ^{131}I in childhood. This result has important public health implications in the case of exposure to radioactive iodines in childhood that may occur after radiation accidents or during medical diagnostic and therapeutic procedures. Indeed, stable iodine supplementation in iodine-deficient populations may reduce the subsequent risk of radiation-related thyroid cancer in these situations.

REFERENCES

(1) United Nations Scientific Committee on the Effects of Atomic Radiation (UNSCEAR). Sources and effects of ionizing radiation. New York (NY): United Nations; 1994.

(2) Shore RE. Issues and epidemiological evidence regarding radiation-induced thyroid cancer. Radiat Res 1992;131:98–111.

(3) Ron E, Lubin JH, Shore RE, Mabuchi K, Modan B, Pottern LM, et al. Thyroid cancer after exposure to external radiation: a pooled analysis of seven studies. Radiat Res 1995;141:259–77.

(4) Ron E. Cancer risks from medical radiation. Health Phys 2003;85:47–59.

(5) United Nations Scientific Committee on the Effects of Atomic Radiation (UNSCEAR). Sources and effects of ionizing radiation—Vol. II Effects. New York (NY): United Nations; 2000.

(6) Kazakov VS, Demidchik EP, Astakhova LN. Thyroid cancer after Chernobyl. Nature 1992;359:21.

(7) Baverstock K, Egloff B, Pinchera A, Ruchti C, Williams D. Thyroid cancer after Chernobyl. Nature 1992;359:21–2.

(8) Tronko ND, Epstein Y, Oleinik V, et al. Thyroid gland in children after the Chernobyl accident (yesterday and today). In: Nagataki S, ed. Nagasaki Symposium on Chernobyl: Update and Future. Elsevier Science, B.V. Amsterdam (The Netherlands); 1994:3–46.

(9) Tsyb AF, Parshkov EM, Ivanov VK, Stepanenko VF, Matveenko EG, Skoropad YD. Disease indices of thyroid and their dose dependence in children and adolescents affected as a result of the Chernobyl accident. In: Nagataki S, ed. Nagasaki Symposium on Chernobyl: Update and Future. Elsevier Science, B.V. Amsterdam (The Netherlands); 1994:9–19.

(10) Stsjazhko VA, Tsyb AF, Tronko ND, Souchkevitch G, Baverstock KF. Childhood thyroid cancer since accident at Chernobyl. BMJ 1995;310:108.

(11) Abelin T, Averkin JI, Egger M, Egloff B, Furmanchuk AW, Gurtner F, et.al. Thyroid cancer in Belarus post-Chernobyl: improved detection or increased incidence? Soz Praventivmed 1994;39:189–97.

(12) Likhtarev IA, Sobolev BG, Kairo IA, Tronko ND, Bogdanova TI, Oleinic VA, et al. Thyroid cancer in the Ukraine. Nature 1995;375:365.

(13) Astakhova LN, Anspaugh LR, Beebe GW, Bouville A, Drozdovitch VV, Garber V, et al. Chernobyl-related thyroid cancer in children of Belarus: a case-control study. Radiat Res 1998;150:349–56.

(14) Jacob P, Kenigsberg Y, Zvonova I, Goulko G, Buglova E, Heidenreich WF, et al. Childhood exposure due to the Chernobyl accident and thyroid cancer risk in contaminated areas of Belarus and Russia. Br J Cancer 1999;80:1461–9.

(15) Shibata Y, Yamashita S, Masyakin VB, Panasyuk GD, Nagataki S. 15 years after Chernobyl: new evidence of thyroid cancer. Lancet 2001;358:1965–6.

(16) Davis S, Stepanenko V, Rivkind N, Kopecky KJ, Voilleque P, Shakhtarin V, et al. Risk of thyroid cancer in the Bryansk oblast of the Russian Federation after the Chernobyl power station accident. Radiat Res 2004;162:241–8.

(17) Yamashita S, Shibata Y, eds. Chernobyl: a decade. Elsevier, Amsterdam (The Netherlands); 1997.

(18) Cardis E, Amoros E, Kesminiene A. Observed and predicted thyroid cancer incidence following the Chernobyl accident—evidence for factors influencing susceptibility to radiation induced thyroid cancer. In: Thomas G, Karaoglou A Williams, ed. World Scientific Publishing, Singapore; 1999: p. 395–404.

(19) Shakhtarin VV, Tsyb AF, Stepanenko VF, Orlov MY, Kopecky KJ, Davis S. Iodine deficiency, radiation dose, and the risk of thyroid cancer among children and adolescents in the Bryansk region of Russia following the Chernobyl power station accident. Int J Epidemiol 2003;32:584–91.

(20) Astakhova LN, Cardis E, Shafarenko LV, Gorobets LN, Nalivko SA, Baverstock KF, et al. Additional documentation of thyroid cancer cases (Belarus): report of a survey, International Thyroid Project. 1995;95/001; International Agency for Research on Cancer, Lyon (France); 1995.

(21) Cardis E, Okeanov AE. What's Feasible and Desirable in the Epidemiologic Follow-Up of Chernobyl. 1996; First International Conference of the European Commission, Belarus, the Russian Federation and the Ukraine on the radiological consequences of the Chernobyl accident (Minsk, Belarus, 18–22 March 1996):835–50.

(22) Gavrilin YI, Khrouch VT, Shinkarev SM, Krysenko NA, Skryabin AM, Bouville A, et al. Chernobyl accident: reconstruction of thyroid dose for inhabitants of the Republic of Belarus. Health Phys 1999;76:105–19.

(23) Stepanenko VF, Voilleque PG, Gavrilin YI, Khrouch VT, Shinkarev SM, Orlov MY, et al. Estimating individual thyroid doses for a case-control study of childhood thyroid cancer in Bryansk Oblast, Russia. Radiat Prot Dosimetry 2004;108:143–60.

(24) Gavrilin YI, Khrouch VT. Validation of semi-empirical model of the thyroid gland internal irradiation dose formation and selection of areas (x) at estimating thyroid doses for adults of rural regions [in Russian]. Bulletin of Public Information Centre on Atomic Energy, 1999;11:33–41 and 54.

(25) Lozovsky LN. Iodine on soils of Belarussia [in Russian]. 1971; Doctoral Thesis. Moscow, MSU, 223.
(26) Vinogradov AP. Geochemical situation in the areas of thyroid goiter [in Russian]. Izvestia Akademii nauk SSSR, ser geogr i geofiz 1946;10:341–56.
(27) Kovalsky, VV. Biological role of iodine [in Russian]. In: Biological role of iodine. Eds. Kovalsky V.V., Blokhina R.I., Katalymov M.V., Kolomijtseva M.G., Litvin I.I., Rish M.A., Veslukhin R.V. Moscow, Kolos, 1972: 32.
(28) BEIR V. Committee on the Biological Effects of Ionizing Radiation. The effects on population of exposure to low levels of ionizing radiation. National Academy of Sciences, Washington (DC); 1990.
(29) Direct estimates of cancer mortality due to low doses of ionising radiation: an international study. IARC Study Group on Cancer Risk among Nuclear Industry Workers. Lancet 1994;344:1039–43.
(30) Preston DL, Shimizu Y, Pierce DA, Suyama A, Mabuchi K. Studies of mortality of atomic bomb survivors. Report 13: Solid cancer and noncancer disease mortality: 1950–1997. Radiat Res 2003;160:381–407.
(31) EPICURE (Computer Package). Hirosoft International; 2002.
(32) Parkin DM, Kramarova E, Draper GJ, Masuyer E, Michaelis J. Neglia J, et al, eds. International Incidence of Childhood Cancer, Vol. II. IARC Scientific Publication No. 144, International Agency for Research on Cancer, Lyon (France); 1998.
(33) Astakhova LN, ed. Children's thyroid gland: consequences of the Chernobyl accident [in Russian]. Ministry of Public Health of Belarus, Minsk; 1996.
(34) Gembicki M, Stozharov AN, Arinchin AN, Moschik KV, Petrenko S, Khmara IM, et al. Iodine deficiency in Belarusian children as a possible factor stimulating the irradiation of the thyroid gland during the Chernobyl catastrophe. Environ Health Perspect 1997;105 Suppl 6:1487–90.
(35) Nauman J, Wolff J. Iodide prophylaxis in Poland after the Chernobyl reactor accident: benefits and risks. Am J Med 1993;94:524–32.
(36) Zanzonico PB, Becker D. Effects of time of administration and dietary iodine levels on potassium iodide (KI) blockade of thyroid irradiation by 131I from radioactive fallout. Health Phys 2000;78:660–7.

NOTES

This study was made possible by contracts FI4C-CT96–0014 and ERBIC15-CT96–0308 from the European Union (Nuclear Fission Safety and INCO-Copernicus Programmes) and a contract from the Sasakawa Memorial Health Foundation (Chernobyl Sasakawa Health and Medical Cooperation Project). The Study Group is grateful to the Ministries of Public Health and the Regional Departments of Health in Belarus and the Russian Federation for support of the study, to the former head doctor of Gomel Specialised Dispensary (Dr. V. Vorobey) and the head doctor of Mogilev Diagnostic Centre (Dr. T. Krupnik) for their assistance and that of their staff in organizing interviews and clinical examinations of study subjects, and the ZAGS and address bureaus in Gomel and Mogilev regions for assistance in selecting and tracing subjects.

We especially thank all of the study subjects who agreed to participate in the study and are grateful to the study interviewers. We also gratefully acknowledge the contributions of Drs. A. Ye. Okeanov, N. Bazoulko (Minsk, Belarus), A. Konogorov (Canada), and E. Amoros (France) who participated in the feasibility study and took part in the design and start of implementation of this study; Dr. V. Pitkevitch (deceased), who assisted in the development of the dosimetry questionnaire; Dr. V. Stepanenko (MRRC of RAMS, Obninsk, the Russian Federation) for helpful discussions concerning the content of the dosimetry questionnaire; Drs. A. Bratilova (St. Petersburg, the Russian Federation) and S. Shinkarev (Moscow, the Russian Federation), who contributed to the development and testing of the dose reconstruction method; Drs. Keith Baverstock (University of Kuopio, Finland) and Silvia Franceschi (IARC, Lyon) for useful discussion and comments either in the design and/or conduct of the study; Mrs. N. Krutovskikh and H. Tardy (Lyon, France) for assistance with the verification of data from the questionnaires; and Ms. L. Richardson and Dr. I. Deltour for useful discussions about the results and their presentation.

Manuscript received September 24, 2004; revised January 19, 2005; accepted April 5, 2005.

課題論文5　Tanaka S, et al：BMJ, 2015 ［歯科疾患］

日本の小児における副流煙曝露と乳歯う触の発生：
一般住民ベースのケース・コントロール研究

重要単語 (Abstractより)		
❶	deciduous teeth	乳歯
❷	population based retrospective cohort study	一般住民ベースのケース・コントロール研究
❸	main outcome measure	主要アウトカム
❹	Cox regression	Cox回帰
❺	hazard ratio	ハザード比
❻	propensity score	傾向スコア
❼	prevalence	有病率
❽	95% confidence interval	95%信頼区間

講義内容

確率分布	交絡調整方法	誤差の表示	仮説検定とp値
	・プロペンシティスコア ・VanderWeele-Shpitserの基準	・標準偏差 ・パーセンタイル ・標準誤差 ・95%信頼区間	・帰無仮説，対立仮説 ・優越性，非劣性 ・非劣性マージン ・交互作用の検定 ・片側検定，両側検定 ・αエラー，βエラー ・有意水準 ・サンプルサイズ
単変量分布	多変量分布（回帰）	データの型に応じた指標	
・正規分布	・線型モデル	・平均 ・平均の差，回帰係数	
			疫学
・二項分布	・ロジスティック回帰 ・条件付きロジスティック	・発生リスク ・リスク比，オッズ比	・コホート研究 ・ケース・コントロール研究 ・比，率，割合 ・交絡 ・誤分類 ・バイアスと感度解析
・Poisson分布	・Poisson回帰	・発生率 ・発生率比	
・指数分布	・Cox回帰*，指数回帰	・生存曲線，ハザード ・ハザード比	
	誤差が階層構造の確率分布	メタアナリシス	臨床試験
	・変量効果モデル，Bayesモデル	・公表バイアス ・ファンネルプロット ・不均一性 ・リスクオブバイアス評価ツール ネットワークメタアナリシス ・直接比較，間接比較 ・間接比較への依存度 ・直接比較と間接比較の一貫性 ・ランキングの解釈	・主要エンドポイント ・ランダム化 ・ITTの原則 ・プロトコール逸脱 ・有害事象，副作用 ・中間解析 ・サブグループ解析 ・GCP，倫理指針 ・データの品質管理・保証

＊正確にはセミパラメトリックモデルで，確率分布ではない

RESEARCH

OPEN ACCESS

Secondhand smoke and incidence of dental caries in deciduous teeth among children in Japan: population based retrospective cohort study

Shiro Tanaka, Maki Shinzawa, Hironobu Tokumasu, Kahori Seto, Sachiko Tanaka, Koji Kawakami

Department of Pharmaco-epidemiology, Graduate School of Medicine and Public Health, Kyoto University, Yoshida-Konoe-cho, Sakyo-ku, Kyoto 606-8501, Japan
Correspondence to: K Kawakami kawakami.koji.4e@kyoto-u.ac.jp
Additional material is published online only. To view please visit the journal online (http://dx.doi.org/10.1136/bmj.h5397)
Cite this as: *BMJ* 2015;351:h5397
doi: 10.1136/bmj.h5397
Accepted: 22 September 2015

ABSTRACT

STUDY QUESTION
Does maternal smoking during pregnancy and exposure of infants to tobacco smoke at age 4 months increase the risk of caries in deciduous teeth?

METHODS
Population based retrospective cohort study of 76 920 children born between 2004 and 2010 in Kobe City, Japan who received municipal health check-ups at birth, 4, 9, and 18 months, and 3 years and had information on household smoking status at age 4 months and records of dental examinations at age 18 months and 3 years. Smoking during pregnancy and exposure of infants to secondhand smoke at age 4 months was assessed by standardised parent reported questionnaires. The main outcome measure was the incidence of caries in deciduous teeth, defined as at least one decayed, missing, or filled tooth assessed by qualified dentists without radiographs. Cox regression was used to estimate hazard ratios of exposure to secondhand smoke compared with having no smoker in the family after propensity score adjustment for clinical and lifestyle characteristics.

STUDY ANSWER AND LIMITATIONS
Prevalence of household smoking among the 76 920 children was 55.3% (n=42 525), and 6.8% (n=5268) had evidence of exposure to tobacco smoke. A total of 12 729 incidents of dental caries were observed and most were decayed teeth (3 year follow-up rate 91.9%). The risk of caries at age 3 years was 14.0% (no smoker in family), 20.0% (smoking in household but without evidence of exposure to tobacco smoke), and 27.6% (exposure to tobacco smoke). The propensity score adjusted hazard ratios of the two exposure groups compared with having no smoker in the family were 1.46 (95% confidence interval 1.40 to 1.52) and 2.14 (1.99 to 2.29), respectively. The propensity score adjusted hazard ratio between maternal smoking during pregnancy and having no smoker in the family was 1.10 (0.97 to 1.25).

WHAT THIS STUDY ADDS
Exposure to tobacco smoke at 4 months of age was associated with an approximately twofold increased risk of caries, and the risk of caries was also increased among those exposed to household smoking, by 1.5-fold, whereas the effect of maternal smoking during pregnancy was not statistically significant.

FUNDING, COMPETING INTERESTS, DATA SHARING
This study was supported by a grant in aid for scientific research 26860415. The authors have no competing interests or additional data to share.

Introduction

Dental caries is a continuing problem worldwide. Among all causes of disability adjusted life years evaluated in the Global Burden of Disease 2010 Study, the global prevalence of untreated caries was the highest, with no decreasing trends between 1990 and 2010, and its global burden is ranked 80th.[1] In developed countries, the prevalence of caries in deciduous teeth remains high (20.5% in children aged 2 to 5 years in the United States[2] and 25.0% in children aged 3 years in Japan),[3] and established measures for caries prevention in young children is limited to sugar restriction, oral fluoride supplementation, and fluoride varnish.[4]

The cause of caries involves various physical, biological, environmental, and lifestyle factors—for example, cariogenic bacteria, inadequate salivary flow, insufficient exposure to fluoride, and poor oral hygiene,[5] and the crucial event in the clinical course is the initial acquisition of *Streptococcus mutans*. However, the efficacy of caries prevention by chlorhexidine, which effectively eliminates *S mutans*, is inconclusive. Randomised controlled trials in adults and school children have shown that chlorhexidine is not effective, and the American Dental Association does not recommend its use.[6] However, a two year randomised controlled trial of 334 preschool children aged 4 and 5 years found a small but significant reduction of dental caries in deciduous teeth with chorhexidine use.[7] *S mutans* is usually transmitted from mothers and possibly from cross infection among children in nursery environments.[8] The risk of acquisition is particularly high from 19 to 31 months of age, referred to as a window of infectivity.[9] Therefore the effects of preventing or delaying the acquisition of *S mutans* before or during the window of infectivity remain unknown.

WHAT IS ALREADY KNOWN ON THIS TOPIC

The prevalence of caries in deciduous teeth in developed countries remains high

Established measures for caries prevention in young children is limited to sugar restriction, oral fluoride supplementation, and fluoride varnish

Cross sectional studies have suggested associations between exposure to secondhand smoke and caries in deciduous and permanent teeth, but data from cohort studies are limited to one study in Sweden

WHAT THIS STUDY ADDS

Exposure to tobacco smoke at 4 months of age was associated with an approximately twofold increased risk of caries in deciduous teeth

The risk of caries was also increased by 1.5-fold among those exposed to smoking in the household, whereas the effect of maternal smoking during pregnancy was not statistically significant

Although these findings cannot establish causality, they support extending public health and clinical interventions to reduce secondhand smoke

Secondhand smoke may directly influence teeth and microorganisms.[10] The adverse effects of secondhand smoke include inflammation of the oral membrane and impaired salivary gland function[11] and a decrease in serum vitamin C levels[12] as well as immune dysfunction. Children exposed to passive smoking also have lower salivary IgA levels and higher levels of sialic acid with higher activity.[12] Sialic acid enhances agglutination of *S mutans*, leading to the formation of dental plaque and caries.[13] In addition to the direct effects of secondhand smoke, inhibition of the morphology and mineralisation of dental hard tissue in the offspring of rats exposed to passive smoking was also reported.[14] The global prevalence of those exposed to secondhand smoke is estimated to be 40% of children and more than 30% of non-smokers.[15] Cross sectional studies have suggested associations between secondhand smoke and caries in deciduous and permanent teeth,[10 16-18] ut data from cohort studies are limited to the registry of 18 142 teenagers in Sweden.[19] In that study, maternal smoking during early pregnancy and exposure to secondhand smoke from mothers were linked to an increased risk of increments in caries during the ages of 13 to 19 years, whereas these associations may be confounded by unmeasured lifestyle factors such as tooth brushing.[20] Hence it is still uncertain whether a reduction in the prevalence of exposure to secondhand smoke among children would contribute to caries prevention. We investigated maternal smoking status during pregnancy and before the window of infectivity as risk factors for the incidence of caries in deciduous teeth in a cohort of 76 920 Japanese children, taking lifestyle factors of the children into consideration.

Methods
Settings and study design
The Kobe Offspring Study was designed as a population based retrospective cohort study using records of municipal health check-ups in Kobe City, Japan. In Japan, health check-ups are mandatory for women of childbearing potential and children up to 3 years old according to the Maternal and Child Health Act.[21] We had access to deidentified data on health check-ups from 31 March 2004 to 1 April 2014 after approval by the Planning and Coordination Bureau of Kobe.

Kobe City is the sixth largest city in Japan, with a population of about 1.5 million, and is the capital city of Hyogo Prefecture on the southern side of the main island of Japan. According to vital statistics for 2013 there were 90 216 births in Kobe between 2004 and 2010 (see supplementary figure 1). All women of childbearing age and children from pregnancy to 3 years of age residing in Kobe City participated in the health check-up programme. We included children who were born between 2004 and 2010 with available information on associated smoking at age 4 months and records of dental examinations at 18 months and 3 years. In the study protocol, we estimated the cohort size based on the annual number of participants, but the sample size calculation based on statistical considerations was not relevant owing to the retrospective design of the study.

Patient involvement
There was no direct patient involvement in this study. The datasets used for analysis did not include names and identity numbers of citizens.

Measurements
The health check-up programme in Kobe City consisted of completing a standardised pregnancy notification form, neonatal health check-ups, and advice provided during home visits and health check-ups of infants at ages 4, 9, and 18 months and 3 years at healthcare centres of ward offices or designated clinics. Personal and physical data on pregnancy provided by the mother included maternal age at birth, planned and actual date of delivery, height, body weight, occupation, birth order and gestational age of the infant, and multiple births. Personal, physical, and laboratory data from the infant's birth to 3 years of age included gestational age at birth; abnormalities during pregnancy and at delivery; body weight; height; head and chest circumference; physical, neurological, ophthalmological, and dental examinations; hearing tests; urinary protein level; and occult blood by a dipstick test.

Information on lifestyle factors was based exclusively on information from standardised parent reported questionnaires, which mothers were required to fill out at every health check-up. Exposure to secondhand smoke from pregnancy to 3 years of age was assessed as: maternal smoking during pregnancy (never, former, or current smoker), daily number of cigarettes smoked during pregnancy, presence of smokers in the household during pregnancy, smoking status of parents and family members when the infant was 4 months of age (non-smoker, smoking away from child, or smoking in front of child), and presence of smokers in the family at 9 months, 18 months, and 3 years. Information on third hand smoke was not available. In the current analysis we defined household smoking as smoking by family members in the household when the infant was 4 months old, and we defined exposure to tobacco smoke as smoking by family members in front of the infant at age 4 months. Other lifestyle factors included the number of family members in the household; people involved in parenting and childcare; use of a babysitter or nursery; mental status of the mother, assessed by a picture face scale with five levels from a smile to a tearful face; frequency of alcohol consumption during pregnancy; sleeping hours or sleep duration of the child; dietary habits of the child, such as breast feeding and bottle feeding and frequency of eating sweets and drinking juice; and oral care, such as tooth brushing alone or by parents.

Assessment of dental caries
Qualified dentists assessed the oral conditions of the children at 18 months and 3 years of age through visual examination and not radiography. They classified each tooth into one of seven types: normal, decayed, missing, filled, treated by diammine silver fluoride, observation required, or treated by a dental sealant. We counted teeth treated by diammine silver fluoride as well as decayed teeth as decayed. Incidence of dental caries was defined as the occurrence of at least one decayed,

missing, or filled tooth. Other records of dental examinations included the caries activity test (0 to 4 points, 4 points indicating most active), presence of plaque, abnormal conditions of soft tissues and occlusion, and treatment with fluoride varnish.

Statistical analysis

The primary outcome was time to the first incidence of caries in deciduous teeth. Secondary outcomes were the first incidence of caries in mandibular or maxillary anterior teeth or molars and numbers of decayed, missing, or filled teeth at 18 months and 3 years, using the DMF (decayed, missing, filled) index. We used the difference between birth date and the first date of assessment when dental caries was diagnosed as failure time, and the difference between birth date and the last date of assessment (18 months if assessment at 3 years was not done) as censored time. The Kaplan-Meier method was used to estimate the risks of caries at 3 years of age. We expressed the effects of secondhand smoke on the incidence of caries as hazard ratios with 95% confidence intervals, estimated by Cox regression adjusted for a linear term of the propensity score. The proportional hazards assumption was confirmed with log-negative log graphs. We compared the numbers of decayed, missing, or filled teeth using mixed models adjusted for a linear term of the propensity score. For each infant we calculated the propensity score, defined as the conditional probability of a child being exposed to secondhand smoke at 4 months of age given several confounders (see box), using logistic regression and single mean imputation for missing covariates.

Sensitivity analyses

We performed four sensitivity analyses: Cox regression analysis restricted to first born singletons, which accounts for the effects of clustering of children within the same family; Cox regression analysis excluding children with a propensity score below the first centile and above the 99th centile, which ensures strict overlap of propensity scores of different groups; and Cox regression analysis further adjusting for the covariates of number of teeth at 9 months, fluoride varnish treatment at 18 months and 3 years, tooth brushing alone at 18 months and 3 years, tooth brushing by parents at 18 months and 3 years, bottle feeding at 4 months and 9 months, baby food intake at 9 months, age at start of baby food, frequency of eating sweets at 18 months and 3 years, eating sweets irregularly at 18 months and 3 years, and drinking juice every day at 18 months and 3 years, which adjusts for post-exposure covariates as potential confounders; and exponential regression analysis handling the time to event data as interval censored, which accounts for the fact that time to events were not known exactly.

All reported probability values were two sided, and we considered P<0.05 to be statistically significant. An academic statistician conducted all analyses using SAS software version 9.4 (SAS Institute, Cary, NC).

Results

The database of the health check-up programme in Kobe City consisted of records of 145 318 participants in the health check-up programme in Kobe City between 2004 and 2014. We initially identified 82 543 infants born between 2004 and 2010 who received a health check-up at 4 months of age. Information about exposure to smoking at 4 months was available for 82 409 (99.8%) children and the records of a dental examination were available for 76 920 (93.2%) of these children (see supplementary figure 1). Thus the analysis population used for time to event analysis consisted of the 76 920 children. Background characteristics differed significantly for mother's age, smoking and alcohol consumption, gestational week, and birth weight between those included and excluded in this analysis. The differences were, however, generally small (see supplementary table 1).

Tables 1 and 2 describe the baseline characteristics and lifestyles of the 76 920 children, categorised into three groups according to details of family smoking at age 4 months: family members did not smoke, family members smoked away from the infant; and infant was exposed to secondhand smoke. Prevalence of smoking in the household (family members who smoked when the infant was 4 months old) was 55.3% (42 525/76 920), and most smokers were the fathers (see supplementary table 2). Among them, 5268 (6.8%) children had evidence of exposure to tobacco smoke—that is, at least one family member smoked in their

---

Potential confounders

Maternal factors
- Maternal age at birth
- Alcohol consumption during pregnancy
- First birth
- Multiple birth
- Pre-eclampsia
- Anaemia
- Threatened abortion
- Gestation weeks
- Caesarean section
- Vacuum extraction
- Mental status four months post partum

Infant factors
- Birth year of child
- Sex of child
- Nuchal cord
- Asphyxia
- Jaundice and transfusion
- Convulsion
- Incubator
- Oxygen inhalation
- Weight at birth
- Height at birth
- Head circumference at birth
- Chest circumference at birth
- Bottle feeding

Other factors
- People involved in parenting
- Support by family, friends, and neighbours

RESEARCH

Table 1 | Background data on 76 920 infants according to smoking status of family members and exposure to tobacco smoke at 4 months of age. Values are numbers (percentages) unless stated otherwise

Characteristics	Not exposed to secondhand smoke (n=34 395)	Exposed to only household smoking (n=37 257)	Exposed to tobacco smoke (n=5268)
Mean (SD) maternal age at delivery (years)*	32.5 (4.2)	30.5 (4.9)	30.0 (5.2)
Maternal age ≥35 years*	6892 (27.5)	4743 (18.1)	640 (17.8)
Maternal smoking during pregnancy*	2062 (8.4)	6176 (24.1)	879 (25.0)
Maternal alcohol consumption during pregnancy:*			
Occasional	4410 (17.9)	4242 (16.6)	725 (20.7)
Daily	147 (0.6)	147 (0.6)	37 (1.1)
Girl	51 151 (48.7)	55 402 (48.7)	7828 (48.6)
First birth*	40 060 (45.7)	12 144 (49.7)	1002 (30.3)
Multiple birth*	275 (1.1)	205 (0.8)	18 (0.5)
Pre-eclampsia	777 (2.3)	970 (2.6)	148 (2.8)
Anaemia	3653 (10.6)	3935 (10.6)	556 (10.6)
Threatened abortion	3822 (11.1)	4073 (10.9)	586 (11.1)
Gestational weeks:†			
22-27	54 (0.2)	67 (0.2)	10 (0.2)
28-36	1978 (5.9)	2160 (6.0)	271 (5.4)
36-43	31 212 (93.9)	33637 (93.8)	4762 (94.4)
Mean (SD) birth weight (g)	3008.9 (418.8)	2995.8 (416.6)	3026.1 (415.4)

*Data missing for 33% of infants.
†Data missing for 4% of infants.

Table 2 | Characteristics of 76 920 children according to smoking status of family members and exposure to tobacco smoke at 4 months of age. Values are numbers (percentages) unless stated otherwise

Characteristics	Not exposed to secondhand smoke (n=34 395)	Exposed to only household smoking (n=37 257)	Exposed to tobacco smoke (n=5268)
Mean (SD) No of teeth at 9 months	3.5 (2.2)	3.6 (2.2)	3.6 (2.2)
Treated by fluoride varnish at 18 months	29 783 (99.4)	31 758 (99.3)	4246 (99.1)
Tooth brushing:			
Own self at 18 months	27 370 (80.2)	28 884 (78.3)	3817 (73.5)
Own self at 3 years	27 781 (87.7)	29 847 (87.0)	4034 (83.2)
Parents at 18 months	26 175 (76.7)	26 365 (71.4)	3368 (64.8)
Parents at 3 years	28 497 (90.0)	29 100 (84.8)	3661 (75.5)
Plaque present:			
18 months	7045 (20.7)	8320 (22.6)	1406 (27.2)
3 years	4924 (15.7)	6450 (19.0)	1175 (24.5)
Feeding method:			
Bottle at 4 months	13 456 (39.9)	17 163 (47.4)	2696 (52.8)
Bottle at 9 months	12 136 (35.9)	14 972 (41.3)	2160 (43.0)
Baby food at 9 months	31 334 (92.7)	33 187 (91.6)	4462 (88.8)
Mean (SD) age at start of baby food (months)	5.6 (0.8)	5.4 (0.8)	5.4 (0.9)
Mean (SD) frequency of eating sweets at 18 months (daily)	1.5 (0.6)	1.5 (0.6)	1.6 (0.7)
Mean (SD) frequency of eating sweets at 3 years (daily)	1.5 (0.6)	1.5 (0.6)	1.6 (0.6)
Consumption of sweets:			
Irregularly at 18 months	9743 (28.3)	12 568 (33.7)	2009 (38.1)
Irregularly at 3 years	10 106 (29.4)	12 344 (33.1)	1896 (36.0)
Daily juice consumption:			
18 months	12 424 (36.3)	16 964 (45.9)	2553 (49.1)
3 years	13 291 (42.0)	16 870 (49.2)	2428 (50.1)
Use of babysitter or nursery:			
4 months	592 (1.7)	740 (2.0)	160 (3.0)
18 months	8071 (23.6)	9420 (25.5)	1629 (31.4)
3 years	13 915 (44.0)	15 806 (46.2)	2511 (51.8)

*1% to 14% of infants had missing data on each item.

presence. Prevalence of household smoking at age 3 years in the three groups was 4.9%, 68.4%, and 76.2%, respectively (see supplementary table 2). The mothers of children who were exposed to smoking tended to be younger, and around 25% of those whose infants were exposed to secondhand smoke during pregnancy (table 1). Abnormalities at delivery, gestational age, and birth weight did not differ significantly across the three groups (table 1). More than 99% of children received fluoride varnish at 18 months. Four month old children with family members who smoked had their teeth brushed less frequently by themselves or by parents. The frequency of eating sweets was similar across the three groups, but exposure to smoke was associated with higher proportions of bottle feeding, drinking juice every day, and use of a babysitter or nursery (table 2).

Of the 76 920 children, 70 711 (91.9%) attended a dental examination at 3 years of age. There were significant differences in mother's age, child's sex, first born status, and maternal anaemia at delivery between those who were followed for three years and those who were not, including smoking status at four months (see supplementary table 3). Overall, 12 729 cases of dental caries were observed, with 12 579 related to decayed teeth. The mean DMF index (the numbers of decayed, missing, or filled teeth) was 0.06 (2.5 centile: 0, median: 0, 97.5 centile: 0) at age 18 months and 0.61 (2.5 centile: 0, median: 0, 97.5 centile: 6) at age 3 years. Unadjusted three year risks of caries calculated by the Kaplan-Meier method were 18.0% in total and 14.0% for infants in households where no family members smoked, 20.0% when family members smoked away from infants, and 27.6% when infants were exposed to tobacco smoke at age 4 months (table 3). The propensity score adjusted hazard ratios of having family members who smoked away from or in front of children compared with having no smoker in the family were 1.46 (95% confidence interval 1.40 to 1.52, P<0.01) and 2.14 (1.99 to 2.29, P<0.01), respectively. Similar associations were observed for different sites (mandibular or maxillary, anterior teeth or molars). Sensitivity analysis indicated

Table 3 | Propensity score analysis of exposure to secondhand smoke at age 4 months and incidence of caries

Variables	Not exposed to secondhand smoke (n=34 395)	Exposed to only household smoking (n=37 257)		Exposed to tobacco smoke (n=5268)	
		Hazard ratio (95% CI)	P value	Hazard ratio (95% CI)	P value
Incidence of any caries (unadjusted) (%):	4453 (14.0*)	6925 (20.0*)		1351 (27.6*)	
Unadjusted	Ref	1.54 (1.48 to 1.61)	<0.01	2.35 (2.19 to 2.52)	<0.01
Propensity score adjusted†	Ref	1.46 (1.40 to 1.52)	<0.01	2.14 (1.99 to 2.29)	<0.01
Sensitivity analysis‡	Ref	1.71 (1.56 to 1.87)	<0.01	2.92 (2.48 to 3.43)	<0.01
Sensitivity analysis§	Ref	1.46 (1.40 to 1.52)	<0.01	2.13 (1.99 to 2.29)	<0.01
Sensitivity analysis¶	Ref	1.32 (1.24 to 1.40)	<0.01	1.77 (1.58 to 1.98)	<0.01
Sensitivity analysis**	Ref	1.40 (1.35 to 1.46)	<0.01	1.94 (1.83 to 2.07)	<0.01
Incidence of caries in maxillary anterior teeth (unadjusted) (%):	2882 (9.0*)	4602 (13.3*)		892 (18.2*)	
Crude	Ref	1.55 (1.47 to 1.62)	<0.01	2.24 (2.07 to 2.43)	<0.01
Propensity score adjusted†	Ref	1.48 (1.41 to 1.56)	<0.01	2.10 (1.94 to 2.28)	<0.01
Sensitivity analysis‡	Ref	1.71 (1.57 to 1.87)	<0.01	2.94 (2.49 to 3.45)	<0.01
Sensitivity analysis§	Ref	1.46 (1.40 to 1.52)	<0.01	2.14 (2.00 to 2.30)	<0.01
Sensitivity analysis¶	Ref	1.32 (1.24 to 1.41)	<0.01	1.77 (1.58 to 1.99)	<0.01
Sensitivity analysis**	Ref	1.45 (1.38 to 1.52)	<0.01	1.99 (1.84 to 2.15)	<0.01
Incidence of caries on maxillary molars (unadjusted) (%):	1361 (4.3*)	2297 (6.7*)		478 (9.8*)	
Crude	Ref	1.60 (1.49 to 1.71)	<0.01	2.43 (2.18 to 2.71)	<0.01
Propensity score adjusted†	Ref	1.51 (1.41 to 1.62)	<0.01	2.23 (2.00 to 2.49)	<0.01
Sensitivity analysis‡	Ref	1.71 (1.56 to 1.87)	<0.01	2.95 (2.50 to 3.48)	<0.01
Sensitivity analysis§	Ref	1.46 (1.40 to 1.53)	<0.01	2.16 (2.01 to 2.32)	<0.01
Sensitivity analysis¶	Ref	1.32 (1.24 to 1.40)	<0.01	1.78 (1.59 to 2.01)	<0.01
Sensitivity analysis**	Ref	1.49 (1.39 to 1.60)	<0.01	2.16 (1.94 to 2.40)	<0.01
Incidence of caries on mandibular anterior teeth (unadjusted) (%):	287 (0.9*)	494 (1.4*)		112 (2.3*)	
Crude	Ref	1.60 (1.38 to 1.85)	<0.01	2.58 (2.07 to 3.22)	<0.01
Propensity score adjusted†	Ref	1.50 (1.29 to 1.74)	<0.01	2.36 (1.88 to 2.95)	<0.01
Sensitivity analysis‡	Ref	1.71 (1.57 to 1.87)	<0.01	2.96 (2.51 to 3.50)	<0.01
Sensitivity analysis§	Ref	1.47 (1.40 to 1.53)	<0.01	2.17 (2.01 to 2.33)	<0.01
Sensitivity analysis¶	Ref	1.32 (1.24 to 1.41)	<0.01	1.79 (1.59 to 2.01)	<0.01
Sensitivity analysis**	Ref	1.50 (1.30 to 1.75)	0.89	2.35 (1.88 to 2.94)	<0.01
Incidence of caries on mandibular molars (unadjusted) (%):	2062 (6.5*)	3666 (10.7*)		768 (16.0*)	
Crude	Ref	1.72 (1.62 to 1.82)	<0.01	2.70 (2.47 to 2.95)	<0.01
Propensity score adjusted†	Ref	1.58 (1.49 to 1.67)	<0.01	2.39 (2.18 to 2.61)	<0.01
Sensitivity analysis‡	Ref	1.71 (1.56 to 1.87)	<0.01	2.95 (2.50 to 3.48)	<0.01
Sensitivity analysis§	Ref	1.46 (1.40 to 1.53)	<0.01	2.17 (2.02 to 2.33)	<0.01
Sensitivity analysis¶	Ref	1.32 (1.24 to 1.41)	<0.01	1.79 (1.59 to 2.01)	<0.01
Sensitivity analysis**	Ref	1.54 (1.46 to 1.63)	<0.01	2.24 (2.06 to 2.43)	<0.01

*Estimated by Kaplan-Meier method.
†Adjusted for birth year of child, maternal age, alcohol consumption during pregnancy, smoking status during pregnancy, sex, first birth, multiple birth, pre-eclampsia, anaemia, threatened abortion, gestational weeks, caesarean section, vacuum extraction, nuchal cord, asphyxia, jaundice and transfusion, convulsion, incubator, oxygen inhalation, weight, height, head and chest circumference at birth, weight at 4 months, bottle feeding at 4 months, people involved in child care at 4 months, support by family, friends, or neighbours at 4 months, and mother's mental status at 4 months.
‡Restricted to first born singletons.
§Children with a propensity score below first centile or above 99th centile were excluded.
¶Further adjusted for number of teeth at 9 months, treatment with fluoride varnish at 18 months and 3 years, tooth brushing alone at 18 months and 3 years, tooth brushing by parents at 18 months and 3 years (%), bottle feeding at 4 months and 9 months, baby food at 9 months, age at start of baby food, frequency of sweets at 18 months and 3 years, eating sweets irregularly at 18 months and 3 years, and drinking juice every day at 18 months and 3 years.
**Exponential regression analysis handling time to event data as interval censored.

that these associations were robust against the influence of behaviour patterns from the age of 4 months to 3 years. Supplementary table 4 provides propensity score adjusted risk ratios for caries at 18 months and 3 years (that is, analysis as binary outcomes). Children with family members who smoked had significantly more decayed, missing, or filled teeth than those with no smokers in the family. The mean DMF index at 18 months was 0.03 (2.5 centile: 0, median: 0, 97.5 centile: 0) with no family members who smoked, 0.07 (2.5 centile: 0, median: 0, 97.5 centile: 0, P<0.01) with family members who smoked away from infants, and 0.11 (2.5 centile: 0, median: 0, 97.5 centile: 2, P<0.01) with infants exposed to tobacco smoke at age 4 months. The mean DMF index at 3 years in the three groups was 0.44 (2.5 centile: 0, median: 0, 97.5 centile: 5), 0.72 (2.5 centile: 0, median: 0, 97.5 centile: 7, P<0.01), and 1.07 (2.5 centile: 0, median: 0, 97.5 centile: 9, P<0.01), respectively.

Table 4 shows associations between maternal smoking during pregnancy and incidence of caries. The crude risk of caries among children exposed to maternal smoking during pregnancy was higher than that of those who were not exposed (crude hazard ratio 1.14, 95% confidence interval 1.00 to 1.30, P=0.05), but this association was weakened in the propensity score adjusted analysis (adjusted hazard ratio 1.10, 95% confidence interval 0.97 to 1.25, P=0.14). The mean DMF index at 18 months was 0.04 (2.5 centile: 0, median: 0, 97.5 centile: 0) for infants exposed to secondhand smoke, 0.04 (2.5 centile: 0, median: 0, 97.5 centile: 0, P=0.59) for infants exposed to only maternal smoking during pregnancy, 0.07 (2.5 centile: 0, median: 0, 97.5 centile: 0, P<0.01) for infants exposed to only household smoking at 4 months, and 0.7 (2.5 centile: 0, median: 0, 97.5 centile: 0, P<0.01) for infants exposed to secondhand smoke during pregnancy and at 4 months. The mean DMF index at 3 years was 0.42 (2.5 centile: 0, median: 0, 97.5 centile: 5), 0.46 (2.5 centile: 0, median: 0, 97.5 centile: 8, P=0.74), 0.72 (2.5 centile: 0, median: 0, 97.5 centile: 7, P<0.01), and 0.84 (2.5 centile: 0, median: 0, 97.5 centile: 6, P<0.01), respectively.

Discussion

In this population based retrospective cohort study of 76 920 Japanese children, exposure to tobacco smoke was associated with an approximately twofold increased risk of caries in deciduous teeth. The risk of caries was also increased, by 1.5-fold, among infants exposed to smoking in the household, whereas the effect of maternal smoking during pregnancy was only 1.1-fold. Differences in behaviour patterns were apparent between those exposed to and not exposed to smoking, such as lack of tooth brushing and irregular consumption of sweets. We confirmed our findings through sensitivity analysis using information about behaviour patterns during the ages of 4 months to 3 years, but we cannot completely exclude the possibility of bias due to residual confounding.

Secondhand smoke was operationally defined in previous studies as exposure to smoking by one or both parents or family members, maternal smoking during pregnancy, or high serum cotinine levels. We used three definitions for secondhand smoke—maternal smoking during pregnancy, smoking in the household when the infant was aged 4 months, and exposure to tobacco smoke at age 4 months. Kobe City published guidelines for prevention of secondhand smoke in 2004 and recommended separation of smoking areas at home as well as in the workplaces. In this study, fewer infants at age 4 months were exposed to tobacco smoke than those exposed to smoking in the household, possibly reflecting the wide spread separation of smoking areas at home, but the effects on the risk of caries were significant even for smoking in the household. These findings are consistent with past cross sectional studies in which 10 out of 11 studies found significant positive associations between secondhand smoke and caries of deciduous teeth.[10] On the other hand, only a few studies[22-24] have examined the effects of maternal smoking during pregnancy. Two studies from the National Health and Nutrition Examination Survey reported that the incidence density ratios of maternal smoking during pregnancy were 1.54 (P=0.02)[22] and 3.85 (P=0.054)[23] among children aged 2 to 5 or 6 years, whereas the prevalence ratio of caries between 3 year old Japanese children with and without exposure to maternal smoking was 1.78 (P<0.05).[24] These results are opposite to our findings. However, it is notable that in the National Health and Nutrition Examination Survey (NHNES) the effects of maternal smoking and household smoking may be confounded[22 23] because exposure to maternal smoking during pregnancy would be correlated with household smoking after childbirth, which was not handled separately in the NHNES analysis. Other differences in design include availability of data on oral care and dietary habits, which could be important confounders,[20] and cross sectional or cohort design. Taken together, further research is needed for a definitive conclusion, although our findings suggest that the effects of maternal smoking during pregnancy are weaker than those of exposure to secondhand smoke after childbirth.

The estimated hazard ratios of exposure to tobacco, around 1.5-fold to twofold higher, are small but may be important from a public health viewpoint. The three year risk of caries in this cohort was 18.0%. This estimate is slightly lower than the averages in the United States[2] and Japan,[3] and the high utilisation of fluoride varnish, tooth brushing, and dental examinations may have contributed to the reduction in risk of caries. However, more than half of the children in this cohort had family members who smoked, and most smokers were their fathers. These results can be considered representative of children in large cities in Japan, given the high participation rate in this study. Indeed, exposure to secondhand smoke is widespread among children worldwide, at a rate of 40%, which is higher than any other age categories.[15] The associations between secondhand smoke and risk of caries would support extending public health and clinical interventions to reduce secondhand smoke. For example, education on the harm of secondhand smoke might

RESEARCH

Table 4 | Propensity score analysis of maternal smoking during pregnancy and incidence of caries

Variables	Not exposed to secondhand smoke during pregnancy and at 4 months (n=22 554)	Exposed to only maternal smoking during pregnancy (n=2062)		Exposed to only household smoking at 4 months (n=22 060)		Exposed to secondhand smoke during pregnancy and at 4 months (n=7055)	
		Hazard ratio (95% CI)	P value	Hazard ratio (95% CI)	P value	Hazard ratio (95% CI)	P value
Incidence of any caries (unadjusted) (%):	2848 (13.5*)	290 (15.1*)		4164 (20.2*)		1516 (23.1*)	
Crude	Ref	1.14 (1.00 to 1.30)	0.05	1.60 (1.52 to 1.69)	<0.01	1.89 (1.77 to 2.02)	<0.01
Propensity score adjusted†	Ref	1.10 (0.97 to 1.25)	0.14	1.52 (1.44 to 1.60)	<0.01	1.71 (1.59 to 1.83)	<0.01
Sensitivity analysis‡	Ref	1.16 (0.93 to 1.43)	0.18	1.75 (1.58 to 1.93)	<0.01	2.05 (1.82 to 2.30)	<0.01
Sensitivity analysis§	Ref	1.10 (0.97 to 1.26)	0.14	1.51 (1.43 to 1.59)	<0.01	1.74 (1.62 to 1.87)	<0.01
Sensitivity analysis¶	Ref	1.04 (0.87 to 1.25)	0.65	1.30 (1.21 to 1.40)	<0.01	1.46 (1.32 to 1.62)	<0.01
Sensitivity analysis**	Ref	1.09 (0.97 to 1.23)	0.16	1.46 (1.39 to 1.53)	<0.01	1.61 (1.51 to 1.72)	<0.01
Incidence of caries in maxillary anterior teeth (unadjusted) (%):	1897 (9.1*)	178 (9.3*)		2802 (13.6*)		976 (14.8*)	
Crude	Ref	1.03 (0.88 to 1.21)	0.67	1.58 (1.49 to 1.68)	<0.01	1.75 (1.61 to 1.90)	<0.01
Propensity score adjusted†	Ref	1.01 (0.86 to 1.18)	0.93	1.51 (1.42 to 1.61)	<0.01	1.61 (1.48 to 1.75)	<0.01
Sensitivity analysis‡	Ref	1.15 (0.93 to 1.43)	0.19	1.75 (1.59 to 1.93)	<0.01	2.05 (1.82 to 2.31)	<0.01
Sensitivity analysis§	Ref	1.10 (0.97 to 1.26)	0.15	1.52 (1.44 to 1.60)	<0.01	1.75 (1.62 to 1.88)	<0.01
Sensitivity analysis¶	Ref	1.04 (0.86 to 1.24)	0.70	1.31 (1.21 to 1.41)	<0.01	1.46 (1.32 to 1.62)	<0.01
Sensitivity analysis**	Ref	1.01 (0.86 to 1.17)	0.94	1.48 (1.39 to 1.57)	<0.01	1.57 (1.45 to 1.70)	<0.01
Incidence of caries in maxillary molars (unadjusted) (%):	856 (4.1*)	84 (4.4*)		1335 (6.5*)		543 (8.3*)	
Crude	Ref	1.08 (0.86 to 1.36)	0.51	1.63 (1.49 to 1.78)	<0.01	2.11 (1.89 to 2.36)	<0.01
Propensity score adjusted†	Ref	1.04 (0.83 to 1.31)	0.71	1.54 (1.41 to 1.69)	<0.01	1.91 (1.70 to 2.14)	<0.01
Sensitivity analysis‡	Ref	1.16 (0.93 to 1.43)	0.19	1.75 (1.58 to 1.93)	<0.01	2.06 (1.82 to 2.32)	<0.01
Sensitivity analysis§	Ref	1.10 (0.96 to 1.25)	0.18	1.52 (1.44 to 1.60)	<0.01	1.75 (1.63 to 1.88)	<0.01
Sensitivity analysis¶	Ref	1.04 (0.87 to 1.25)	0.68	1.30 (1.21 to 1.40)	<0.01	1.46 (1.32 to 1.63)	<0.01
Sensitivity analysis**	Ref	1.04 (0.83 to 1.31)	0.71	1.53 (1.40 to 1.67)	<0.01	1.87 (1.67 to 2.09)	<0.01
Incidence of caries in mandibular anterior teeth (unadjusted) (%):	182 (0.9*)	18 (0.9*)		307 (1.5*)		102 (1.6*)	
Crude	Ref	1.09 (0.67 to 1.77)	0.74	1.73 (1.44 to 2.08)	<0.01	1.81 (1.42 to 2.31)	<0.01
Propensity score adjusted†	Ref	1.04 (0.64 to 1.68)	0.89	1.60 (1.33 to 1.93)	<0.01	1.57 (1.22 to 2.02)	<0.01
Sensitivity analysis‡	Ref	1.15 (0.93 to 1.43)	0.20	1.75 (1.59 to 1.93)	<0.01	2.07 (1.83 to 2.33)	<0.01
Sensitivity analysis§	Ref	1.10 (0.96 to 1.26)	0.16	1.52 (1.44 to 1.60)	<0.01	1.76 (1.63 to 1.89)	<0.01
Sensitivity analysis¶	Ref	1.04 (0.87 to 1.25)	0.68	1.30 (1.21 to 1.41)	<0.01	1.47 (1.33 to 1.64)	<0.01
Sensitivity analysis**	Ref	1.04 (0.64 to 1.68)	0.89	1.61 (1.33 to 1.94)	<0.01	1.58 (1.23 to 2.03)	<0.01
Incidence of caries in mandibular molars (unadjusted) (%):	1289 (6.2*)	144 (7.6*)		2132 (10.5*)		848 (13.1*)	
Crude	Ref	1.24 (1.04 to 1.49)	0.02	1.77 (1.64 to 1.90)	<0.01	2.27 (2.07 to 2.49)	<0.01
Propensity score adjusted†	Ref	1.18 (0.99 to 1.41)	0.07	1.62 (1.50 to 1.74)	<0.01	1.94 (1.76 to 2.13)	<0.01
Sensitivity analysis‡	Ref	1.15 (0.93 to 1.43)	0.19	1.75 (1.58 to 1.93)	<0.01	2.06 (1.83 to 2.32)	<0.01
Sensitivity analysis§	Ref	1.10 (0.96 to 1.26)	0.16	1.52 (1.44 to 1.60)	<0.01	1.75 (1.63 to 1.89)	<0.01
Sensitivity analysis¶	Ref	1.04 (0.86 to 1.25)	0.70	1.30 (1.21 to 1.40)	<0.01	1.47 (1.32 to 1.63)	<0.01
Sensitivity analysis**	Ref	1.17 (0.98 to 1.39)	0.08	1.58 (1.48 to 1.70)	<0.01	1.86 (1.70 to 2.04)	<0.01

*Estimated by Kaplan-Meier method.
†Adjusted for birth year of child, maternal age, alcohol consumption during pregnancy, smoking status during pregnancy, sex, first birth, multiple birth, pre-eclampsia, anaemia, threatened abortion, gestational weeks, caesarean section, vacuum extraction, nuchal cord, asphyxia, jaundice and transfusion, convulsion, incubator, oxygen inhalation, weight, height, head and chest circumference at birth, weight at 4 months, bottle feeding at 4 months, people involved in child care at 4 months, support by family, friends, or neighbours at 4 months, and mother's mental status at 4 months.
‡Restricted to first born singletons.
§Children with a propensity score below first centile or above 99th centile were excluded.
¶Further adjusted for number of teeth at 9 months, treatment with fluoride varnish at 18 months and 3 years, tooth brushing alone at 18 months and 3 years, tooth brushing by parents at 18 months and 3 years (%), bottle feeding at 4 months and 9 months, baby food at 9 months, age at start of baby food, frequency of sweets at 18 months and 3 years, eating sweets irregularly at 18 months and 3 years, and drinking juice every day at 18 months and 3 years.
**Exponential regression analysis handling time to event data as interval censored.

increase if dentists became aware of the risk of caries due to secondhand smoke as well as tobacco consumption of their clients. However, further investigation is necessary to conclude whether a smoking prevention programme would reduce the risks of caries, since the size of effects of secondhand smoke was not large. Propensity score analysis allowed adjustment for confounders in this study, but residual bias due to unmeasured confounders, although potentially small, cannot be ruled out.

Limitations of this study
These findings must be interpreted in the context of study limitations. Firstly, information on smoking status was obtained by questionnaires completed by mothers, and biomarkers such as serum cotinine levels were not available in this study. In particular, the prevalence of maternal smoking during pregnancy may be underreported. It is also difficult in an epidemiological study to separate the effects of secondhand smoke from those of third hand smoke—the residual contamination from

tobacco smoke that remains on a variety of indoor surfaces. Secondly, oral conditions were not necessarily assessed by paediatric dentistry. Thirdly, as we carried out an observational study rather than a randomised trial, it is impossible to establish causality. In addition to the possibility of unmeasured confounders, we cannot entirely exclude the potential of bias owing to missing covariates. We calculated the propensity score with the use of single imputation, but multiple imputation outperforms single imputation theoretically. However, we expect that it would not make much difference in this situation. Fourthly, the portion of children exposed to smoke only during pregnancy was relatively small and therefore the non-significant results for maternal smoking may be due to low statistical power to detect a small effect. Finally, given the substantial variability in the prevalence of caries, exposure to secondhand smoke, and lifestyle across countries, our results may not be generally applicable to populations with different environmental and lifestyle factors. For example, fluoridation of water in the community has not been carried out in Japan since 1972, although fluoride varnish (table 2) and fluoride toothpaste is common. Furthermore, sugar intake for each person also varies across countries (for example, 48 g/day in Japan, 84 g/day in the US, and 107 g/day in Britain in 2011).[25]

Conclusion

Exposure to secondhand smoke at 4 months of age, which is experienced by half of all children of that age in Kobe City, Japan, is associated with an increased risk of caries in deciduous teeth. Although these findings cannot establish causality, they support extending public health and clinical interventions to reduce secondhand smoke.

We thank the Child and Family Bureau and Public Health and Welfare Bureau of Kobe City for providing the health check-up data and advice; C Wilunda and C Hongyan (Kyoto University) for their advice; and K Fujii (Kyoto University) for secretarial assistance.

Contributors: ShT performed statistical analysis and had full access to all the data in the study and takes responsibility for the integrity of the data and the accuracy of the data analysis. MS, HT, and KK contributed to the design and conduct of the study. SK and SaT contributed to the writing of the manuscript. KK is the principal investigator and the guarantor of the study. The sponsor of the study had no role in the study design, data collection, data analysis, data interpretation, or writing of the report.

Funding: This study was supported by a grant in aid for scientific research 26860415.

Competing interests: All authors have completed the ICMJE uniform disclosure form at www.icmje.org/coi_disclosure.pdf and declare: no support from any organisation for the submitted work; no financial relationships with any organisations that might have an interest in the submitted work in the previous three years; no other relationships or activities that could appear to have influenced the submitted work.

Ethical approval: This study was exempt from obtaining individual informed consent based on the Ethical Guidelines for Epidemiological Research by Ministry of Health, Labour, and Welfare. The study protocol was approved by the Ethics Committee, Kyoto University Graduate School and Faulty of Medicine (E2045). We managed the data based on the Act of Personal Information Protection in Kobe City and take responsibility for their integrity.

Data sharing: No additional data available.

Transparency: The lead author (KK) affirms that the manuscript is an honest, accurate, and transparent account of the study being reported; that no important aspects of the study have been omitted; and that any discrepancies from the study as planned (and, if relevant, registered) have been explained.

This is an Open Access article distributed in accordance with the Creative Commons Attribution Non Commercial (CC BY-NC 4.0) license, which permits others to distribute, remix, adapt, build upon this work non-commercially, and license their derivative works on different terms, provided the original work is properly cited and the use is non-commercial. See: http://creativecommons.org/licenses/by-nc/4.0/.

1. Marcenes W, Kassebaum NJ, Bernabé E, et al. Global burden of oral conditions in 1990-2010: a systematic analysis. *J Dent Res* 2013;92:592-7.
2. Dye BA, Tan S, Smith V, et al. Trends in oral health status: United States, 1988-1994 and 1999-2004. *Vital Health Stat* 2007;(248):1-92.
3. Ministry of Health, Labour and Welfare. Survey of dental diseases 2011. www.mhlw.go.jp/toukei/list/62-23.html.
4. Chou R, Cantor A, Zakher B, Mitchell JP, Pappas M. Preventing dental caries in children <5 years: systematic review updating USPSTF recommendation. *Pediatrics* 2013;132:332-50.
5. Rethman MP, Beltrán-Aguilar ED, Billings RJ, et al.; American Dental Association Council on Scientific Affairs Expert Panel on Nonfluoride Caries-Preventive Agents. Nonfluoride caries-preventive agents: executive summary of evidence-based clinical recommendations. *J Am Dent Assoc* 2011;142:1065-71.
6. Du MQ, Tai BJ, Jiang H, Lo EC, Fan MW, Bian Z. A two-year randomized clinical trial of chlorhexidine varnish on dental caries in Chinese preschool children. *J Dent Res* 2006;85:557-9.
7. Selwitz RH, Ismail AI, Pitts NB. Dental caries. *Lancet* 2007;369:51-9.
8. Alves AC, Nogueira RD, Stipp RN, et al. Prospective study of potential sources of Streptococcus mutans transmission in nursery school children. *J Med Microbiol* 2009;58(Pt 4):476-81.
9. Caufield PW, Cutter GR, Dasanayake AP. Initial acquisition of mutans streptococci by infants: evidence for a discrete window of infectivity. *J Dent Res* 1993;72:37-45.
10. Hanioka T, Ojima M, Tanaka K, Yamamoto M. Does secondhand smoke affect the development of dental caries in children? A systematic review. *Int J Environ Res Public Health* 2011;8:1503-19.
11. Strauss RS. Environmental tobacco smoke and serum vitamin C levels in children. *Pediatrics* 2001;107:540-2.
12. Avşar A, Darka O, Bodrumlu EH, Bek Y. Evaluation of the relationship between passive smoking and salivary electrolytes, protein, secretory IgA, sialic acid and amylase in young children. *Arch Oral Biol* 2009;54:457-63.
13. Dong Q, Wu H, Dong G, Lou B, Yang L, Zhang L. The morphology and mineralization of dental hard tissue in the offspring of passive smoking rats. *Arch Oral Biol* 2011;56:1005-13.
14. Levine MJ, Hertzberg MC, Levine MS, Ellison AS, Stinson MW, Li HC. Specificity of salivary bacterial interactions: role of terminal sialic acid residues in the interactions of salivary glycoproteins with streptococcus sanguis and streptococcus mutans. *Infect Immun* 1978;19:107-15.
15. Oberg M, Jaakkola MS, Woodward A, Peruga A, Prüss-Ustün A. Worldwide burden of disease from exposure to second-hand smoke: a retrospective analysis of data from 192 countries. *Lancet* 2011;377:139-46.
16. Aligne CA, Moss ME, Auinger P, Weitzman M. Association of pediatric dental caries with Second-hand smoking. *JAMA* 2003;289:1258-64.
17. Majorana A, Cagetti MG, Bardellini E, et al. Feeding and smoking habits as cumulative risk factors for early childhood caries in toddlers, after adjustment for several behavioral determinants: a retrospective study. *BMC Pediatr* 2014;14:45.
18. Nakayama Y, Mori M. Association of environmental tobacco smoke and snacking habits with the risk of early childhood caries among 3-year-old Japanese children. *J Public Health Dent* 2015;75:157-62.
19. Julihn A, Ekbom A, Modéer T. Maternal overweight and smoking: prenatal risk factors for caries development in offspring during the teenage period. *Eur J Epidemiol* 2009;24:753-62.
20. Alm A, Wendt LK, Koch G, Birkhed D. Oral hygiene and parent-related factors during early childhood in relation to approximal caries at 15 years of age. *Caries Res* 2008;42:28-36.
21. Ministry of Health, Labour and Welfare. The Maternal and Child Health Act 2014. http://law.e-gov.go.jp/htmldata/S40/S40HO141.html.
22. Iida H, Auinger P, Billings RJ, Weitzman M. Association between infant breastfeeding and early childhood caries in the United States. *Pediatrics* 2007;120:e944-52.
23. Shulman JD. Is there an association between low birth weight and caries in the primary dentition? *Caries Res* 2005;39:161-7.
24. Tanaka K, Miyake Y, Sasaki S. The effect of maternal smoking during pregnancy and postnatal household smoking on dental caries in young children. *J Pediatr* 2009;155:410-5.
25. Food and Agriculture Organization of the United Nation. FAOSTAT 2011. http://faostat.fao.org/site/609/default.aspx#ancor.

© BMJ Publishing Group Ltd 2015

Web appendix: supplementary information

演習問題の解答と解説

I 代表的なグラフ

問題1

1 Abstract（抄録）の方法（Methods）に記載があります.
- P：276＋1300 patients who were younger than 15 years at the time of the Chernobyl nuclear power plant accident.
- E and C：radiation exposure whose doses were estimated based on their whereabouts and dietary habits at the time of the accident and in following days, weeks, and years
- O：thyroid cancer through 1998

2 95％信頼区間

3 d

サンプルサイズが4以上であれば（ふつうはそうですよね），平均±標準偏差＞95％信頼区間＞平均±標準誤差

問題2

1 b

a, cの場合，脳卒中発生時点は正確にはわかりません（区間打ち切りといいます）. dではすべての脳卒中を把握できない可能性があります.

2 d

3 b

dはCox回帰のための仮定です（第7講参照）.

4 a

半数以上の対象者がイベントを起こしていないと，生存確率は50％以下になりません.

II 臨床試験の統計解析

問題1

両側検定（two-sided）です.
Methods（方法）の統計解析の最後の行に記載があります（All statistical tests were two-sided）.

問題2

1 b

2 a

3 d

有意水準が5％であればcは正しいのですが，有意水準は必ずしも5％とは限りません.

4 a

5 a

6 d

サンプルサイズが不足していた可能性もあります.

7 c

検出限界以下の値が打ち切りですから，生存時間解析（第7講参照）と同じ方法を用いることができます.

III 臨床試験のデザイン

問題1

非劣性マージンが1.11の場合は非劣性が示されず，1.21の場合は非劣性が示されます.

問題2

1 d

2 b

3 d

4 a, b, c
ただし，a は必ずしも好ましいことではありません．

V メタアナリシス

問題1

1 それぞれ114件と33件
Summary（抄録）のFindings（結果）に記載があります（We screened 114 potentially eligible studies and identified 33 randomised controlled trials）．

2 変量効果モデル
Summary（抄録）のMethods（方法）の最後の行に記載があります（a random-effects network meta-analysis within a Bayesian framework）．

3 スポンサーシップバイアス
製薬企業がスポンサーとなって試験を実施することによるバイアスのこと．公表バイアス，パフォーマンスバイアス，報告バイアスに関連します（第19講，第30講を参照）．

VI ネットワークメタアナリシス

問題1

1 d
不一貫性が強い場合，間接比較を考慮して解析すると直接比較よりも信頼区間が広がることがあるため，c は誤りです．

2 c
不均一性とは，試験間で治療効果の大きさが異なることです．

3 b

VII コホート研究とケース・コントロール研究

問題1
家族歴，遺伝要因，人種など

問題2
いえません．小さながんまでスクリーニングできるようになり，予後のよい患者が増えた可能性があります．

問題3

1 a

2 b

3 a

4 d

5 b

6 38.7倍（＝1/0.02586倍）

7 38.7乗（＝1/0.02586乗）

VIII プロペンシティスコア

問題1

1 a
このような場合は，比較可能性が全くないので交絡を調整することは原理的にできません．

2 b
ロジスティック回帰やCox回帰でサンプルサイズが小さく，説明変数の数に比べイベント数が少ないと，すべての交絡因子を回帰モデルに入れられないことがあります．目安として，説明変数1つあたり5〜10以上のイベントが必要といわれています．

3 a
中間因子が交絡因子となっている場合の統計解析については，本書では解説しませんでしたが特殊な統計手法が必要です．